Drugs
and
Therapy

A Handbook of Psychotropic Drugs

Drugs and Therapy

A Handbook of Psychotropic Drugs

Second Edition

Alvin K. Swonger, Ph.D.
Associate Professor of Pharmacology and
Toxicology, College of Pharmacy, University
of Rhode Island, Kingston

Larry L. Constantine, L.C.S.W.
Assistant Professor of Human Development and
Family Relations, University of Connecticut
School of Family Studies, Storrs; Family
Therapist, Acton, Massachusetts

Little, Brown and Company
Boston/Toronto

There are among us a few whose capacity to extend themselves in warmth and in love is truly exceptional:

Adolph and Sandy Alla
Roger and Carolyn Miller
John and Pat Remmers
Howie and Jane Stockwell

Contents

Preface   xi

I. Drugs in Therapeutic Perspective

1. Drugs in the Therapeutic Encounter   3
   CASE HISTORY/THE DRUG-THERAPY INTERFACE/THE NEW PSYCHOTHERAPIST

2. Psychopathology, Drugs, and Disease   11
   PSYCHOLOGICAL HEALTH AND PSYCHOPATHOLOGY/THE ETIOLOGY OF
   PSYCHOPATHOLOGY/ORGANIC PROCESS/PSYCHOLOGICAL PROCESS/
   INTERPERSONAL SYSTEMIC PROCESS

3. Drugs, Learning, and Psychotherapy   27
   LEARNING AND PSYCHOTHERAPY/NEUROLOGIC BASES OF LEARNING/DRUGS AND
   LEARNING

II. Foundations of Drug Action: Neuropharmacology

4. Introduction to Functional Neuroanatomy   47
   PERIPHERAL NERVOUS SYSTEM/CENTRAL NERVOUS SYSTEM

5. The Physiology of Nerve Cells   61
   CYTOLOGY/THE CELL MEMBRANE/CONDUCTION AND TRANSMISSION

6. Neurotransmission   69
   MECHANISMS OF SYNAPTIC TRANSMISSION/ACUTE DRUG INTERACTIONS WITH
   SYNAPTIC TRANSMISSION/ADAPTIVE CHANGES IN SYNAPTIC MECHANISMS/
   ACETYLCHOLINE/NOREPINEPHRINE/DOPAMINE/EPINEPHRINE/SEROTONIN/
   GABA/GLYCINE/GLUTAMATE AND ASPARTATE/HISTAMINE/PEPTIDE
   NEUROREGULATORS/CYCLIC NUCLEOTIDES

7. Principles of Pharmacology   113
   RECEPTORS/DOSE-RESPONSE RELATIONSHIP/ROUTES OF ADMINISTRATION/THE
   BLOOD-BRAIN BARRIER/DRUG METABOLISM AND ELIMINATION/DRUG
   INTERACTIONS/MULTIPLICITY OF EFFECTS

III. Drug Use, Drug Abuse

8. Clinical Psychopharmacology   125
   RATIONAL PSYCHOTHERAPEUTICS/DIAGNOSIS/KNOWLEDGE OF THE PSYCHIATRIC
   PROBLEM/PSYCHIATRIC SIDE EFFECTS/DRUG ACTIONS AND INTERACTIONS/
   POLYPHARMACY: PROS AND CONS/PSYCHOLOGICAL FACTORS IN DRUG RESPONSE/
   THERAPEUTIC DESIGN

9. Drug Abuse   145
   WHAT IS IT?/PHARMACOLOGIC ASPECTS/PSYCHOLOGICAL ASPECTS/DRUG ABUSE
   EDUCATION

IV. Drugs and Arousal State

10. The Physiology of Sleep and Arousal   161
    THE DIFFUSE THALAMIC SYSTEM/THE RETICULAR ACTIVATING SYSTEM/
    ELECTROENCEPHALOGRAPHY/DUAL-AROUSAL THEORY/SLEEP AND DREAMING/
    SLEEP DISORDERS

11. Sedative-Hypnotics   183
    GENERAL PHARMACOLOGY/EARLY SEDATIVE-HYPNOTICS/BARBITURATES/
    NONBARBITURATE HYPNOTICS/SLEEP AIDS/IMPLICATIONS FOR PSYCHOTHERAPY

12. Alcohol: The Nonprescription Sedative-Hypnotic   195
    INCIDENCE/ACUTE PHARMACOLOGY/CHRONIC TOXICITY/TOLERANCE AND
    DEPENDENCE/ALCOHOL-INDUCED DISORDERS/DRUG INTERACTIONS/DISULFIRAM/
    TREATMENT OF ALCOHOL WITHDRAWAL/INTERPERSONAL AND SYSTEMIC
    INVOLVEMENT IN ALCOHOLISM/IMPLICATIONS FOR PSYCHOTHERAPY

13. Stimulants   211
    XANTHINES/CATECHOLAMINE-RELEASING STIMULANTS/ATTENTION DEFICIT
    DISORDERS/COCAINE/NICOTINE/IMPLICATIONS FOR PSYCHOTHERAPY

14. Psychedelics   227
    CLASSIFICATIONS/LSD/PCP/OTHER TRUE PSYCHEDELICS/CANNABIS/IMPLICATIONS
    FOR PSYCHOTHERAPY

V. Psychiatric Disorders and Drugs

15. Neuroanatomic Bases of Emotion   239
    GENERAL FUNCTIONS OF THE LIMBIC SYSTEM/FUNCTIONS OF SPECIFIC LIMBIC
    STRUCTURES

16. Psychosis and Antipsychotic Drugs   253
    CLASSIFICATION OF PSYCHOSES/NEUROBIOLOGIC THEORIES OF SCHIZOPHRENIA/
    ANTIPSYCHOTIC DRUGS: HISTORY, MECHANISMS, CLINICAL INDICATIONS, AND
    ADVERSE EFFECTS/PHENOTHIAZINES/RAUWOLFIA ALKALOIDS/BUTYROPHENONES/
    THIOXANTHENES/ATYPICAL NEUROLEPTICS/INTERACTIONS OF NEUROLEPTICS/
    MATTERS OF STRATEGY/IMPLICATIONS FOR PSYCHOTHERAPY

17. Anxiety and Anxiolytics   273
DIAGNOSTIC CLASSIFICATION OF ANXIETY DISORDERS/MEPROBAMATE/
BENZODIAZEPINES: MECHANISMS, COMPARISONS, AND MATTERS OF STRATEGY/
HYDROXYZINE/IMPLICATIONS FOR PSYCHOTHERAPY

18. Depression and Antidepressants   285
DIAGNOSTIC CLASSIFICATIONS OF DEPRESSION/DICHOTOMOUS CONCEPTS OF
DEPRESSION/NEUROCHEMICAL THEORIES OF DEPRESSION/TRICYCLIC
ANTIDEPRESSANTS: MECHANISMS, EFFECTIVENESS, COMPARISONS, DOSAGE
SCHEDULES, ADDITIONAL USES, PREDICTING RESPONSIVENESS/MONOAMINE
OXIDASE INHIBITORS/ATYPICAL ANTIDEPRESSANTS/STIMULANTS AS
ANTIDEPRESSANTS/IMPLICATIONS FOR PSYCHOTHERAPY

19. Manic-Depressive Disorder and Lithium   305
MANIC-DEPRESSIVE DISORDER/LITHIUM: INDICATIONS, MECHANISMS, MATTERS OF
STRATEGY, ADVERSE REACTIONS, IMPLICATIONS FOR PSYCHOTHERAPY

VI. *Motor Function and Drugs*

20. The Extrapyramidal Motor System   315
CORPUS STRIATUM/THE CEREBELLUM/SUMMARY OF FUNCTIONS/DUAL-PROCESS
THEORY OF RESPONSE EXECUTION

21. Disorders of the Extrapyramidal System   321
PARKINSONISM AND ANTIPARKINSONIAN AGENTS/HUNTINGTON'S DISEASE/OTHER
ORGANIC MOTOR DYSFUNCTIONS/PSEUDOPARKINSONISM/TARDIVE DYSKINESIAS/
AKATHISIAS AND ACUTE DYSTONIC REACTIONS/FUNCTIONAL MOTOR DISORDERS/
IMPLICATIONS FOR PSYCHOTHERAPY

VII. *Pain and Its Drug Management*

22. Neurophysiology of Pain and Temperature   333
NEUROPHYSIOLOGY OF PAIN/IMPLICATIONS FOR PSYCHOTHERAPY/
NEUROPHYSIOLOGY OF TEMPERATURE

23. Narcotic Analgesics   339
HISTORY/ACTIONS ON THE CNS/ENDOGENOUS MORPHINE-LIKE SUBSTANCES/
PERIPHERAL ACTIONS/INTOXICATION, TOLERANCE, AND DEPENDENCE/NARCOTIC
ABUSE/MORPHINE ANALOGS/METHADONE TREATMENT PROGRAMS/IMPLICATIONS
FOR PSYCHOTHERAPY

24. Nonnarcotic Analgesics   347
SHARED PHARMACOLOGIC PROPERTIES OF ASPIRIN-LIKE DRUGS/SALICYLATES/
OTHER ASPIRIN LIKE DRUGS/IMPLICATIONS FOR PSYCHOTHERAPY

25. Headaches and Neuralgia   355
MIGRAINE AND CLUSTER HEADACHES/MUSCLE TENSION HEADACHES/NEURALGIAS/
IMPLICATIONS FOR PSYCHOTHERAPY

VIII. Drugs and Consciousness

26. Neuroanatomy of the Cerebral Cortex   363
ORGANIZATION OF THE CORTEX/SENSORY AND MOTOR FUNCTIONS/ASSOCIATIVE
CORTEX/LATERALIZATION OF FUNCTION

27. Toward a Neurophysiologic Basis of Mind   373
LAMINAR ORGANIZATION, CELL TYPES, AND EXTRINSIC CONNECTIVITY/A MODEL OF
THE CEREBRAL CELL COLUMN

28. Epilepsy and Antiepileptic Drugs   387
PHYSIOLOGIC BASIS OF EPILEPSY/TYPES OF EPILEPSY/EEG DIAGNOSIS OF EPILEPSY/
HYDANTOINS/BARBITURATES/OXAZOLIDONES/SUCCINIMIDES/
BENZODIAZEPINES/VALPROIC ACID/IMPLICATIONS FOR PSYCHOTHERAPY

Appendix A
Psychotropic Drugs in Top 200 of All New and Refill Prescriptions
in 1972 and 1981   403

Appendix B
Some Adverse Reactions of Potential Psychotherapeutic Significance   405

Appendix C
Case History   411

Appendix D
Drug Report   413

Index   415

Preface

Seven years of use of the first edition of *Drugs and Therapy* by students and practitioners has convinced us of the reality of the need we perceived for a resource book exploring the interface between drug and nondrug therapy. The second edition retains as its focus the goal of addressing that need.

The experience gained from using the book ourselves, and observing its use by students and clinicians, has indicated both strengths and weaknesses in the first edition. In planning and producing this edition, we have made every effort to retain and build on the strengths and to correct the weaknesses. Our fundamental orientation toward an integrative systems approach remains a basic organizing principle of the book. It is intended that the organization of the book serves to strengthen important lines of association: the interactions of the organic, psychological, and interpersonal levels of organization in mental health and illness and the relationships between normal brain functions, psychopathology, and treatment.

Other features retained from the first edition include the treatment of drugs in classes, concise summaries of implications for psychotherapy, the drug synopses at the end of relevant chapters, and the appendix of psychiatric side effects.

The synopses briefly summarize salient aspects of medically important drugs in the class being discussed. It is impossible to include more than a small fraction of all the members of a given class; consequently, some criteria, at more or less arbitrary points, have been used to select agents to be synopsized. The synopses are limited to agents in current use medically. Social drugs and agents of mere heuristic interest are excluded. Agents with important research uses are included if they also have current therapeutic applications. Psychotropic drugs that appear under the relevant headings in the *AMA Drug Evaluations* and/or among the 200 most prescribed drugs (see Appendix A) are found in the appropriate synopses.

A drug synopsis identifies the agent by its preferred *generic* name, followed by a list of synonyms (if any) and trade names. Only the most commonly used trade names are given. The chemical group or subgroup and drug class appear next. Major and/or unusual applications are identified, followed by data regarding dosages.

Dosage data presented in drug synopses are for reference only and ARE NOT for medical purposes either as a guide to or as a check against drug administration.

Unless otherwise indicated, dosages are in milligrams (mg) and represent the total adult daily *oral* dose, which may in clinical practice be divided among several administrations. Where a single range is indicated, this represents upper and lower limits of *normal* clinical use as compiled from numerous sources. A single figure indicates a *typical* dosage. Wherever possible, the data from several sources have been used to derive a typical range and a range of extremes. The psychotherapist may wish to consult with the prescribing physician if a client is receiving doses outside the extreme range or markedly different from typical or normal dosage. The information and rationale used by the physician in arriving at dosage may be useful to the psychotherapist.

This edition features a complete revision of the content and approach in the chapters pertaining to drug classes. The psychopathologic conditions for which psychotropic drugs are employed are described more fully, with special emphasis on variables that help to predict responsiveness to drug treatment or to dictate drug selection. Neurochemical and neuroanatomic mechanisms of drug action are highlighted. More information is provided regarding psychiatric and other side effects, such as period of maximal risk, to aid the clinician in recognizing and assessing the impact of such symptoms. There is more focus on comparisons within classes that often provide the basis for decisions about drug selection. As the quantity of information has expanded, so has the effort to cluster detail into patterns. The many tables and illustrations serve as aids in visualization or as easily accessible data sources.

Among the topics added are acute and adaptive neurochemical mechanisms of drug action, receptor mechanisms, new transmitter substances, rational psychotherapeutics, sleep disorders, alcohol-drug interactions, alcohol toxicities and alcohol-induced disorders, psychobiologic theories of schizophrenia and depression, diagnostic classifications of psychiatric disorders, pain and its drug management, and a neurophysiologic model of consciousness.

The second edition also provides an expanded discussion of the following subjects: drugs used in chronic organic brain syndrome; cocaine; the septal region of the brain; PCP; marijuana; extrapyramidal disorders and drugs; and antiepileptic medications. New drug entries have been added, and data on older drugs, especially those that were new at the time of the first edition, have been updated.

The first edition was approximately a year and a half from conception to publication; the second edition has, in a real sense, been in preparation ever since the publication of the first. Both of us are notorious squirrels.

When the book is employed by one of us (A.K.S.) as a text, the following are provided to students as course performance objectives:

1. You should be able to specify information about drug classes and individual drugs that relates to overall psychotherapy: (a) clinical indications and uses; (b) mechanisms of therapeutic effect in relation to normal brain function; (c) abuse liability; (d) adverse effects (especially psychiatric); and (e) interactions with other drugs, diet, or psychotherapy. Evaluation method: periodic multiple choice quizzes.
2. You should be able to specify and recognize organic conditions that produce psychiatric manifestations that are often mistaken for psychopathologic conditions. Evaluation method: case history (see Appendix C, for example).
3. You should be able to utilize standard reference sources to ascertain the likelihood that a given drug being employed by a client is producing psychiatric side effects or a substance-induced disorder. Evaluation method: drug report (see Appendix D, for example).
4. You should be able to evaluate drug information in formulating reasoned viewpoints concerning matters of psychopharmacology that relate to your professional activities. Evaluation method: take-home essay examination.

These performance objectives are offered here as a guide both to the student and to the practitioner who is using the book as a means of sharpening professional skills.

We are especially indebted to Elsie Castro Swonger, who painstakingly prepared over thirty original illustrations; to Richard Sheinaus, who drew the illustrations taken from Swonger's *Nursing Pharmacology* (Boston: Little, Brown, 1978); to Julie Stillman, Priscilla Hurdle, and the staff of Little, Brown and Company, who transmogrified a caterpillar of a manuscript into a butterfly of a book; and to our students, who engendered the challenge and inspiration to provide a resource worthy of their curiosities.

A.K.S.
L.L.C.

Dosage data presented in this book are for reference only and are not for medical purposes either as a guide to or as a check against drug administration.

Drugs in Therapeutic Perspective

I

℞

An interface is the area where two systems meet and interact. This book begins with an interface between the world of the psychotherapist, whose work is with people, and the world of the psychopharmacologist, whose work is with the drugs that may treat or torment those people. Part One deals with drugs that affect the mind and psychotherapy, an interpersonal change-directed process. The inquiry begins with the problem that arises when drugs enter into the encounter between a nonmedical therapist and his or her client. The rationale and framework for inquiry are established in the first chapter through case examples and an explanation of the factors in the interface. An attempt is made in the second chapter to build an integrative perspective on psychopathology and its alleviation through drugs or therapy or both. Emotional and behavioral problems are seen as the outcome of numerous interacting and even mutually causal processes— organic processes, psychological processes, and systemic processes—which can cripple and limit people. The demonstrated and the possible interactions between drugs and learning in psychotherapy are elaborated in the third chapter.

Medical issues are not of interest to the medical professions alone, for they often have a major effect on the work of the nonmedical psychotherapist. Although drugs and drug therapy are generally assumed to be the sole province of psychiatrists, to be truly effective, the nonmedical therapist needs a good working knowledge of psychopharmacology and a readiness to work cooperatively with a physician. The therapist should know, for example, that withdrawal from addiction to a minor tranquilizer can be a major problem and should be medically supervised. It is essential for the therapist to know that alcohol, barbiturates, and minor tranquilizers have characteristics and effects in common, and that minor tranquilizers, even when legitimately obtained, often become drugs of abuse.

A routine check on the medication of new clients, including a telephone conversation with the prescribing physician, could reveal important drug-related issues early in therapy and help to establish a good professional working relationship with the physician. A therapist who is especially knowledgeable about drugs might suspect the possibility that some apparently psychogenic symptoms could be adverse drug reactions and might, as a matter of course, check the medication the client is receiving in an index of psychiatrically significant adverse drug reactions.

Foreknowledge can be essential, since drug-related issues can complicate the therapeutic encounter with unexpected swiftness.

1

Drugs in the Therapeutic Encounter

1

℞

Two family therapists, just completing their internships in a nonmedical, clinical training program and working together as a team for the first time, had been with their clients the Jays (a pseudonym) for not quite a quarter of an hour and were already facing their first crisis. Gerry, a 20-year-old son living at home with his parents, temporized in the dining room while the therapists, who were in the living room with the parents, tried to get the session started. Gerry was the identified patient. Previously diagnosed as everything from a "behavior problem" to "paranoid schizophrenic," Gerry had been in and out of special schools since he was 10 years of age.

When at last Gerry joined his father and mother, he and his father immediately began a sullen, sniping fight in which neither addressed the other directly. The mother acted as an ineffective mediator. Each found ample reason to point out why the other should be regarded as the cause of problems, but saw no reason to talk with the other. One of the therapists suggested to the father and son that they not talk with each other directly, and, since they *were* not doing so, why look at each other? In that they were sitting in chairs that more or less faced each other, why not sit back to back to reduce the prospect of their looking at each other, much less talking to each other? With some reluctance the two began to try out this suggestion.

No sooner had Gerry turned his back on his father and lowered himself into the chair than he jumped up, clearly agitated and confused.

"I don't like this," he said stumblingly. He seemed to be panicked at the idea of turning his back on his father. "I don't like this at all!... I'm, ah, leaving."

While Gerry started up the stairs, the father accusingly addressed the therapists, "I hope you know what you're doing! He's an epileptic, as you well know. And on medication."

Actually, the therapist knew of neither the epilepsy nor the medication, such "medical" details having been omitted by the social caseworker who had briefed them for the referral.

This unexpected intrusion of medical problems raised many questions for the nonmedical psychotherapists, the immediate ones including: What was the medication? What effects was it likely to have on Gerry's behavior within and outside of therapy? What was the risk of triggering a seizure in therapy? How much was this risk reduced by the medication? How would the medication and the epilepsy limit Gerry's participation in therapy? What effect did Gerry's illness have on the family and what effect did his family experience have on his illness? Could any of his supposedly psychological problems be attributable either to the epilepsy or to its treatment with drugs? Where did the medication regimen fit into the family process? Did either the drugs or the illness place limits on what might be accomplished in therapy with Gerry?

In this case, consultations between the therapists and the family physician and also between the therapists and a specialist answered some of the questions while subsequent interviews with the family answered others. Gerry was receiving phenytoin and primidone, both effective antiepileptics with little likelihood of significant behavioral side effects at moderate doses. His thrice daily medication regimen proved to have a significant systemic role, for it required Gerry, whose management of time was random, to adhere to the clock. It also provided him with a means of exerting power over his parents in that he could refuse or neglect to take his medication, thereby threatening them with the possibility of bringing on renewed epileptic attacks, although he had in fact been free of seizures for several years under this medication. Portions of the family therapy were later directed to the family's disparate styles for management of time and to ways of preventing future antagonistic confrontations.

Although Gerry's medication turned out to play a minor role in the then current problems, his epilepsy was found to be central to the problem. The condition, possibly resulting from birth trauma (anoxia and forceps delivery reported but not independently confirmed), involved a temporal lobe focus. This form, sometimes known as psychomotor epilepsy, may be associated with paroxysmal outbursts of bizarre and aggressive behavior, sudden changes in mood, as well as paranoid ideation, all of which were recorded in Gerry's case record. Interestingly, although medication kept him free of *identified* seizures, his EEG (Chap. 10) continued to be "strikingly abnormal ... with left occipitotemporal paroxysmal, slow, and spiky activity." Thus, it is possible that some of Gerry's behavior problems could have been associated with subictal states, that is, focal brain activity below the level of seizures. There was a very small but still distinct possibility that a seizure might be triggered by an acutely emotional situation, which had occurred in the past. During therapy, this risk would have to be taken into account.

The epilepsy, with its requirement for continuous medication, was of profound symbolic importance to the father, who saw in it the collapse of any hope that his son would grow up to attain a success that he himself had never been able to attain. A second focus during family therapy was therefore on the involvement of these images in the problems between father and son; ultimately, both of them began to see Gerry's disablement put in a more realistic perspective.

Drugs once more entered the therapy sessions, when it became evident that the father was not just an occasional drinker but was engaging in daylong drinking bouts and had already been labeled alcoholic by the military. He drank to drown his disappointment, and he resolved his paradoxical preoccupation with power in this manner. Now there were more questions: Is it possible to conduct therapy with someone who is drunk? If it is possible, will it be successful? Should the alcohol abuse be terminated first or the therapy be started first?

In this case, the alcohol problem was temporarily bypassed by arranging to catch the father for therapy shortly after his longest workday, when he could be expected to be sober. (Eventually he entered and completed a detoxification program and went into a follow-up therapy group for alcoholic patients.)

This was to be only the first of many cases in which drugs and medical issues intruded on the therapist-client relationship. Although most nonmedical psychotherapists have had inadequate training and experience with drugs, drugs are a frequent issue in their work.

The Drug-Therapy Interface

Psychotherapists and Psychotropics

We believe along with others that there is justification in regarding psychotherapy as a distinct emergent profession that crosses traditional disciplinary divisions and whose practitioners evidence considerable commonality even though their various and different credentials seem to set them apart from each other. In the public mind, the professions most closely associated with psychotherapy are psychiatry, clinical psychology, and psychiatric social work. Though we would certainly agree that this book may be useful to psychiatrists, we are more directly addressing their nonmedical colleagues.

In addition to clinical psychologists and psychiatric social workers, we address ourselves to marriage and family counselors, child guidance workers, pastoral counselors,

certain sociologists, community mental health professionals, school guidance counselors, social case workers of many kinds, psychiatric nurses and very possibly other
nurses, family therapists, various psychologists—indeed to all who may need to understand psychotherapeutic principles and whose work may involve facilitating essential
personal changes that will lead to a healthy mental and interpersonal life.

When we write of drugs, unless we state explicitly to the contrary, we are referring to
psychotropic drugs, i.e., the drugs that have as a primary action "an effect on psychic
function, behavior, or experience" [2]. We include the qualifier *primary* because many
drugs not generally classed as psychotropic, e.g., the antihistamines, may have such
actions as side effects. The root of the term *psychotropic* means, literally, "mind-turn-
ing" (i.e., changing or attracted to the mind).

Psychotropic drugs may be divided into a number of major classes based on action
and therapeutic use. For the purposes of this book, psychotropic drugs are divided into
12 classes. Each drug class may contain several distinct chemical groups. The 12 classes
are (1) sedative-hypnotics (Chaps. 11, 12), (2) stimulants (Chap. 13), (3) psychedelics
(Chap. 14), (4) antipsychotics (Chap. 16), (5) anxiolytics (Chap. 17), (6) antidepressants (Chap. 18), (7) antimanics (Chap. 19), (8) extrapyramidal drugs (Chap. 21),
(9) narcotic analgesics (Chap. 23), (10) nonnarcotic analgesics (Chap. 24), (11) drugs
used to treat headaches (Chap. 25), and (12) antiepileptics (Chap. 28). There are, of
course, many other drugs and drug classes with central nervous system (CNS) effects
of greater or lesser magnitude. Our selection is based on relevance to psychotherapy
and the psychotherapist. For example, we do not cover as classes the anorexics (appetite suppressors), anesthetics, or antihistamines, except as examples of these fall into
the 12 drug classes that are of primary significance to the purposes of this book.

The *sedative-hypnotics* include the many barbiturates and other agents that either
sedate or induce sleep, depending on the dosage. The so-called minor tranquilizers, so
widely prescribed that some among them, such as Miltown and Equanil (meprobamate), Librium (chlordiazepoxide), and Valium (diazepam), have become household
words, may also legitimately be classed as sedative-hypnotics, though more often they
are called anxiolytics. *Anxiolytics* are employed to reduce anxiety. *Stimulants,* such as
amphetamine, cocaine, and caffeine, have effects that are essentially the reverse of
sedative-hypnotics. *Neuroleptics,* sometimes referred to as major tranquilizers or antipsychotic agents, are effective in ameliorating symptoms of psychosis, especially
schizophrenia, without producing significant sedation. The major chemical group
within the neuroleptics is the phenothiazines, which include the important drug
chlorpromazine (Thorazine). *Antidepressants,* as the name implies, alleviate some
kinds of depression. Major groups in this class are the monoamine oxidase (MAO)
inhibitors, such as tranylcypromine (Parnate), and the tricyclics, for example, imipramine (Tofranil) and amitriptyline (Elavil). The *psychedelics* include lysergic acid
diethylamide (LSD), psilocybin (an active principle in the "sacred mushroom" *Psilocybe mexicana*), and tetrahydrocannabinol (THC), the psychoactive component in
marijuana. *Antiepileptics,* an example of which is the extensively used drug phenytoin
(Dilantin), prevent epileptic seizures when administered chronically. *Anticonvulsants*
are related agents that stop prolonged epileptic attacks that are in progress.

Antiparkinsonians comprise a group of drugs useful in treating Parkinson's disease
and related conditions involving the extrapyramidal motor system. *Lithium* is a unique
agent employed in treating the manic-depressive syndrome. It may also be a genuinely
prophylactic treatment, preventing recurrences of the manic-depressive cycles. A
number of specialized agents have been useful in treating migraine and cluster headaches and for neuralgia, a painful and debilitating nerve disorder.

Under current laws, the psychotherapist who is not also a physician can neither prescribe nor administer most psychotropic drugs. (The exceptions would be social drugs, such as caffeine, and over-the-counter drugs; even then, there might be room for allegations of unlicensed medical practice.) Why then should the nonmedical psychotherapist have any more than a superficial knowledge of psychotropic medication?

The first reason is simply that psychotropic drugs, both licit and illicit, prescribed and self-administered, are ubiquitous. If we count caffeine, nicotine, cannabis, and alcohol, virtually all clients in psychotherapy are likely to use or to have used psychotropic drugs. Even excluding these, an unknown but undoubtedly high percentage of clients seeking psychotherapy will be using some psychotropic drug. In one study of the general population, one in six women and one in fourteen men indicated they had used a prescription psychotropic drug as often as daily in the preceding year [1]. In recent years, the steepest rise in psychotropic drug prescriptions has been in the antianxiety drugs, or anxiolytics, accounting for more than 80 million prescriptions in the United States in 1970 and over 100 million in 1980.

General practitioners write the bulk of psychotropic prescriptions. Physicians are also one of the major sources of referrals to therapists in both private and agency practices. But various studies indicate that the general public is most likely to take its problems to a physician first. It is not uncommon for physicians to prescribe medication, especially sedative-hypnotics or minor tranquilizers, and make a referral for psychotherapy only when difficulties persist. Clients may spontaneously seek psychotherapy while still on medication, because they have found the medication inadequate.

The growing popularity of comprehensive service and multimodal approaches to treatment make it very possible that psychotherapy will have to be coordinated with drug therapy. For psychotherapists working in hospitals or other institutional settings, this combination may well be the rule rather than the exception.

Drug abuse and nonabusive self-administration of drugs constitute another major area in which drugs enter into the encounter of the psychotherapist with the client. This category is especially large in that it includes alcohol and the other social drugs, as well as the sedative-hypnotics and anxiolytics.

Drug Therapy and Psychotherapy

The ultimate aim of all drug therapy should, of course, be the elimination of the need for the drug, although this may be an impossibly high aim in the case of certain chronic disorders like parkinsonism and epilepsy. More and more, though, the general trend is to prescribe psychotropic drugs as, at best, temporary measures—to diminish symptoms rapidly, to promote a good outlook to therapy, and even to aid in building the client-therapist relationship. In other words, drugs are prescribed as supportive adjuncts to psychotherapy.

Controlled scientific research on drug therapy and psychotherapy presents an interesting picture. From early studies, drugs alone would appear to be significantly better than traditional psychotherapy alone; this was reported in four of five studies reviewed by May [4]. Psychotherapy with drugs was significantly more effective than psychotherapy alone (reported in six of eight studies); but there is little difference between drugs alone and drugs with psychotherapy. Statistically speaking, no interactive effects between the drug and nondrug modes were found; that is, the relationships were simply additive. At least in the context of most of these studies—primarily short-term studies of hospitalized populations in which the drugs were major tranquilizers and the therapies were "traditional"—drugs would seem to add more to therapy than therapy to drugs. Some finer aspects of such drug-therapy interactions will be explored in Chapter 8.

Here, we are merely interested in the encounter between drugs and psychotherapy, which includes positive as well as negative effects. Throughout this book, there are cautions about the possible interference or disadvantages of drugs in psychotherapy, but this is done only to confront the practicing professional with issues and questions, with dilemmas and difficulties, to be faced and explored, not with the intention of providing answers or taking a stance on drug therapy versus psychotherapy. There are no clear-cut general answers. We have had experience with individual cases in which the use of drugs appeared clearly justified and beneficial and with others in which the use of drugs seemed definitely harmful. But few situations correspond to either extreme, and in every case the unique and individual circumstances of each client must be considered.

The impact of the psychotherapy on drug therapy is as manifold as the converse. It is well established that the effectiveness of medication is influenced by the patient's attitude toward it. By assuming benefit and promoting a positive attitude to legitimately prescribed psychotropic medication, the psychotherapist can increase the probability of beneficial results. The opposite effect has been demonstrated as well: A therapist can certainly interfere with the effectiveness of good drug therapy; this could be a profound disservice to the client.

More generally, the meaning of the drug and drug-taking to the client is an important factor in the drug-therapy interface and it is a potentially important area of influence by the psychotherapist. Drugs may be viewed as alien or unnatural by some clients, an invasion of their personal and bodily integrity. Others may see drugs as a quick cure and preferable to the slow process of working through problems. Drugs may often compromise a client's sense of responsibility or personal involvement in his or her problems, the problem and its solution appearing, logically, to be chemical. By making the patient responsible for his or her own medication, this effect may be counteracted. By highlighting the client's benefits from drugs but putting these benefits in a realistic perspective, the therapist can promote a utilitarian attitude to psychotropic medication that leads neither to dependence nor to premature rejection. Chapter 8 will continue with this topic.

Areas of Inquiry

The therapist's areas of inquiry can be divided into five broad informal areas, although the categories may well overlap: (1) drugs as causative agents in psychopathology, (2) drug side effects, (3) drug abuse, (4) neurologic implications, and (5) interactions with the psychotherapeutic process.

1. What symptoms or manifest psychopathologies might be drug-induced? For example, schizoid and paranoid behaviors may result from the use of amphetamine. Administration of LSD may constitute a psychotrauma that, in rare cases, appears capable of triggering acute or even chronic psychotic behavior. A more equivocal example is that of the alleged "amotivational syndrome" associated with extensive cannabis use. Personality changes have been attributed to the use of certain drugs (e.g., ethosuximide). Chronic alcohol abuse can produce neurologic damage that may be expected to have behavioral ramifications.

2. What bodily or subjective mental complaints may actually be side effects of drugs? The side effects of psychotropic medication and other medication may become part of the clinical picture and be confused with psychosomatic symptoms. Tics and muscular

spasms may be side effects of some drugs in certain individuals; the drug-caused symptom may even become integrated into the psychological and interpersonal problems of the client in a way that appears to reverse causes. Depression, which has many causes and serves many purposes, may also be caused or precipitated by a variety of drugs, including the widely used minor tranquilizers. Even peripherally acting drugs may produce psychic manifestations, for example, anxiety associated with hypertensive crisis. (Psychiatric side effects of drugs are summarized in appendix B.)

3. How does psychotropic drug abuse affect therapy? Does ending abuse take precedence over other psychotherapeutic goals? Should the therapist insist on cessation as a prerequisite to therapy? If not, what impact will continued use have on the efficacy and efficiency of psychotherapy? What direct and indirect roles does abuse have in the client's problems? It should be recognized that any drug can be abused, and nearly every psychotropic drug has been abused. This includes currently illicit drugs such as heroin, legitimate prescription drugs such as barbiturates and minor tranquilizers, and social drugs, including caffeine and nicotine.

4. What does the client's drug therapy or use suggest regarding actual neuropathologies? How may these be related to apparent psychopathologic symptomatology? A past preference for, or positive response to, certain drugs with anticonvulsant properties may suggest the possibility of brain lesions and subseizure brain activity in a nonepileptic client. Should either the client's physician or a neurologist be consulted? Is a referral in order? It is also possible for psychotropic medication to mask neurologic problems. Nor can the psychotherapist assume that because a drug was prescribed by a physician, a thorough neurologic investigation was conducted. (This subject of neuropathology is discussed in more detail in Chap. 2.)

5. How might the client's being on a drug, whether prescribed or self-administered, interact with the course of psychotherapy? In what ways might drug therapy enhance or reinforce psychotherapy? In what ways might drugs interfere? The therapist must consider, for example, the effects of drug use on the client's ability to learn, to assimilate new information about himself or herself, and to retain new behaviors and manifest them when not under medication. (These issues are explored in greater detail in Chap. 3.) On the other hand, drug control of epileptic-like states of emotional disturbance could significantly simplify the course of psychotherapy. Clients who would otherwise be too agitated, anxious, or depressed to benefit from a particular mode of psychotherapy may be able to improve more or faster when drugs are a part of the total clinical approach.

Another example will illustrate further aspects of these areas of inquiry in the drug-therapy interface.

A clinical psychologist had been asked by Tom Borno to see his wife, Anne, whose "performance" at home (as he put it) had been steadily declining. He suspected her of drinking excessively (she had once had a drinking problem), but could find no direct evidence. He described her as "forgetful" and complained that sometimes when he returned home from work she would be "completely dysfunctional" and would "rage at" him for prolonged periods. He knew she had seen a doctor on several recent occasions, ostensibly about her "emotional problems," but Tom perceived no improvement. Therefore, he had taken it upon himself to find an alternative course.

Initially resentful, the wife rapidly warmed to the psychologist, who began focusing on themes of power in her marriage, her oppression by her husband, and lack of personal fulfillment—all very real issues in her life. The client traced her troubles back several years, describing a rising tension and dissatisfaction with her marriage. Increasing consciousness of women's issues, which for many had opened opportunities, only made her more aware of the frustrations of her narrow life and the limitations imposed by her husband's dominance. Complaining of tension, she had obtained from her physician a prescription for a tranquilizer, i.e., an anxiolytic. This seemed to help some but was never enough. She and her therapist worked for several months, making some progress, but it was far short of what the therapist was hoping for.

When the therapist began to explore what the tranquilizers meant to her client, she learned that Anne took them daily in high-to-normal dosages, but added "an extra tablet or two" whenever she anticipated particularly difficult times, especially with her husband. A check with the Bornos' family physician revealed that he had stopped prescribing for the client nearly a year earlier, when he had learned that she was using two prescriptions, one from another local physician. It eventually turned out that she had been obtaining diazepam on three prescriptions from three different physicians, each of whom had no knowledge of the patient's "shopping around." At this point, the psychologist shifted the focus of therapy to the drug abuse and persuaded the client to collaborate with a physician.

Diazepam, as she was using it, can have among possible side effects both amnesic symptoms and, in certain individuals at some dosages, a paradoxical rage reaction. The physician confirmed that adverse reactions to the drug were possible, and he was instrumental in persuading the client to stop taking the drug. He managed the withdrawal while the clinical psychologist intensified her work around the power struggle in the client's marriage.

In retrospect, Tom Borno's suspicion that his wife might be alcoholic was not far wrong, for in many ways the prescription anxiolytic was playing a role in her life very much like that of alcohol in the life of the alcoholic person.

The New Psychotherapist

What may be needed is a psychotherapist whose perspective is little short of universal, who is not only an effective psychotherapist in his or her chosen modalities and methodologies but is also fully conversant with the psychotropic drugs, their effects and uses, and their relationship to medical or organic factors in mental health. In theory, this is the function of the psychiatrist, who is both a physician and a psychotherapist. There are, however, too few psychiatrists in proportion to the other psychotherapeutic professionals, all of whom combined probably do not meet the needs of society today.

Thus, it will probably be necessary for nonmedical therapists to step, albeit cautiously, into this breach and increasingly become involved in matters previously regarded as medical. This cannot be an entirely unilateral endeavor; closer relationships than ever between nonmedical psychotherapists and the medical profession are called for. An astute psychotherapist may suspect an organic basis for some aspects of a client's problem but will have served the client poorly unless he or she arranges a consultation with or referral to a qualified physician to confirm or disprove this suspicion. The possibilities of this cooperative interdependence are illustrated in the case history that follows.

Chucky was a 9-year-old boy whose parents requested help on referral from the school where the boy was considered "hyperactive" and a major behavior problem. The entire family entered family therapy, and it was soon evident that whatever the origins of the boy's restless and disruptive behavior it had become a part of the family life. Soon after therapy began, Chucky's physician gave him methylphenidate (Ritalin), a stimulant that paradoxically is effective in many cases of hyperkinesis. (See further discussions in Chap. 13.) In true hyperkinesis, there is a lack of ability to maintain focused attention. This, combined with disruptive behavior, might have seriously interfered with the effectiveness of the family therapy in Chucky's case and prevented dealing with numerous family problems. Under one theory of hyperkinesis, a developmental failure results in a deficit of reafferent stimuli of the sort one gets from rhythmic activity and motion. Even before the drug therapy was begun, the psychotherapist found that Chucky was attentive and not disruptive for substantial periods when he was allowed to rock or pivot energetically in his chair, and he would relax completely if rocked or stroked rhythmically by the therapist or one of his parents. This suggested a direct way of dealing with the hyperkinesis and it revealed a general lack of affectionate physical contact among members of the family. In the past, fights and wrestling matches among the children seemed to have been the substitute for affectionate contact. The therapist could, now that he had determined this, try to promote affectionate contact among the family members.

Later, through the family, the physician was asked if he would gradually reduce the medication at a time the boy and his family felt was appropriate. This was worked out as part of the therapy process. By this stage, the situation in the family had changed enough so that Chucky was able to maintain his improved behavior and outlook both in school and at home. This is an example of cooperative medical-nonmedical intervention. The physician's prescription probably simplified the family therapy. In turn, the family therapy eliminated the need for drug maintenance.

Selected References and Further Readings

1. Brecher, E. M. *Licit and Illicit Drugs.* Boston: Little, Brown, 1972.
2. Hinsie, L. E., and Campbell, R. J. *Psychiatric Dictionary,* (4th ed.). New York: Oxford University Press, 1970.
3. Hurst, L. A. Genetic Factors. In B. J. Wolman (Ed.), *Handbook of Clinical Psychology.* New York: McGraw-Hill, 1965.
4. May, P. R. Psychotherapy and Ataraxic Drugs. In A. E. Bergin and S. L. Garfield (Eds.), *Handbook of Psychotherapy and Behavior Change: An Empirical Analysis.* New York: Wiley, 1971.

Psychopathology, Drugs, and Disease

2

Psychotherapy begins when a client who has a problem visits a therapist for help. During the first interview, the client may say: "Something is wrong. I feel lousy, depressed. I can't seem to work any more, and people are saying I have been acting funny. I don't understand what it is all about. I don't know what I could do to change things." These are all the bases we need to define the appeal for help.

The client has specified that there is indeed a *problem* ("Something is wrong"), a problem that may have both immediate and ultimate causal components. The problem lies in part or is in part manifest in *affect* ("I feel lousy, depressed") and in *behavior* or functioning ("I can't seem to work any more, and people are saying I have been acting funny"). Our client confesses that he or she lacks *insight* into the problem ("I don't understand what it is all about") and does not believe he or she has the means of *self-change* ("I don't know what I could do to change things").

The five elements of the problem situation as defined by this client are therefore (1) the *problem* or "psychopathology" itself, (2) feeling or mood (*affect*), (3) *behavior* or functioning, (4) *insight*, and (5) the inability for *self-change*. These elements of the problem situation are given varying degrees of attention or emphasis by the practitioners in the various schools and modalities of therapy, providing one basis for comparing and contrasting therapies, including drug therapy. For example, behavioral therapy or behavior modification, as the terms obviously imply, focuses primarily on *behavior,* giving only secondary attention, if any, to *affect* or *insight.* The "supportive interviewing" sometimes employed by counselors or social workers deals with *affect* first, *behavior* second, and *insight* third. By contrast, traditional psychoanalysis places the greatest emphasis on *insight* as a route to the "real underlying" problem and its "root causes." In the final analysis, the differences among therapies and their underlying theories are a matter of emphasis rather than absolute exclusion of any of the five cited factors. Moreover, truly effective therapists of almost any persuasion doubtlessly deal with all facets directly or indirectly.

The possible outcomes of psychotherapy provide an even more evident contrast in terms of the elements of the client's problem. The client might well say at some future date, "Well, I feel better, but I still can't get any work done." This would be an indication that the therapist had successfully addressed *affect* but probably nothing else. Conceivably, the therapist might be rewarded with, "I don't know what you did, but everything is A-OK now!"—an indication that the therapist has not, and perhaps need not, have provided any *insight.*

The use of psychotropic drugs in psychotherapy may also be examined in relation to the elements of the problem. Antidepressants, anxiolytics, and lithium are essentially directed at the alteration of affect; that is, they represent direct means of altering or regulating mood. Neuroleptics are directed at the level of functioning, disrupting the florid symptomatology of schizophrenia. Similarly, hypnotics are used to treat the functional disability of insomnia, and stimulants are used to treat the attention deficit in hyperkinetic children. Methadone maintenance of narcotic addicts also focuses on improvement in the capacity to function in society. Disulfiram use in alcoholism, it might be argued, helps to support commitment to self-change. The use of lysergic acid diethylamide (LSD) in alcohol treatment programs aims at facilitating insight. There are as yet no definitely established examples in which drug psychotherapy addresses underlying pathophysiology. Chemical interventions in schizophrenias may deal with a biochemical component of the pathophysiology of the disorder but probably do not address the cause or causes. In order to explore and define the encounters and interactions between drug therapy and nondrug, nonmedical psychotherapy, we will first build a systematic framework for the conduct of our inquiry in a manner that does not specifically exclude any particular viewpoint or school of thought.

Psychological Health and Psychopathology

We begin our inquiry into the nature of psychotherapy in what may be thought a most unusual area—with the nature of psychological health. This beginning enables us to reveal something of our biases regarding a disease orientation to psychotherapy as opposed to a health orientation to psychotherapy. Strangely, the mental health professions have defined and delved into psychopathology but have almost excluded a definition of mental health, the assumed end of their endeavors. It is our contention that a failure to delineate clearly the objectives of therapy in terms of what constitutes psychological health is dereliction of duty.

The Nature of Psychological Health

What is mental health? First, psychologically healthy persons feel good about themselves as persons, which is essential, though almost certainly not quite enough. This self-regard has two components: self-esteem or a positive evaluation of self, and self-acceptance or acceptance of even negative aspects of self. This is the minimum that is expected of a healthy person. A healthy person may feel depressed or anxious at times, perhaps even for extended periods, but no one seriously doubts his ability to transcend the situation if it is tractable. He knows he is a "good person."

Second, the psychologically healthy person shows a high degree of flexibility in interpersonal relations. Such a person has a relatively large internal repertoire of behaviors with which to meet interpersonal contingencies and comparatively few blocks that might prevent the full utilization of this repertoire. In his ability to choose freely from a wide range of behaviors, the mentally healthy person is what Bower [2] has described as "psychologically robust," able truly to meet "the slings and arrows" of interpersonal life. This ability, of course, ranges, in various individuals, from little or no flexibility through many varied options.

Finally, the psychologically healthy person would be able to function effectively in real social systems, systems that require the ability to function either autonomously *or* dependently, as the situation demands. Compared with dependence, independence has traditionally been valued as a more mature mode of interpersonal functioning. Following the emergence of the "third force," or humanistic psychology, and under the influence of the more progressive developmentalists, a third mode of functioning has been recognized as being even more psychologically adaptive. The independent person who *must* be autonomous has a handicap compared with the independent person who can also be dependent; for example, nurses are all too familiar with the patient who has great difficulty in the hospital environment because he or she cannot tolerate being dependent. *Interdependence,* or *synergic autonomy,* is a rich and balanced mixture of dependence and independence, with the ability to function, as appropriate, in either mode. *Synergy* refers to the transcendence of dichotomies (such as dependence versus independence) and is recognized as an element in the perceptions of psychologically healthy individuals [7, 10]. In truth, in all real interpersonal systems, individuals can be neither fully autonomous nor fully dependent; thus, synergic autonomy is a more realistic and effective mode of functioning.

In our view, then, the three primary components of psychological health are self-regard, interpersonal flexibility, and interdependent functioning. Self-regard is a quality of the person viewed in isolation, an internal, personal, or "intrapsychic" characteristic. Behavioral flexibility is an interpersonal or interactive characteristic. Interdependence, or synergic autonomy, is a systemic, systems-theoretical construct. We shall have other occasions to make use of this triple perspective of intrapersonal, interpersonal, and metapersonal points of view.

The reader will note that our definition of psychological health is not closely aligned with any one school of psychology. It is an attempt at something empirical and not many levels removed from physical, demonstrable reality—or at least a person's direct experience of this reality. It does not get into high levels of abstraction such as "successful resolution of the Oedipal conflict" to define health, nor does it involve the high degree of value judgment in such concepts as "adequate impulse control" or "repression of antisocial tendencies." Ours is a kind of minimal definition and therefore one that will be unsatisfactory to many therapists, but which also, for the same reason, has many attractions.

Now it is legitimate to wonder how psychotropic medication can improve self-esteem, enhance behavioral repertoires, or promote synergic autonomy. This question will be taken up in Chapter 3 after a fuller exploration of the coin's obverse—psychopathology.

The Nature of Psychopathology

In the terms just introduced, *psychopathology* is or is manifested in an absence or loss of good feelings about oneself, and/or in a truncated or inadequate interpersonal repertoire, and/or in an inability to function interdependently. Again, we are not relating our definition to any one nosology of the many alternative medical and nonmedical psychological theories, but rather we are attempting a metaperspective that "steps out of" these specialized (and often conflicting) points of view. The client in psychotherapy is simply a person who is "not doing well" in any of the three senses outlined above. If we have not covered all the bases, we have certainly touched the most important ones.

In starting with psychological health and using a nonmedical metaperspective, we are not in any way denying the reality of medical aspects to psychological health or the existence of possibly distinct and certainly classifiable patterns or syndromes of ineffective behavior. General paresis is a real disease with a demonstrable impact on behavior and mental life, for example. While general paresis is a disease, from a mental health perspective it does not constitute a distinct syndrome. Indeed, syphilis was once known as "the great masquerader" because it manifested itself in so many symptoms. On the other side of the coin, the pattern of behaviors identified as schizophrenia means different things to British psychiatrists and to American psychiatrists [3]. The British classify many more patients as schizophrenic than do the Americans.

But we need not settle the question of which syndromes are due to chance and which are true entities, which psychiatric labels are diseases and which are only labels, in order to consider the origins, in general, of psychopathology. We are less concerned with those few specific exceptions that seem established as falling clearly into the medical domain because they have been proved to be caused by a physical pathogen, trauma, or tumor. Nor are we so concerned with those clearly in the purely behavioral realms. Rather, our concern lies with the majority of psychological problems that almost certainly have many possible and even concurrent sources.

The Etiology of Psychopathology

Etiology of a disease refers to the origins and causes that lead to it. When the diseases are forms of psychopathology, etiologic knowledge is, in general, limited. The inadequacies stem from many sources, among them: the organization of psychology and psychotherapy into schools of thought, the difficulty of developing substantive data, and an all-too-common lack of interest in etiology and diagnosis among practitioners. With limited, conflicting, mutually exclusive points of view from which to define and describe etiology, the "schools" of thought do not build on each other's understanding. It is difficult to evaluate data when the syndromes are subtle, the sources manifold, and the disease sometimes not even existing as a discrete entity. The problem of indifference to accurate diagnosis of the unique etiology in an individual case may in part be professional shoddiness or inadequacy, but it seems mostly a result of the common belief among psychotherapists that each has *the* cure for almost any problem, whatever its origins, either because of loyalty to the tenets of a particular therapeutic school of thought or because of a feeling that he or she is "eclectic."

The etiology of psychopathologic symptoms is not merely a pivotal point in the interface between psychotropic drugs and psychotherapy. A broadly based working knowledge of this area is the mark of a true professional psychotherapist and may even spell the difference between cure and disaster. Consider the following case known to the authors:

A 35-year-old woman with a history of neurotic complaints and symptomatology complained to her physician about periods of dizziness, intense anxiety, and blackout. He referred her to a therapist. After becoming discouraged with the lack of progress with her first therapist, the woman visited a second therapist, and thence to group therapy. At no point in this sequence of referrals and patient-initiated efforts to seek help was an adequate neuropsychodiagnostic workup undertaken. The patient suddenly and unexpectedly died 6 months after the initial approach to the physician. Autopsy revealed the presence of a malignant brain tumor.

The maximally effective psychotherapist needs to be cognizant of organic as well as nonorganic factors in psychopathologic etiology. The etiology of what we see as psychological symptoms can involve complex combinations of factors in the following categories:

1. Organic process (in which the determinants are physiologic-anatomic), including genetic defects, diseases, and physical trauma, e.g., minimal brain dysfunction (MBD), psychomotor epilepsy, and inherited predispositions for the emergence of schizophrenic behavior.
2. Psychological or personal processes (in which the determinants are in individual experience), including personal trauma and chronic psychological irritants, conditioning (reinforcement paradigms), and personality organization.
3. Interpersonal systemic process (in which the determinants are in a system qua system), including the effect of labeling, amplification of deviation in family and social systems, and overall family strategies that generate and maintain manifest psychopathology.

The general case involves elements in all three areas—organic process, psychological process, and interpersonal systemic process—interwoven in ways that may often render them analytically inseparable. We shall, however, discuss these individually before presenting a viewpoint of their interweaving.

Organic Process: Genetic Factors

The genetic component in "mental illness" has been the focus of extensive inquiry [5], generating much excitement and even controversy. That there is, for example, a genetic factor in "the schizophrenias" has been fairly well established [3]. Quotation marks are used because it is not at all clear that there is a distinct disease entity properly called schizophrenia. There may be many kinds of schizophrenia, some of which "look alike"; that is, individuals manifesting the same behavior may have very different problems and some "schizophrenics" may in fact have the same problem ("disease") as others with different manifest symptoms. This relationship between clinical symptoms and etiological syndromes such as schizophrenia has been inadequately treated in the literature.

Overall, the research on the genetic factors in mental illness indicates the need for a number of qualifications. (1) It is almost certain in the case of schizophrenia (and probably for many other syndromes for which a genetic factor can be demonstrated) that the inherited factor is polygenic, that is, associated with a gene combination and possibly with a number of distinct combinations. Thus, there is not a simple pattern of inheritance. (2) The heritability of schizophrenia (the best studied example) is low; that is, genetics accounts for only a small portion of the observed variance in the occurrence of the pattern. (3) At best, the inherited factor can be viewed as a predisposition or susceptibility to the "disease" that must be potentiated or exacerbated by environmental factors for the pattern to become manifest. An important question in this respect is whether a predisposition to a particular pattern of behavior with a small heritability (namely, schizophrenia) is distinct from the heritability of personality in general. One might simply say that schizophrenic behavior is more likely to develop in some people with certain personality patterns, which are themselves of only low heritability. It would seem that the burden of proof is on the proposition that these are different concepts; that is, the null assumption is that they are one and the same. (4) The systems theoretic concept of "equifinality" appears to apply to the question of genetic factors in psychological problems. Equifinal processes have different initial conditions and different courses of events, but a common outcome. There is no reason a particular pattern of symptoms that we observe and classify as problematic could not result from various totally different but equifinal processes. In view of the long history of scientific failure to establish a clear and simple etiology for most mental problems, this would seem to be a most apt explanation.

Organic Process: Neuropsychodiagnosis

Neuropsychodiagnosis refers to the process of determining the existence, nature, and extent of organic etiology in manifest psychopathology. It is a complex, subtle, and generally neglected art that can at best be given cursory coverage here. A comprehensive book on the subject by Leonard Small [11] is essential reading for all practicing psychotherapists.

Psychotherapists, even psychiatrists, often neglect diagnosis, especially the diagnosis of organicity, i.e., organic factors in psychopathology. A diagnosis that is mere nosologic classification labels clients, boxing them in, oversimplifying their uniqueness, and perhaps even reinforcing symptomatic patterns. Then, too, there is something final and faintly ominous about the implication of an organic basis in a particular case, though this is founded on false assumptions that organicity implies intractability, or worse, the inappropriateness of psychotherapy. There is always the question of what the psychotherapist is to do with the information even if he or she can determine the organic factors in a particular case.

Nevertheless, the psychotherapist is obligated to be aware of organic processes and to be competent to assess the likelihood or extent of possible organicity in specific cases of psychopathology. Numerous studies involving comprehensive screenings of psychiatric patients have uncovered evidence of previous undiagnosed neurologic involvement in up to half of these patients [11]. In general, it would appear that far more clients who reach a psychotherapist have undiagnosed but diagnosable organic problems than it is comfortable to believe.

Furthermore, the psychotherapist has much to gain from a thorough insight into the organic factors in a case. The nature of the organic problem, once known, can shape the treatment plan, suggesting productive and unproductive directions for therapy and placing realistic limits on what may be accomplished. Or the organic basis may be amenable to direct treatment with drugs, thus simplifying the psychotherapeutic task and greatly improving the outlook. Knowledge of the organic etiology may suggest useful adjuncts or even alternatives to psychotherapy, such as remedial education or special rehabilitation to strengthen specific mental functions. If it is thought that organic factors are at the basis of the client's problem, a different kind of therapy may be employed; for example, the use of art, imagery, and dance therapy if the client is found to have an aphasia that limits the effectiveness of "talking therapy" (see Chap. 3).

The neuropsychodiagnosis of organicity requires the integration of numerous subtle cues, so-called soft signs that suggest the possibility but do not demonstrate the existence of an organic basis. Small [11] outlines a collection of specific signs that may be used to determine whether a consultation or referral for a thorough neurologic workup is indicated. These are summarized below in material adapted from Small [11, pp. 202–203; 215–216].

Grounds for Suspecting Neurologic Implications

A. Birth injuries, prolonged birth, forceps delivery, report of anoxia, low Apgar rating at birth; other head injuries or trauma, especially involving loss of consciousness or paralysis; high fevers, prolonged anesthesia, poisonings, and certain diseases; persistent learning difficulties, school problems, or behavior disorders

B. Paroxysmal phenomena involving any sense modality, loss of balance, dizziness, altered states of consciousness (e.g., feelings of depersonalization or unreality, confusion, perplexity), memory losses or automatic behavior

C. Psychological test results with variation among specific functions exceeding expected variation, e.g., on the Wechsler scales; pronounced "organic indications" on the Bender or projective tests; mixed cortical hemisphere dominance as evidenced by different tests of lateralization

D. Disturbing emotional states that cannot be clearly connected to psychological and systemic processes, precipitating circumstances, or meaning to the client; for example, anxiety, depersonalization, déjà vu experiences, depression, hypochondriasis without discernible precedents

E. A sudden emotional change that cannot be ascribed to specific precipitating circumstances, accompanied by sleep disturbances, ravenous hunger and/or thirst, metabolic disorders, or shifts in sexual appetite

F. Gradual alteration in vision, hearing, touch, motor control, balance, or so-called overlearned skills such as typing or playing of musical instruments

G. Language disturbances and difficulties in spoken or written form (aphasias); difficulty in placing objects in relation to each other without impairment of vision or motor control (construction apraxia); difficulty in performing purposeful movements in the absence of paralysis (apraxia); impairment of the ability to recognize and identify objects in the absence of sensory defects (agnosias)

H. Impairment of recall, disorders of orientation, intellectual deficits, disturbances of drive (including hyperactivity and apathy), and disorders in attention

The organic problems that are most likely to be encountered by the psychotherapist are those that are most likely to be assumed to have purely psychological or interpersonal systemic origins, that is, that have the "softest" signs and look most like other forms of psychopathology. Most prominent among these are minimal brain dysfunction, epilepsy and epileptiform subictal activity (to be discussed in Chap. 27), and mild mental retardation. Others include organically based depression, the so-called positive spike pattern (Chap. 27), chronic organic brain syndrome, various presenile dementias, and schizophrenia, although the incomplete demonstration of the organic basis of the last-mentioned and its complexity and variability equivocate its inclusion here. A partial list of organic problems that may result in psychopathology is presented in Table 2-1.

Minimal Brain Dysfunction (MBD) is a catchall term for a wide variety of symptoms and disorders that are believed, but have not been proved, to have their basis in localized brain damage or dysfunction. The alternative, less appropriate term *minimal brain damage* reflects a previously held belief that all such cases involve overt brain damage. It is now felt that in many cases of MBD, the viability of individual neurons is intact, but the cells have failed to interrelate in such a way as to provide the function normal for that particular brain region. Most often, MBD is manifest in a disparity in psychological abilities, one or a small number of often highly specific mental capacities being impaired. This is in marked contrast to mental retardation, in which there is a more across-the-board depression of abilities. A prime popular example of MBD is dyslexia, in which the ability to read and assimilate written material is impaired. Minimal brain dysfunction may have a variety of behavioral and emotional correlates, either primary or secondary to the disability. Psychotherapy clients with MBD may show apathy, depression, erratic or "immature" behavior, or low self-esteem because of repeated failures, to mention just a few possibilities. In some ways, it is unfortunate to group so many disparate conditions under this heading (some writers even include hyperkinesis

Table 2-1. Some organic disorders having behavioral manifestations

Name of disorder	Descriptions and genetic component if known
I. Acute organic brain syndrome	Psychiatric or cognitive disturbances of sudden onset caused by physical conditions, including (1) diminished cerebral blood flow; (2) diminished oxygen delivery to the brain; (3) reduced glucose utilization as in hypoglycemia or diabetes mellitus; (4) fluid, electrolyte, or metabolic disturbances; (5) elevated intracranial pressure; (6) elevated temperature; (7) nutritional deficiencies; and (8) excessive doses of depressant drugs
II. Chronic organic brain syndrome	Psychiatric or cognitive disturbances of gradual onset in elderly patients because of senile brain damage, cerebral arteriosclerosis, or trauma (polygenic)
III. Presenile cerebral degenerative dementias	
A. Alzheimer's disease	Diffuse cerebral atrophy, indistinguishable from chronic organic brain syndrome associated with senility except that onset is comparatively premature (polygenic)
B. Pick's disease	Demarcated cerebral atrophy (dominant autosomal)
IV. Extrapyramidal degenerative diseases	
A. Wilson's disease	Degeneration of lenticular nuclei possibly related to abnormal copper metabolism, marked by hyperemotionality (autosomal, probably recessive)
B. Huntington's chorea	Chronically developing mental deterioration with choreiform movements and personality change (single autosomal dominant gene)
C. Creutzfeldt's disease	Corticostriatospinal degeneration and spastic pseudosclerosis
V. EEG abnormalities	
A. Grand mal epilepsy	Seizures involving convulsions and loss of consciousness (possibly single or irregular dominant gene)

B. Petit mal epilepsy — Seizures involving lapses or clouding of consciousness without convulsions (possibly single dominant gene)

C. Temporal lobe epilepsy — Seizures of the temporal lobe, often accompanied by psychopathologic manifestations

D. Subictal epilepsy — Epilepsy of subseizure intensity, manifested subtly in behavior

E. Positive-spike potential syndrome — A neurologic syndrome with variable behavioral concomitants

VI. Minimal brain dysfunction — Diverse symptomatologies presumably related to brain damage or dysfunction

VII. Mental retardation — Impaired intellect

VIII. Endocrine malfunctions

A. Graves' disease — Hyperfunctioning of the thyroid gland; psychological manifestations are nervousness, hyperexcitability, restlessness, insomnia, and emotional instability

B. Myxedema — Hypofunctioning of the thyroid gland; most prominent psychological manifestation is physical and mental lethargy; in severe cases, memory impairment and psychoses may occur

C. Cushing's syndrome — Hyperfunctioning of the adrenals; psychiatric disturbances occur frequently

D. Addison's disease — Adrenal insufficiency; weakness and fatigue are early symptoms; dizziness and depression may occur

E. Hypoglycemia — May be due to hyperinsulinism (overreaction of pancreas to glucose ingestion) or poor diet (alcoholism, delayed meals, fasting, crash diets); symptoms include confusion, tremor, anxiety, irritability, hunger, nausea, dullness, apathy, agitation, restlessness, disorientation, impaired perception, altered states of consciousness, and seizure

IX. Chromosomal abnormalities — e.g., Down's syndrome (trisomy of chromosome 21); mongolism marked by deficits in physical and intellectual development

X. Infections — e.g., syphilis, encephalitis, meningitis

XI. Substance-induced disorders — Acute and chronic toxic psychoses, intoxication, and withdrawal

XII. Substance-use disorders — Abuse and dependence

under MBD), since it hardly clarifies either diagnosis or therapy; however, the use of a term implying organic involvement may help to remove some of the blame often heaped on the victim of MBD for academic failure and other school or work problems. It is unfortunate that this relabeling is necessary to reduce blame; even the absence of organicity does not imply the willing complicity of the client.

Serious *mental retardation* is not likely to reach the psychotherapist undiagnosed. Milder retardation is more likely to go undiagnosed or even to be mislabeled as autistic or schizophrenic. Correct diagnosis is difficult and probably requires special training. In mental retardation, therapy must make provision for this and use approaches that are appropriate to the client's level of intellectual functioning. Behavioral techniques, learning divided into small, simple units, psychodramatic and play therapy, emotional ventilation, reassurance, and reality-oriented, goal-directed approaches are all suggested by Small [11]. Work with moderately or more severely retarded clients should be regarded as a professional specialization. Although approximately half of the patients in this category receive psychotropic drug medication, the evidence that any drug choice improves baseline cognitive functioning is inadequate. Neuroleptics are the most widely used drugs in mental retardation. They can be effective in reducing undesirable behaviors, such as aggressive outbursts or self-mutilation, but also further impair learning, performance, and cognition.

Depression and grief-like reactions can be a side effect of numerous physical conditions, among them, multiple sclerosis, arteriosclerosis, paresis, tumors in the corpus callosum, and subdural hematoma. Also, certain drugs may induce depression, including the corticosteroids, sulfonamides, and vitamin B_{12}, as well as the psychotropic drugs phenobarbital (Chap. 11), chlorpromazine (Chap. 16), and others, all listed in Appendix B. The psychotherapist should be alert to these possibilities and conduct inquiries into disease history and drug use.

Among the elderly, *chronic organic brain syndrome* (chronic OBS) is common, affecting one out of every six persons over the age of 65. As much as half the geriatric population of hospitals and nursing homes have chronic OBS [9]. The symptomatology is highly variable, including anxiety, agitation, paranoid behavior, depression, apathy, or withdrawal, depending on the individual's psychological makeup, but the basic syndrome consists of memory defects, disorientation, and intellectual impairment. The phrase "primary degenerative dementia, senile onset" is also used to describe this condition and is usually qualified as uncomplicated, with delirium, delusions, or depression.

Patients later proved at autopsy to have chronic OBS have been misdiagnosed as schizophrenics or primary depressives, among others. Although chronic OBS may, like the acute form, be caused by trauma such as injury, drug intoxication, and severe alcoholism, the vast majority of cases are associated with cerebral arteriosclerosis or senile brain damage, a pattern of unknown etiology. *Arteriosclerosis* is a generic term covering several types of pathologic changes in blood vessels. The most common form is called atherosclerosis. In this disease, accumulations of lipids cause a thickening of the blood vessel wall, resulting in a narrowing of the vessel diameter, resistance to blood flow, elevated blood pressure, inelasticity of the vessel, and poor exchange of nutrients and wastes between the blood and tissues such as the brain. Senility, on the other hand, is caused by diffuse changes in the brain that accompany aging. Among the changes noted in the human brain with aging are a decrease in volume and weight of brain tissue related to a loss of proteins and lipids, decreased glucose utilization, increased vascular resistance, reduced neuronal populations in certain brain regions, and accumulation of lipofuscins. Virtually identical correlates are reported in Alzheimer's presenile psychosis, so that many researchers and clinicians now refer to chronic OBS associated with senility as senile dementia, Alzheimer type.

Chronic OBS, being irreversible, is often approached with pessimism by psychotherapists; however, psychotherapy has been underutilized with these elderly clients. Supportive individual and group therapy can be highly beneficial for the psychiatric symptomatology. Group therapy also creates a setting for positive social interaction among otherwise withdrawn, isolated, or alienated persons. Involvement of the entire family in family therapy is useful in promoting readaptation of the family system to the elderly person's impaired capacities. Almost the entire range of psychotropic drugs covered in this book have been used in chronic OBS. Because paradoxical reactions are common and side effects that may be of little consequence in younger persons are often critical in an older person, all psychotropic drugs must be used cautiously. Sometimes side effects develop in these patients at low doses of psychotropics, and they more frequently exhibit paradoxical reactions, such as excitement rather than sedation when taking barbiturates. It should be noted that many elderly patients with apparent OBS have an underlying medical condition such as chronic heart failure or bronchitis, treatment of which removes the behavior disorder.

The objectives of chemotherapy for chronic OBS center on (1) symptomatic relief of psychiatric disturbances and (2) improvement of cognitive functioning. In the first respect, neuroleptics, especially thioridazine, are useful for emotional disturbances, anxiolytics for anxiety, and tricyclics for depression, all at lower-than-normal doses. Sedative-hypnotics are avoided whenever possible because they tend to aggravate cognitive impairment. Five classes of drugs have been employed for baseline cognitive impairment, but three of these classes have failed to exhibit even good promise of potential value. Stimulants (methylphenidate, pentylenetetrazole, and magnesium pemoline) have not demonstrated long-term effectiveness. Cerebral vasodilators (e.g., papaverine) give a poor response and have dangerous cardiovascular effects. Vitamins, minerals, and hormones have shown no evidence of value. The two most promising approaches are the use of cerebral metabolism stimulators and transmitter precursors (levodopa, 5-hydroxytryptophan, choline). Dihydroergotoxine, a combination of three ergot compounds, is the only stimulator of cerebral metabolism currently available in the United States. Well-controlled studies support claims of the effectiveness of dihydroergotoxine (Hydergine) based on both physician and subjective assessment. There is some evidence that elevating brain levels of acetylcholine is of value, but there is as yet no adequate pharmacologic method for accomplishing this reliably.

Psychological Process

The late Eric Berne had an apt and general metaphor for the psychological etiology of emotional and behavioral problems. He likened the individual's accumulation of experiences, which shapes personality and psychological functioning, to the stacking of coins, layer by layer. The stack may become crooked or unstable because some of the coins are not centered well or are bent. The stack can be skewed as much by the repetition of many small misalignments as by one major disruption of the stack. Although the analogy does not do justice to the robustness of the human organism, it does note the importance of both chronic irritants and traumatic events.

We refer to as psychological process those processes happening within a person or happening *to* a person. Although the various psychological schools give differing emphasis to events that are internal (intrapsychic or intrapersonal) as opposed to those that occur between individuals (interpersonal), psychological theories have in common their ultimate view that the problem, the pathologic state, is *in* the individual rather than resident in any other conceptual or real structure.

Organic process, whether genetic, congenital, or otherwise, can be thought of as the wiring for the complex emotional and behavioral machinery that can become the individual; and the psychological process can be thought of as the programming that will be stored within that machinery.

Drug therapy fits well within most theoretical frameworks in psychology, since drugs are clearly agents acting within the individual. The antagonisms between psychology and drug therapy that have occurred would have to be interpreted within specific theoretical frameworks, which would be beyond the scope of this discussion.

Interpersonal Systemic Process: Family and Society

A system is an organization of interacting parts exhibiting coherent behavior. The behavior of a system is determined not merely by the behavior of its individual parts, but also by its structure, namely, the totality of interrelationships among parts. A system is thus more than the sum of its parts, which is more than adequate justification for making systems the unit of analysis. The processes discussed under this heading are distinguished from those of the last section in that the latter involve or at least imply linear (sequential, classic, or Newtonian) causality, while systemic processes are circular or mutually causal (the Gibbsian paradigm).

Recognition of the role of the family in psychopathology goes back at least as far as Freud's early, linear formulations, though the founder of psychoanalysis chose to focus on individual personality as determined by family rather than the family as a unit. The failure of early investigators to take advantage of the corroborative sources of the family led to some anomalous findings and theories of long standing. Freud, for example, simply assumed that parent-child incest could not conceivably be as common as his patients reported; *therefore,* their reports must be manufactured out of childhood wishes for sexual involvement with their parents. But recent inquiries involving non-clinical, noncriminal populations have revealed that actual incest is probably much more common than previously imagined. Freud's analysis of Schroeber, on which his theory of paranoia is based, is also illustrative of the importance of real data on the real family system. A recent analysis of Schroeber's father's writings suggest that many if not all the patient's persecutory allegations were not imagined, that his father was in fact an invasive martinet.

Beginning in contemporary times with the work of Don Jackson and others of the so-called Palo Alto group and Nathan Ackerman in New York, the role of the family system in the promotion and maintenance of supposedly individual problems has been steadily elucidated. We now know that the "identified patient" (or individual client) and his or her particular behaviors serve a real purpose in his family, that the entire family system often functions inadvertently to keep the identified patient in that role and to facilitate continued symptoms, and that an induced improvement in his or her symptoms is often followed by a compensatory outbreak of symptoms in some other family member. Perhaps the most fundamental contribution of the family systems theorists and of family therapy is to implicate the entire system, its coherent functioning as an entity, as opposed to specific members. Thus, it now appears to be inadequate to look for causes of children's behavior in that of their parents; each is cause and outcome of the other in a mutually determined system. Adequately controlled outcome research has yet to be completed, but the cumulative evidence strongly suggests that intervention in this family system as a unit—changing the most significant interpersonal system in which individuals are embedded—is often the most efficient means of accomplishing significant change in affected individuals.

We must also implicate the entire social system in which individuals participate. Even families do not exist in a vacuum. Social psychology and epidemiologic studies have clearly indicated that class and community are important explanatory variables in the incidence of psychological problems. More recently, the so-called ecologic perspective [1] has emerged, recognizing the involvement of a person's complete social network as contributory to the continuation, if not the causes, of behavioral and emotional difficulties.

We must also include in pathogenic processes of the social system such positive feedback loops as the effects of labeling a person as "hyperkinetic," "neurotic," or "schizophrenic," for example, and such pervasive contextual shapers as institutionalization [12].

Models of human functioning and dysfunctioning that view behavior as inextricably embedded in a complete system of individuals rather than in some one person or a currently interacting pair include family systems theories as well as ecologic or network perspectives. Completely developed theories are notably lacking, but among the better-rounded examples we would have to include Minuchin's [8] and Kantor and Lehr's [6] typal theories and psychopolitical model, although there are many other specialized or partial theories in this area. An insider's purview may be obtained from Ferber, Mendelsohn, and Napier [4].

Etiology: A Systemic Overview

All these processes—organic, psychological, and interpersonal systemic—are seen to interact, manifest psychopathology being the current end product of their involuted interplay. The pure and simple cases of an entirely systemic process or an organic defect with no systemic involvement, for example, are probably rare. The following scenario exemplifies the complex interplay of factors we are suggesting:

Harold was the second of four children. Both his birth and that of his older brother, Peter, had been unusually protracted. Anoxia and prolonged pressure had resulted in minor undetected brain damage in Harold's case, causing focal electrical activity in the temporal lobe. Subictal activity—below the threshold of a true seizure—in this region can be very difficult to diagnose or detect and may be manifest only in slight biases toward sudden specific behavior sequences. Harold's organic problem was to remain undiscovered. His parents had always regarded him as "difficult." Even as an infant, he had had sudden temper tantrums when mildly frustrated and occasionally without apparent reason. These, in turn, frustrated and angered his parents. As their efforts at control proved fruitless, they increasingly withdrew affection and simply isolated Harold when he was unmanageable.

By his middle childhood years, Harold was openly labeled as the "troublemaker" in his family, a role he accepted and filled with growing effectiveness. This gave him a sense of special status to compensate for his parents' clear preference for Peter, "a somewhat slow, quiet, but well-behaved" child. By this time, Harold's temper, thoroughly learned and elaborated, generally provided a quick diversion from any serious contention among other family members whenever Harold could take sides. Even in his own eyes, Harold was the "cause" of family problems. In school, he was first labeled a "behavior problem," justifying special treatment by teachers and administrators, which, combined with his "bad boy" status among peers, further entrenched him in antisocial behavior patterns. Later he was relabeled by the school as "hyperactive" and placed on amphetamines, which did not seem to help his "hyperactivity." He was soon removed from amphetamine therapy, and the temporary abatement of his tantrums passed unnoticed. (The amphetamines have some anticonvulsant effects and were once employed as antiepileptics.)

He appeared to be a likely candidate for juvenile delinquency. Instead, under an insistent internal drive to be accepted positively by his peers at least, Harold gradually learned to avoid confrontation and anger-provoking situations and to "manage" the subictal states by recognizing their onset and withdrawing temporarily from other people.

His shift to nonaggression was seen by all to be a dramatic maturation into a "good boy," though he began to show more "neurotic" symptoms, such as excessive scratching. With Harold's withdrawal as "scapegoat," the rest of his family began to have more violent arguments among themselves. When he started school at a nearby community college, Harold found that without strong role expectations from this new social system, he was better able to maintain new and more rewarding interpersonal behaviors. Weekends with his family, however, became increasingly difficult for him and left him "emotionally exhausted." As the first term progressed, he experienced increasing difficulty in studying. It was for this that he sought help as a young adult.

There are many possible sequels. It may be that the psychologist whom he is presently seeing at college is an incredibly astute clinician attuned to subtle cues in neuropsychodiagnosis. In this case, there will be a referral for a neurologic workup, and eventually Harold will be placed on an effective regimen of appropriate antiepileptic medication with perhaps a cautious supplement of an anxiolytic. Simple drug therapy will alleviate the subictal states manifested as sudden and inappropriate outbursts of temper or the need for rapid retreat from social situations. However, Harold is also burdened with deeply entrenched negative feelings about himself and with ingrained patterns of dysfunctional behavior of long standing. These he would carry with him into his new family of procreation should he be satisfied temporarily by the improvement brought about by drug therapy.

Individual psychotherapy by itself could eventually modify many of these learned behaviors and improve Harold's self-image, but it would be working uphill against the forces of his family of origin. This course alone would be unlikely to have any significant effect on his subictal states; thus, Harold would always be saddled with an unexplained irritability and perhaps be limited in potential by labels such as "unstable" or "odd."

The college psychologist might instead have a family systems orientation and involve Harold's entire family in family therapy. This could be a more efficient way to bring about immediate changes in Harold's interpersonal functioning with the added possible side benefit of preventive effects for the rest of the family. Insight into family dynamics for Harold and his siblings might in itself be sufficiently advantageous to justify this approach. But, again, without diagnosis and drug treatment, Harold's subictal focal activity would remain intact.

Overview

It should be self-evident by now that *only a comprehensive therapeutic perspective is adequate.* Psychotherapy must be prepared to deal with genetic and other organic factors, with individual personality, experience, and behavior, and with social and systemic processes, as well as the interactions among all of these.

In summary, then, we have a picture in which potentiating genetic factors—some merely possible, some established—and neurophysiologic realities of trauma and disease are mediated by personal-interpersonal experience, modifying and modified by social and family systems to yield what we, in retrospect, judge to be mental health or mental illness. A simpler view cannot do justice to the full weight of evidence from many fields.

Viewed in this nonsimplistic perspective, differential diagnosis is a subtle, if not intractable, demand. Different problematic syndromes comprise varying mixes of the origins discussed. Worse, individuals could manifest the same symptoms traceable to completely different causal patterns. The consistent failure of research to find background characteristics with any significant correlation with a specific syndrome when whole populations are studied supports this contention. The question is more than academic, for the origins of a "dysfunctional" pattern of behavior probably affect the efficiency and effectiveness of agents chosen for intervention.

Some of the evidence for genetic factors in mental illness, especially schizophrenia, has been used erroneously to justify drug therapy. Such arguments must be examined carefully. Even should some particular syndrome be found to be entirely of genetic origin, this would not invalidate nondrug psychotherapy, any more than congenital birth defects of the motor system invalidate the use of physical therapy to compensate for or even to correct specific difficulties. Conversely, behavioral or emotional problems traceable entirely to the dynamics of the family system of origin could still legitimately be treated with appropriate drugs. Aside from what we agree are essential ethical and philosophical issues beyond the scope of this treatise, the questions in every case are those of efficiency and effectiveness. Intuitively, one expects these to be related to underlying causal factors, but there is certainly no solid evidence in the form of differential outcome studies. The psychotherapist must always be concerned with the degree of change induced by any intervention as measured against its cost to the client in time, pain, and money. As to effectiveness, there are several issues. The first is fundamental: Does drug therapy actually bring about or induce change? That is, when do drugs cure and when do they merely ameliorate symptoms? At present, the evidence for amelioration is far more massive than the evidence for actual correction, except with very special agents and applications. Even here, the evidence is inconclusive and the cures impermanent, requiring continued administration. We must also wonder about specificity of drugs to the actual problems presented: Do drugs, as generally employed, address the actual etiologic factors in the client's problems, or do they sometimes mask these factors?

In some sense, these are somewhat unfair questions, for as the strong proponents of drug therapy would maintain, drugs are seldom, if ever, intended to be the sole treatment modality. Unfortunately, however, institutions are sometimes prone to violate good intentions in practice. Our primary interest, however, remains the relationship of psychotropic drugs to nondrug psychotherapy; thus, the questions pertaining to drugs as an independent mode of treatment will be left posed but unanswered.

Selected References and Further Readings

1. Auerswald, E. H. Interdisciplinary Versus Ecological Approach. In W. Gray et al. (Eds.), *General Systems Theory and Psychiatry.* Boston: Little, Brown, 1969.
2. Bower, E. M. Primary Prevention of Mental and Emotional Disorders. In A. V. Bindman and A. D. Spiegel (Eds.), *Perspectives in Community Mental Health.* Chicago: Aldine, 1969.
3. Eisenberg, L. Psychiatric intervention. *Sci. Am.* 229:16–24, 1973.
4. Ferber, A., Mendelsohn, M., and Napier, A. *The Book of Family Therapy.* New York: Science House, 1972.
5. Hurst, L. A. Genetic Factors. In B. J. Wolman (Ed.), *Handbook of Clinical Psychology.* New York: McGraw-Hill, 1965.
6. Kantor, D., and Lehr, W. *Inside the Family: Toward a Theory of Family Process.* San Francisco: Jossey-Bass, 1975.
7. Maslow, A. *Eupsychian Management.* Homewood, Ill.: Irwin & Dorsey Press, 1965.
8. Minuchin, S. *Families and Family Therapy.* Cambridge, Mass.: Harvard University Press, 1974.
9. Prien, R. F. Chronic Organic Brain Syndrome. (No. 0-482-317 [189].) Washington, D.C.: U.S. Govt. Printing Office, 1972.
10. Shostrom, E. *Manual for the Personal Orientation Inventory.* San Diego: Educational and Industrial Testing Service, 1966.

11. Small, L. *Neuropsychodiagnosis in Psychotherapy.* New York: Brunner-Mazel, 1973.
12. Szasz, T. S. *The Manufacture of Madness.* New York: Harper & Row, 1970.
13. Wender, P. H. Minimal Brain Dysfunction: An Overview. In M. A. Lipton et al. (Eds.), *Psychopharmacology: A Generation of Progress.* New York: Raven, 1978.
14. Yesavage, J. A. Pharmacotherapy of the aged central nervous system. *Clin. Neuropharmacol.* 4:199–220, 1979.

Drugs, Learning, and Psychotherapy

3

The front page of an issue of *The Radical Therapist* once carried the headline, "Therapy means change—not oatmeal!" Change—change in perceptions, in outlook, in behavior, in interpersonal style—is the essence of psychotherapy. By definition, then, psychotherapy means learning. This, however, entails learning something much broader in scope than what is implied by "learning theory" or behavioral psychology.

Learning and Psychotherapy

Modes of Learning

How do people learn? Especially, how do they learn such complex and subtle sequences of behavior as are involved in interpersonal life? This question cannot be answered fully. It is not too basic, however, to begin by pointing out the obvious, that people learn what they *do*. They learn the style and behaviors that they experience firsthand. Direct, personal experience in a role or situation is the most important learning mode.

People also appear to learn through emulation; they learn what they see. But obviously at some point the model observed must be translated by the observer into firsthand experience for it to become learned behavior. Learning from *modeled behavior* must be regarded as a secondary learning mode.

Finally, people learn what is expected. Their behavior is shaped by the values, norms, attitudes, and *expectations* of their family and social milieus. We know that children, for example, do conform in some ways to the expectations of their parents; but we also know that children are far more likely to develop behaviors that conform with what they see their parents doing than behaviors that are consistent with what their parents *say* they should do. Therefore, expectations as a mode of learning must fall a poor third behind models and experience.

Learning Styles

Learning requires the ordered intake of information by an organism. Especially as regards the consequences of behavior, the intake process must permit, at some level, the integration of self-experience with the new information being fed back to the organism. When a person is closed to information, learning cannot take place.

A key question for the psychotherapist is, therefore, "How do people take in information?" One answer is, "Differently." People have very individualized ways of taking in information, that is, inputting and integrating it, and hence their learning styles are very personalized. It is possible to induce significant change in some people simply by telling them something about their behavior and its impact on others. For others, taking in information in this straightforward verbal, intellectual way is impossible. With still others, such a direct delivery of information could actually block change. The intake of information is dependent on many factors: *timing* (people are receptive at some times but not at others); *setting* (people may listen to things outside their own home that they could not listen to at home); *mood* (they may feel as though they just cannot take anything in at a particular time); and even the *source* of information (strangers may be able to communicate successfully things that intimates could not).

Discovering and using the unique style by which his client takes in information is a real challenge for the psychotherapist. Some people, for example, find it easier to take in significant information about themselves when it is addressed to a third party than when they are confronted with it directly. There are few general rules, but several major classes of learning style have been identified [7].

There are people whose preferential mode for initially taking in new information, especially about themselves, is *experiential* as opposed to *representational;* that is, they would first have to experience something and then have it explained. Others have just the reverse preference. A preferential mode is a path of least resistance for taking in information. Individuals tend to show a strong preference for one of three primary dimensions in the matter of taking in information. These are: (1) *cognitive,* or intellectual, (2) *affective,* or emotional, and (3) *imagistic,* i.e., when use is made of deeply felt images, metaphors, or symbolism.

Differences in learning style probably account for many of the reasons why particular clients will do better in one kind of therapy or with one therapist than another, since therapists and systems of therapy tend to favor particular methods of delivering information.

The Therapist in the Learning Process

Besides the ongoing self-appraisal of outcome research, which seeks to establish the efficacy of psychotherapy or the differential effectiveness of various modes, recent inquiry has begun to question whether the therapist is even necessary to produce change. It is certainly now evident that personnel lacking the traditional educational requisites may still, by special training or by virtue of personality and life experience, function effectively as psychotherapists. What role, what functions, does the psychotherapist fill in the learning process? Is a therapist indispensable, or may therapeutic change be entirely self-induced? Is a psychotherapist just an overtrained, highly paid friend?

The therapist's problem is essential and unavoidable in the induction of change in any system, whether the system approached is an individual client, a family, or an entire social network. First and foremost, the therapist functions as the needed outsider. The individual literally cannot see himself or herself or his or her own processes. In using any function of the mind for self-scrutiny and exploration, that function itself is excluded from the analysis; the microscope cannot be used to view itself. The externalization of the mind's own mappings of mental and emotional process is bound by a fundamental limitation: The instrument of analysis and purposive modification, one's mind, is the instrument that generated the mapping. Any fallacies and flaws are then doubly reinforced. In any multiperson system, it is easy to appreciate the fact that as long as an individual is participating in the action of that system, he or she cannot understand the system and its workings as a whole, but can have only a limited personalized perspective from his or her particular position in the process. The individual will be least able to apprehend his or her own part in the process in relation to the parts played by others. Only a person at the edge of the action, close enough to see well but not within it, can understand the workings of the complete system [11].

We might consider a family or other interpersonal system to be like a football team in which each of the players has been separately given or has individually evolved his moves in the team's plays. No player in the game knows any complete play, and each sees the game from one perspective at ground level. In contrast, from the pressbox on the 50-yard line, one can see the overall action that reveals the part played by each team member in generating and promoting or opposing the action. This understanding could become accessible to players on the field through mappings in the form of the familiar play diagrams. The team itself could have generated these by piecing together their individual perceptions, provided they had the metalanguage—the play diagrams—in which to "talk" about such a process.

It is possible to demonstrate (and, given rigorous definitions, to prove rigorously) that within any language, including the "languages" of interpersonal sequences or of mental processes, there are things within the language that cannot be correctly described in the language itself, that unresolvable paradoxes result when the description of such a language system is attempted within the same language. A metalanguage, a language in which to talk about the language, which is external to the language under examination, is required. (The problems of communication and paradox and their place in psychopathology and psychotherapy are the subject of a treatise by Watzlawick et al. [27].)

The effective psychotherapist supplies three fundamentally indispensable things to the individual or group in psychotherapy: The therapist is a bystander or observer to the process; the therapist supplies a metalanguage for the understanding of the process; and the therapist is a mirror, feeding back information into the process where it affects the process and makes possible internally generated changes.

Truax and Carkhuff [26], in their summary of findings on the effectiveness of the therapist, identified three characteristics associated with therapeutic effectiveness: nonpossessive warmth, authenticity, and accurate empathy. Nonpossessive warmth involves genuine concern and caring for the individual in an atmosphere of trust in which the therapist's needs for the client (possessiveness) are subordinated. Probably this could be supplied by many kinds of relationships, though there may be a greater probability for the nonpossessive quality in a therapist-client bond. Authenticity, in which the therapist's communications are straightforward, genuine, and congruent in all ways, models high-level interpersonal functioning for the client. Thus, the behavior of the person filling the therapeutic function should exhibit mentally healthy attitudes. Of course, psychotherapists have no special claims to personal mental health.

Accurate empathy corresponds to the effective feedback function that has been mentioned. Truax and Carkhuff [26] addressed individual-oriented psychotherapeutic models, and hence their findings concern accurate feedback of affect and meaning. While accurate empathy may be acquired in many ways, it is aptly described as a skill and one that is sorely lacking in the general population (perhaps in the population of therapists as well). When the feedback function is generalized to include accurate and careful input of complex personal and interpersonal systems processes, we have reached a level at which the role of the trained psychotherapist seems secured. (By the use of training, we are not restricting ourselves to traditional or academic training, however.)

Processes of Self-Change

Prochaska and DiClemente have developed a transtheoretical model of self-change [19] and have employed it as a basis for studying the change processes used by smokers to stop smoking [18]. Their system defines five change processes, each of which can be described at two levels: experiential and environmental. They include conditioning (counterconditioning and stimulus control); contingency control (reevaluation and contingency management); catharsis (corrective emotional experience and dramatic relief); consciousness-raising (feedback and education); and choosing (self-liberation and social liberation). In their study of 886 subjects attempting to stop smoking, they noted that the use of different change processes varied over time as the subjects passed through successive stages of change. Few change processes were utilized during the precontemplative stage; consciousness-raising and self-evaluation were emphasized during the contemplative stage; choosing, conditioning, and contingency control all played a significant role during the action phase, with the latter two continuing to be especially important during the maintenance stage. Relapsers exhibited change modes that appeared as a mix of the contemplative and action phases.

Neurologic Bases of Learning and Memory

Dual-Memory Theories

One issue that has received much attention from learning theorists is the division of memory function into multiple stages. The most common formulation has divided memory into a two-stage process: short-term memory and long-term memory. In addition to these two stages, some theorists make note of one or two additional rapid processes: a sensory register that holds onto sensory inputs for a fraction of a second to allow processing to occur and a reticular facilitation mechanism capable of sustaining a response tendency for a few seconds. The term *short-term memory* generally refers to retention occurring up to a few hours, while *long-term memory* refers to retention after several hours up to many years or a lifetime.

Short-Term Memory

Short-term memory provides the basis for temporary processing of sensory information and provisional response execution. It contributes to the organism's psychological present. The capacity of short-term memory is limited. Presumably, the holding of a new item in short-term memory involves a reduction in the holding of one or more previously acquired items.

Young, who in 1938 postulated the first dualistic theory of memory, proposed that memory might be related to facilitation of particular synapses by electrical activity occurring in reverberatory circuits. Later, in 1951, Young modified his position, attributing only a short-term memory to the activity of reverberatory circuits. Hebb, in 1949, had proposed a similar idea, postulating that short-term memory involved the establishment of electrical circuits, which he called "cell assemblies," which remained active until anatomic modifications, related to long-term memory, could occur.

The idea that short-term memory is based on some kind of electrical facilitation is now well supported by experimental observations. Short-term memory, unlike long-term memory, is disrupted completely by electroconvulsant or chemo-shock. Experimental studies have shown that if a period of learning is immediately followed by electroconvulsant shock treatment or by convulsant or high doses of a stimulant or depressant drug, the learning is not retained when the animal is subsequently retested.

On the other hand, smaller doses of stimulants facilitate short-term memory. This effect has been attributed to the ability of stimulants to increase the electrical activity of neurons throughout the brain. Short-term memory is not impaired by inhibitors of protein synthesis while long-term storage is.

In the realm of verbal retention, several features distinguish short-term memory. Firstly, there is evidence indicating that acoustical representation may be instrumental in verbal short-term memory. Secondly, recall performance falls off rapidly during the short-term phase and only much more slowly during the long-term phase. Thirdly, meaningfulness of verbal material is a variable that influences short-term recall, while no effect of this variable has been demonstrated in long-term memory.

Long-Term Memory

The relatively permanent retention of learned behaviors or associations is provided by long-term memory. While it is generally agreed that this involves some kind of anatomic alteration, the nature of the changes remains obscure. Early theorists were content simply to allude to permanent, anatomic changes. Eccles, in 1951, was the first to propose a detailed hypothetical mechanism for the occurrence of these anatomic alterations. More recently, in 1970, Kety [12], making use of many experimental findings, proposed the following schema:

In the CNS there is a network of fairly random synapses of sufficient complexity for pathways to form and be reinforced between many neurons. Only a minority of these synapses are involved in mediating the primitive and genetically endowed adaptive responses. The aroused state induced by novel or significant stimuli is pervasive and affects synapses throughout the CNS, suppressing most, but permitting or even accentuating activity in those that are transmitting the novel or significant stimuli. The affective state accompanying or reflected in increased turnover of norepinephrine favors the development of persistent facilitatory changes in all synapses currently in a state of excitation or recently active. In the short run, this could be an enhancement of transmitter release at these synapses by an action of norepinephrine on the presynaptic neuron. Long-lasting alterations could be the result of structural changes caused by stimulation by norepinephrine of protein synthesis (by way of the adenyl cyclase system) at recently active synapses. Recently active synapses would be "recognized" by the presence of less calcium ion and more magnesium ion at the outer membrane surface because of the recent ion exchanges accompanying depolarization. The activity of adenyl cyclase is stimulated by the presence of magnesium ion and is inhibited by calcium ion so that adenyl cyclase at recently active neurons would be more susceptible to stimulation by norepinephrine than at other neurons.

Long-term memory is not disrupted by electroconvulsant shock. On the other hand, inhibitors of protein synthesis may prevent consolidation of learning into long-term stores. Moreover, protein synthesis increases during learning. It is important to remember, however, that there remains considerable controversy regarding the effect of protein synthesis inhibitors as well as the role of proteins in long-term memory. A number of alternative postulates have been offered.

Learning Systems in the CNS

A point that is too seldom stressed in writings about the physiology of learning and retention is that these processes occur diffusely throughout the brain. Not all brain regions exhibit an equal degree of plasticity, but plasticity is the distinctive attribute of neural tissue. A number of interrelated but distinguishable systems are involved with regulation of plasticity in the brain. Contrary to the views of some learning and behavioral psychologists, the precepts that characterize plasticity of function in one brain region may differ substantially from the laws governing analogous processes in another brain region. The idea of Skinnerian behaviorism, for example, that all examples of learning can be subsumed under the principles of operant conditioning, is, in our opinion, in error. In Chapter 15 we discuss the exceptional nature of prepared learning, as a special case of conditional behavior. But more than that, the distinctiveness of the principles governing respondent conditioning in general, as well as those governing verbal learning and retention, justify viewing these examples of neural plasticity as separate processes, sharing some features in common with operant learning but nevertheless each distinguishable. In the realm of functional anatomy, it is likewise apparent that one can deal independently with the anatomic regulation of mesodiencephalic plasticity, rhinencephalic plasticity, and neocortical plasticity.

Mesodiencephalic Plasticity

Although the midbrain and diencephalon have enjoyed their share of theorists' interest, their role in learning is less well studied in the laboratory than that of the higher brain centers. Fessard, in 1954, proposed that "heterogeneous pathways" of the reticular formation were the anatomic site where linkage occurs between a conditional stimulus (CS) and an unconditional stimulus (UCS) in respondent conditioning. Similarly, Gastaut, in 1958, suggested that the mesencephalic and thalamic components of the reticular activating system were ideally suited for closure of CS-UCS linkages, since inputs from all sensory pathways reach this area.

Indeed, much conditional learning can occur in completely decorticate animals, particularly respondent conditioning. More complex behaviors are severely impaired, but simple conditional acquisition can take place. One of the definitional distinctions between operant and respondent types of conditioned behaviors is that the respondent type involves elicited or nonvoluntary responses. It is only to be expected, therefore, that this class of learning should be associated for the most part with subcortical brain regions. This is not to say that in the intact animal there is no cortical contribution to respondent conditioning, but rather that the cortical component is not critical.

Certain neurons in the reticular formation (as well as other brain regions) can be conditioned by classic procedures to fire in response to stimuli to which they did not originally respond. This type of cell is referred to as polyvalent in that these cells can respond to stimuli in more than one modality. Some such cells during conditioning modify their firing pattern in such a way that the CS comes to elicit a pattern different from that originally elicited by either the CS or the UCS but similar to that elicited by the combined presentation of CS and UCS together. Cells such as these may participate in the linking of conditional and unconditional stimuli.

Rhinencephalic Plasticity

Plasticity of the rhinencephalon (limbic system) may involve, in part, processes identical to those in the mesodiencephalon. Conditionable polyvalent neurons have been observed, for example, in the hippocampus. In addition, however, another kind of plasticity regulated by subcortical reward and punishment systems characterizes the rhinencephalon. These systems are closely related to the concept of reinforcement and are the anatomic substrates for the learning and retention of operant behaviors.

A technique devised by Olds in the 1950s led to the mapping of the brain in terms of the motivational characteristics of various regions. In this procedure, an electrode is implanted in the region under study, and the animal is given the opportunity to press a

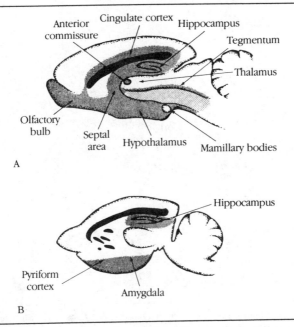

Fig. 3-1. *Medial (above) and lateral (below) sections of a rat brain showing areas where stimulation is rewarding (shaded) or punishing (strippled). Modified from J. Olds. Self-Stimulation Experiments and Differentiated Reward Systems. In H. H. Jasper et al. (Eds.),* The Reticular Formation of the Brain. *Boston: Little, Brown, 1958.*

lever that delivers an electric pulse to that area. If the animal continues to press the lever repeatedly, the area is said to be a reward center, or positive incentive area. A converse approach is to provide the animal with a lever that delays delivery of an electric pulse via an implanted electrode. In this case, repeated lever-pressing indicates that the area is a "punishment" center or aversive area.

A map of the motivational centers of the brain is illustrated in Figure 3-1. Nearly all the neocortex and thalamus is neutral (neither an incentive or aversive area) with respect to self-stimulation. Reward centers include the septal area, portions of the hypothalamus and ventral tegmentum, the anterior thalamus, the medial amygdala, portions of the hippocampus, the medial forebrain bundle, and parts of the caudate, globus pallidus, substantia nigra, and lenticular fasciculus. Aversive areas include much of the dorsal tegmentum, the periventricular gray of the midbrain, the medial caudate, portions of the hippocampus and fornix, the intralaminar nuclei of the thalamus, and the lateral amygdala. It is not necessarily true, however, that all these areas normally function as reward or punishment centers.

The medial forebrain bundle and areas innervated by it, the lateral hypothalamus and the septal area (Fig. 3-2) are the most potent regions with respect to self-stimulation. It has been proposed that the medial forebrain bundle functions as a reward system. Appropriate reinforcers are presumed to activate the medial forebrain bundle, which then signals facilitation of the preceding behaviors.

The lateral hypothalamus supports extremely rapid rates of self-stimulation. A laboratory animal will press a lever to the point of exhaustion for stimulation at this site. On

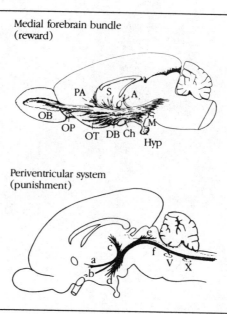

Medial forebrain bundle
(reward)

Periventricular system
(punishment)

Fig. 3-2. *Midline view of a generalized mammalian brain. (Top) Medial forebrain bundle. A, anterior commissure; Ch, chiasm (optic); DB, nucleus of the diagonal band; Hyp, hypothalamus; M, mamillary body; OB, olfactory bulb; OP, olfactory peduncle; OT, olfactory tract; PA, paraolfactory area; S, septum. (Bottom) Periventricular system. a, periventricular nucleus; b, supraoptical nucleus; c, dorsomedial thalamus; d, posterior hypothalamus; e, tectum of midbrain; f, motor nuclei of cranial nerves. From L. Clark et al. The Hypothalamus. Edinburgh: Oliver & Boyd, 1958. By permission of the publisher and The William Ramsay Henderson Trust.*

the other hand, a septal implantation yields a slow but persistent rate of lever-pressing. There is also a distinction between the way in which these sites interact with aversive midbrain stimulation. Stimulation of the lateral hypothalamus increases the rate at which an animal will press a lever to avoid midbrain stimulation, whereas stimulation of the septum decreases the rate at which it will press a lever to avoid midbrain stimulation. These two differences have led us to hypothesize that the lateral hypothalamus is associated with preconsummatory reward, whereas the septum mediates consummatory reward. Preconsummatory reward is associated with an increase and quickening of the behavior associated with the reward, e.g., the first bite of food when the animal is hungry or copulatory behavior in the sexually aroused animal. Consummatory reward, on the other hand, is associated with a cessation of the behavior that brought about the reward, e.g., orgasm or the bite of food that produces a "full" feeling. Thus, lateral hypothalamic stimulation produces a feeling of pleasure with concomitant intensification of drive; septal stimulation produces a feeling of satiation and drive reduction.

Stein [22] has proposed that the so-called periventricular system (PVS) is a negative reward or punishment system. The periventricular system consists of a medially lying column of cells and tracts running from the diencephalon to the medulla (see Fig. 3-2). In the diencephalon, the PVS is a group of fibers that interconnect the dorsomedial nucleus of the thalamus with preoptic and hypothalamic areas. These latter areas give rise to the dorsal longitudinal fasciculus (DLF), a principal descending discharge pathway of the hypothalamus. The DLF gives off fibers to various midbrain and pontine

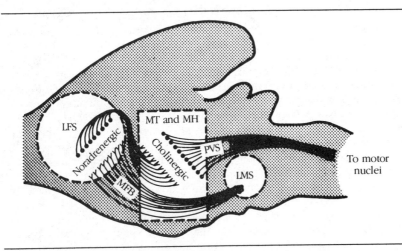

Fig. 3-3. *Hypothetical relationship between reward and punishment mechanisms. A rewarding stimulus releases behavior from suppression by the periventricular system (PVS) in the following sequence of events: (1) activation of medial forebrain bundle (MFB) by stimuli previously associated with reward (or the avoidance of punishment) causes release of norepinephrine into the amygdala and other forebrain suppressor areas (LFS); (2) inhibitory action of norepinephrine suppresses activity of the LFS, thus reducing its cholinergically mediated excitation of the medial thalamus and hypothalamus (MT and MH); (3) decreased cholinergic transmission at synapses in MT and MH lessens the activity in the PVS, thereby reducing its inhibitory influence on motor nuclei of the brainstem. From L. Stein, Chemistry of Purposive Behavior. In J. T. Tapp (Ed.),* Reinforcement and Behavior. *New York: Academic, 1969.*

nuclei and ultimately contributes fibers to the tegmental gray of the pons and the medial reticular gray of the medulla. Together, these areas are called the PVS. All these regions are inhibitory with respect to behavior and aversive with respect to self-stimulation. Figure 3-3 shows a model by Stein, diagramming hypothetically a reciprocal relationship between the reward and punishment systems of the subcortex.

Neocortical Plasticity

Neocortical plasticity appears to involve in part functional activities parallel to those of the mesodiencephalon. Polyvalent neurons are distributed throughout the associative regions of cortex. Also, adrenergic fibers of the median forebrain bundle extend into the granular frontal cortex, so that the subcortical reward system exerts some influence over neocortical plasticity as well as over rhinencephalic plasticity. In addition to these influences, neocortical plasticity is regulated by a system arising in the hippocampus.

Penfield, in 1952, was the first to draw attention to the importance of the hippocampus in memory processes. He proposed that the hippocampus and related temporal cortex were responsible for distribution of information to the neocortex for storage. The evidence for this theory derived originally from observations made by Penfield and others during neurosurgery in human subjects. Bilateral tumor damage or surgical removal of the hippocampus was observed to prevent the storage of any new memory traces or the operation of conscious short-term memory beyond the duration of the immediate attention span. Even unilateral damage on the dominant side produced similar memory deficits with respect to verbal processes. On the other hand, recall of presurgical memories was not impaired at all. Penfield further noted that electrical stimulation of points on the temporal lobe could elicit vivid recollection of detailed memory traces from the subject's past.

In parallel with the greatly expanded role of associative cortex in humans, the memory function of the hippocampus is highly developed only in human beings. In animals with hippocampal lesions, simple conditional responses and sensory discriminations are unimpaired. More complex tasks, and particularly those requiring short-term memory, such as alternation problems, are hindered, but many of the deficits that are seen in hippocampectomized animals are not easily attributable to a short-term memory deficit. The role of the hippocampus as part of a response-inhibitory system, discussed earlier, seems more prevalent in nonhuman species, with a shifting somewhat toward regulation of neocortical plasticity in humans.

The hippocampus apparently influences the neocortex, both by way of the entorhinal cortex and by way of the fornix. The entorhinal cortex lies just posterior to the hippocampus. The fornix is a large fiber bundle that connects the hippocampus to the mamillary bodies of the hypothalamus. A further pathway connects the mamillary bodies to the anterior or limbic thalamus which exerts control over the diffuse thalamic system. Bilateral ablation of the mamillary bodies prevents the laying down of new memories in humans. Korsakoff's syndrome, a disease related to alcoholism, causes neurologic damage to the mamillary bodies and the fornix and is marked by partial retrograde amnesia. Thus, the hippocampal system controls cortical plasticity through its influences on the diffuse thalamic system. The importance of steady-potential shifts in cortical plasticity are described elsewhere (Chap. 9). Since steady-potential shifts are regulated by the diffuse thalamic system, it seems likely that they are involved in the regulation of cortical plasticity by the hippocampus.

The characteristics of cortical plasticity are less well elucidated than those of conditional learning. Verbal and abstract learning, as well as more complex processes such as attitude formation and conscious recall, may be considered principally cortical functions. Although acquisition of verbal behaviors is influenced by reinforcers (and the fornix has been shown to support self-stimulation), verbal learning is less tightly connected with reinforcement than are conditional behaviors. Associations between contiguous verbal items develop regardless of the specific consequences. Cortical learning appears to involve the laying down of patterns of neuronal relationships (or cognitive maps) that delineate in a representational fashion relationships that exist between stimuli. Reinforcers may, however, regulate the ease with which new relationships are established through modulation of steady-potential shifts. Moreover, cortical plasticity relates to reinforcement in the sense that cognitive mapping can be viewed in part as the construction of discriminative stimuli and higher-order generalized laws defining discriminative stimuli that can then be used to govern or influence conditional responses.

Verbal memory is apparently content-addressable, since the speed of recall exceeds what could be reasonably expected from a random-search storage system. The units of semantic memory are concepts, not semantic features or words. Concepts are not built exclusively from simpler concepts as postulated by semantic feature theory, since first-learned concepts are intermediate in generality. There is evidence that verbal memory involves vertical associative processes (successive abstraction) as well as horizontal (nonhierarchical) associations. Vertical associative process involves generation of new concept units to stand for combinations of old concept units.

It can therefore be seen that classical, or respondent, conditioning (the Pavlovian paradigm) and operant learning (the Skinnerian paradigm) are characteristic of the plasticity of different brain systems. Yet another paradigm, which might be termed *patterned* or *associative learning,* is needed to account for human learning and retention above the level of the limbic system. The different paradigms have differing "laws" and the psychotherapist as a change-induction agent must take the differing characteristics into account to be maximally effective. Unfortunately, this multiple paradigmatic approach has not been applied to learning processes in therapy or to research on therapy. As a beginning, it is tempting to view the remarkable success of behavior therapy (the Skinnerian paradigm) in phobias as compared with less spectacular progress in many other problems as relating to a limbic involvement in phobias.

Drugs and Learning

State-dependent Learning

Context and Generalization

All learning is known to be context-dependent and, to varying extents, specialized. Laboratory rats, when trained in a classic Skinnerian bar-pressing paradigm, are often observed to repeat in an almost "superstitious" manner the exact way in which they first pressed the bar to be rewarded, carefully duplicating a sidewise approach to the bar, for example. Similarly, behaviors learned in one setting, such as the laboratory, will not necessarily be spontaneously generalized to other contexts, such as in the field. Human beings are certainly more aware and more complex than laboratory animals, yet to varying degrees they exhibit similar tendencies to fail to generalize fully in many learning processes.

Generalization from one context or setting, one class of experiences, to another is an essential issue for psychotherapy. Ultimately, psychotherapy fails if the client is unable to generalize behaviors learned in therapy to his or her life situations outside that context. All too often, therapists and clients feel that they are making real progress, while others of the client's acquaintance report that they perceive no real changes. The so-called well-analyzed neurotic is the extreme example.

Context dependence argues for therapy in milieus that approximate the life situations to which newly learned behaviors must be generalized. Family unit therapy and sessions in the home setting are examples. But too little is known about what factors influence generalization, either restricting it or increasing the probability and degree of generalization. Knowledge in this area is important, since the therapist cannot be expected to carry the therapy into all-important contexts—work settings, for example.

Drugs as Stimuli

Many psychotropic drugs can act as powerful stimuli on which a subject may be taught to discriminate. For example, an animal can be taught to turn left on a T maze if treated with one drug and right if treated with another, provided sufficient dissimilarity exists. Discrimination does not occur between two drugs of the same class, but can occur between drug and nondrug (placebo) treatment. In general, centrally acting drugs have proved more effective than peripherally acting agents. So effective are drug states as stimuli that only light versus dark appears to be more easily discriminated [16].

Because drug states can function so effectively as stimuli, learning that takes place under the influence of one drug may be transferred only incompletely or not at all to another drug state. This phenomenon is known as *dissociated* or *state-dependent learning.* The drug state appears to be part of the stimulus complex with which behavior is associated, and stimulus generalization to other drug states or the undrugged state may not occur. State-dependent learning has been reported with anesthetics, anticholinergics, narcotics, phenothiazines, amphetamines, alcohol, and marijuana, but it can be expected that state-dependent learning holds for most drugs that have proved effective as discriminative stimuli. These include ether, nitrous oxide, pentobarbital, phenobarbital, secobarbital, amobarbital, chloral hydrate, chlordiazepoxide, meprobamate, atropine, scopolamine, Ditran, nicotine, morphine, pentylenetetrazol, bemegride, amphetamine, mescaline, acetylcholine, norepinephrine, epinephrine, imipramine, haloperidol, and methylphenidate.

Goodwin et al. [9] have reported an experiment demonstrating state-dependent learning in human subjects. The subjects performed memory tasks either while sober or under the influence of alcohol and were later tested for recall in the same or the other condition. Subjects who were intoxicated during both sessions had higher recall than subjects intoxicated only during the first sessions.

Other researchers have verified that state-dependent learning occurs in humans in relation to alcohol [4, 28] and marijuana [5]. Free recall is affected more than recognition [5]. When recall is cued or prompted, the influence of drug-state dependency is reduced or absent [8, 17]. Apparently, drug state is just one of several elements defining context. When other elements are sufficiently distinctive, a change in drug state may not have an overwhelming effect on transfer of learning. When other features of the context are less distinctive, the drug state may have a pronounced impact on transfer of learning.

It should be clear that the phenomenon of state dependency has significant implications for psychotherapists. If the client is taking tranquilizers during therapy, will change or learning resulting from the therapeutic sessions be evidenced in the undrugged state? Conversely, if therapy is undertaken with an alcoholic client, will learning occurring in the therapist's office while the patient is sober have any impact on behavior during a drinking bout? If a patient takes diazepam (Valium) before facing the therapist, will the gains from psychotherapy in the drugged state be transferred to the undrugged state? The suggestion from what we know of a state dependency is that a great deal of what is learned in one drug state is not transferred to a dissimilar drug state. In fact, two separate studies cited by May [14] have demonstrated that therapeutic gains while the client is taking drugs may be tied to the drug condition. Regressions on drug withdrawal were found, as expected, to be selective to certain areas of change.

State-dependent performance of complex behavior patterns can play a role in work habits and productivity. Both caffeine and nicotine are psychotropic drugs commonly used in conjunction with or as part of a work ritual. Work dependent on higher brain functions appears especially capable of becoming strongly associated with the drug-state stimulus complex. Some people find it difficult to function effectively without their cup of coffee or tea. The fact that the xanthines (including caffeine) are CNS stimulants and demonstrably enhance performance adds to the dependence potential. One well-known medical writer gave up cigarettes after collaborating on a report on smoking and health only to find himself unable to write at all for nearly a year. His talent was restored when he resumed the use of nicotine.

What options are available to the psychotherapist to circumvent the impact of state dependency? So far, the research suggests two tactics. One tactic is to work with the client in a variety of dosage states. This might be accomplished by altering the time of therapy sessions in relation to the time of medication. Animal studies have shown that generalization of learning is very high when learning sessions involve a full range of dosage states. This tactic is not useful when the problem is drug abuse, and the drug in question is the drug of abuse. The effort to eliminate all use of the drug must take precedence over efforts to circumvent state dependency. The second tactic suggested by research for minimizing drug interference with learning generalizability is to strengthen the definition of context in terms of nondrug characteristics. When there is a strong similarity between the therapy context and the life circumstance in which recall is required, with respect to nondrug characteristics, the relative importance of drug state as a determinant of context will be lessened. If the psychopathologic behavior exhibited by the patient is situational, identification of the triggering cues could be used to therapeutic benefit. Linking the learning of therapeutic sessions to the same cues could be used to maximize chances that learning would be accessible in the situation that has historically triggered the dysfunctional response.

Drugs as Primary Reinforcers

Drugs may act as primary reinforcers, increasing the frequency of a given behavior. A typical experiment demonstrating the reinforcing properties of drugs involves the recording of lever presses by an animal in a situation in which each lever press or a group of presses delivers a fixed quantity of drugs intravenously. Morphine and morphine-like drugs are effective reinforcers, and it appears that the reinforcing capacity is not related to the production of physical dependence, since (1) reinforcement occurs at doses below those that produce dependence and (2) in a series of narcotic analgesics, there was no correlation between efficacy as reinforcers and the intensity of physical dependence associated with the agent. In a self-administered study, both codeine and methadone were stronger reinforcers than morphine, even though physical dependence associated with these two narcotics is of a lower order.

Among stimulants, only one (pemoline) has been found that is not an effective reinforcer. Methamphetamine, dextroamphetamine, cocaine, caffeine, nicotine, methylphenidate, pipradrol, and tranylcypromine have proved to be effective reinforcers. A number of sedative-hypnotics are effective reinforcers. The neuroleptics, on the other hand, not only fail to support self-administration but may even provide negative reinforcement (an animal will work to avoid injections of these drugs), which is probably significant because neuroleptics are one of the few classes of psychotropic drugs that are seldom, if ever, abused.

The role of psychotropic drugs as primary reinforcers contributes much more to their abuse liability than does their ability to establish physical dependence. Indeed, the latter factor is of no significance in the initial stages of a developing addiction. The psychotherapist who is engaged in therapy with an addict (regardless of whether the drug involved is heroin, alcohol, chlordiazepoxide [Librium], or some other drug) must recognize that drug reinforcement of the drug-seeking and drug-taking behaviors and related behavioral dysfunctions is a powerful force countering change and growth. The therapist must consider whether continued therapy will be fruitful in the absence of the client's commitment and the ability to abstain from use of the drug. Although it is not our contention that the therapist need take this position in all cases, we do feel that he or she should realize that continued drug use by the client may seriously compromise the efforts of the therapist. While there may be much truth in the view that drug abuse can be symptomatic of underlying psychopathologic states, it is also true that abuse of psychotropic drugs is a self-reinforcing dysfunctional activity.

The potential for psychotropic drugs to be primary reinforcers must also be taken into account even when drugs are intentionally used as part of therapy.

Drugs as Unconditional Stimuli

Drugs may also generate secondary reinforcers. Drugs elicit a wide variety of effects in the body, and these effects may serve as unconditional responses for classical conditioning. Conditional stimuli that are consistently paired with a drug effect (unconditional response) may acquire the capacity to elicit in part the effects (conditional response) associated with the drug (unconditional stimulus). There are two practical applications of this principle. First, conditional stimuli may acquire power as secondary reinforcers if the conditional response is pleasurable. In other words, if the conditional stimulus can elicit some of the pleasant effects associated with the drug, it can function as a reinforcer for shaping behavior. The so-called needle habit is an example of this phenomenon: an addict who has exhausted his or her drug supply will continue to go through the ritual of injection, because the act of injection has been associated with the action of the drug.

Second, if the conditional stimulus is paired with a drug that elicits withdrawal or for that matter with normal withdrawal, it acquires the capacity to precipitate withdrawal-like responses. Such conditional stimuli intensify drug-craving and may contribute to maintaining the cycle of drug administration and withdrawal that preoccupies an addict.

Note also that these effects may enter into the use or disuse of any drug that can serve as a primary reinforcer, the barbiturates or stimulants, for example, and aspects of the therapy itself, if closely connected with drug administration, may function as conditional stimuli. Clearly, a foresighted therapist will employ this phenomenon to advantage rather than let it become a part of the problem.

Drug Effects on Learning Paradigms

Most drugs known to have substantial and general effects on learning are of no significance to psychotherapists, since they have no therapeutic uses. For example, inhibitors of protein or ribonucleic acid (RNA) synthesis greatly impair consolidation of learning. Less dramatic but measurable effects, however, are observed in subjects treated with various psychotropic drugs. In general, drugs that cause EEG activation (i.e., stimulants) enhance learning, provided the dose employed is moderate. On the other hand, sedative-hypnotics may produce subtle learning deficits in subhypnotic doses but usually only at doses that also depress motor activity. Tranquilizers produce more selective learning deficits.

A classic drug-screening test that effectively differentiates between neuroleptics and sedative-hypnotics is the conditioned avoidance response paradigm. In this procedure, animals are trained to respond to a signal (usually a buzzer) in order to avoid a subsequent electric current by climbing onto a platform or up a pole or by pressing a lever. Once the conditional response is learned, most dosage levels of a sedative-hypnotic will suppress the conditional response only to about the same extent it suppresses the unconditional response (escape from the shock). On the other hand, neuroleptics suppress the conditional response without blocking the unconditional escape response over a wide range of doses.

Neuroleptics also facilitate extinction of a conditioned avoidance response once the conditional stimulus is no longer paired with the unconditional stimulus (shock). This is of particular significance, since many therapists and researchers consider the conditioned avoidance response paradigm to be an animal analogue of neurotic symptomatology in general and phobic states in particular in human subjects [7]. The fact that neuroleptics have found clinical application almost exclusively in psychotic rather than neurotic patients, however, suggests that the conditioned avoidance response paradigm is better suited as a screening test for antipsychotic than for antineurotic drugs. Not surprisingly, neuroleptics impair acquisition of a conditioned avoidance response, while, in contrast, anxiolytics and barbiturates have been reported to facilitate acquisition.

Just as the conditioned avoidance response has proved to be a very good screening test for antipsychotic drugs, another animal test paradigm, "conditioned suppression," has provided a sensitive screening test for anxiolytics. In this procedure, an animal is first trained to perform operant behavior such as lever-pressing for a food reward. A conditioned emotional response (or "freezing response") is then superimposed by pairing a conditional stimulus (such as a buzzer) with shock until the conditional stimulus by itself elicits the freezing behavior. The freezing response can be quantified in terms of suppression of the operant behavior. This procedure has been viewed as analogous to human episodal panic or anxiety attacks.

A variant of this procedure is one in which the shock is contingent on the operant response itself. As above, the animal is first trained to press a lever for a food reward, and then an additional contingency is added such that some (randomly determined) lever presses also result in shock. This produces a conflict situation in which a single response has both positive and aversive consequences, a situation many consider analogous to conflict situations, such as sexual inhibitions, that occur in patients seen in clinical practice.

In general, anxiolytics, especially the benzodiazepines, are effective in reducing suppression of behavior by the conditional stimulus in the preceding paradigms, although meprobamate is effective only in the response-contingent variant. On the other hand, most neuroleptics are ineffective, regardless of dose, in releasing suppression. The narcotics and reserpine *are* effective in the first paradigm.

Implications for Psychotherapy

In summary: One difficulty in the psychotherapist's assessment of the impact of drugs on therapy is that one cannot know to what extent the learning effects introduced here and pharmacologic effects discussed under preceding sections reinforce or cancel each other. It is thus possible that learning facilitated by the use of meprobamate to reduce anxiety, for example, could prove to be highly state-dependent, and thus would not readily generalize to the nondrug state. And there is always the possibility, mentioned in Chapter 1, of psychotherapy's having a negative impact on useful drug therapy. Ultimately, only an accumulated volume of outcome studies can provide sound answers in the general case, but even this may not completely answer the psychotherapist's dilemma concerning his or her present client.

For the moment we must be satisfied with having pointed out that there are many possible interactive effects between drugs and learning in psychotherapy. Not all these are favorable to the facilitation of real change, which, as we noted at the opening of this chapter, is what therapy is really about.

Selected References and Further Readings

1. Agranoff, B. W., Burnell, H. R., Dokas, L. A., and Springer, A. D. Progress in biochemical approaches to learning and memory. In M. A. Lipton et al. (Eds.), *Psychopharmacology: A Generation of Progress.* New York: Raven, 1978.

2. Beecroft, R. S. *Classical Conditioning.* Goleta, Calif.: Psychonomic Press, 1966.
3. Bergin, A. E., and Garfield, S. L. (Eds.). *Handbook of Psychotherapy and Behavior Change: An Empirical Analysis.* New York: Wiley, 1971.
4. Bustamente, J. A., Jordan, A., Vila, M., Gonzales, A., and Insua, A. State dependent learning in humans. *Physiol. Behav.* 5:793–796, 1970.
5. Darley, D. F., Tinklenberg, F. R., Roth, W. T., and Atkinson, R. C. The nature of storage deficits and state-dependent retrieval under marihuana. *Psychopharmacology* (Berlin) 37:139–149, 1974.
6. Drachman, D. A. Central Cholinergic System and Memory. In M. A. Lipton et al. (Eds.), *Psychopharmacology: A Generation of Progress.* New York: Raven, 1978.
7. Duhl, F., Kantor, D., and Duhl, B. Learning, Space, and Action: A Primer on Family Sculpture. In D. Block (Ed.), *Techniques of Family Psychotherapy: A Primer.* New York: Grune & Stratton, 1974.
8. Eich, J. E., Weingartner, H., Stillman, R., and Gillin, J. C. State-dependent accessibility of retrieval cues in the retention of a categorized list. *J. Verb. Learn. Verb. Behav.* 14:408–417, 1975.
9. Goodwin, D. W., Powell, B., Bremer, D., Hoine, H., and Stern, J. Alcohol and recall: State dependent effects in man. *Science* 163:1358–1360, 1969.
10. Hall, J. F. *Verbal Learning and Retention.* New York: Lippincott, 1971.
11. Kantor, D., and Lehr, W. *Inside the Family: Toward a Theory of Family Process.* San Francisco: Jossey-Bass, 1975.
12. Kety, S. S. The Biogenic Amines in the Central Nervous System: Their Possible Roles in Arousal, Emotion, and Learning. In F. O. Schmitt (Ed.), *The Neurosciences, Second Study Program.* New York: Rockefeller University Press, 1970. Pp. 324–336.
13. Maslow, A. H. *Toward a Psychology of Being.* New York: Van Nostrand, 1961.
14. May, P. R. Psychotherapy and Ataraxic Drugs. In A. E. Bergin and S. L. Garfield (Eds.), *Handbook of Psychotherapy and Behavior Change: An Empirical Analysis.* New York: Wiley, 1971.
15. Olds, J. Pleasure Centers in the Brain. In R. F. Thompson (Ed.), *Physiological Psychology: Readings from Scientific American.* San Francisco: Freeman, 1971.
16. Overton, D. A. Discriminative Control of Behavior by Drug States. In T. Thompson and R. Pickens (Eds.), *Stimulus Properties of Drugs.* New York: Appleton-Century-Crofts, 1971.
17. Petersen, R. C. Retrieval failures in alcohol state-dependent learning. *Psychopharmacology* 55:141–146, 1977.
18. Prochaska, J. O., and DiClemente, C. C. Stages and processes of self change of smoking: Toward an integrative model of change. In manuscript.
19. Prochaska, J. O., and DiClemente, C. C. Transtheoretical therapy: Toward a more integrative model of change. In manuscript.
20. Skinner, B. F. *Contingencies of Reinforcement.* New York: Meridith Corp., 1969.
21. Smythies, J. R. *Brain Mechanisms and Behaviour.* New York: Academic, 1970.
22. Stein, L. Reciprocal Action of Reward and Punishment Mechanisms. In R. G. Heath (Ed.), *The Role of Pleasure in Behavior.* New York: Harper & Row, 1964.
23. Stein, L. Noradrenergic Reward Mechanisms, Recovery of Function, and Schizophrenia. In J. L. McGaugh (Ed.), *The Chemistry of Mood, Motivation, and Memory.* New York: Plenum, 1972.
24. Stein, L. Reward Transmitters: Catecholamines and Opioid Peptides. In M. A. Lipton et al. (Eds.), *Psychopharmacology: A Generation of Progress.* New York: Raven, 1978.
25. Thompson, T., and Pickens, R. *Stimulus Properties of Drugs.* New York: Appleton-Century-Crofts, 1971.
26. Truax, C. B., and Carkhuff, R. R. *Towards Effective Counseling and Psychotherapy: Training and Practice.* Chicago: Aldine, 1967.
27. Watzlawick, P., et al. *Pragmatics of Human Communication.* New York: Norton, 1967.
28. Weingartner, H., and Faillace, L. A. Alcohol state-dependent learning in man. *J. Nerv. Ment. Dis.* 153:395–406, 1971.
29. Zornetzer, S. F. Neurotransmitter Modulation and Memory: A New Neuropharmacological Phrenology? In M. A. Lipton et al. (Eds.), *Psychopharmacology: A Generation of Progress.* New York: Raven, 1978.

Foundations of Drug Action: Neuropharmacology II

℞

The step from pharmacologic interactions with learning processes to neuropharmacology is not unlike the next step one takes after reaching the top of a stepladder, more in the nature of a precipitous plunge than an incremental advance. It is important to have an understanding of this plunge and why such a change in levels is desirable.

In the preceding three chapters, we endeavored to establish the case for the nonmedical psychotherapist's familiarizing himself or herself with psychotropic drugs and their possible interactions with the course of psychotherapy. These chapters established a framework for the analysis of this encounter. One might argue, then, that the only task remaining would be to list the currently used psychotropic drugs, their uses and effects, and their potential interactions with psychotherapy.

Such a rote approach might be adequate were it not for our firm conviction that a new order of professional is called for whose perspective spans psychological, medical, and systemologic viewpoints. But, armed only with a list, the psychotherapist would still be at the mercy of the propaganda of the pharmaceutical companies, which have been known to make claims about the performance of their products that are insupportable on the basis of what is known. Moreover, the knowledge gained from a superficial survey of psychopharmacology would be subject to rapid obsolescence, as the rate of new drug development is fairly rapid.

In contrast, the psychotherapist who understands the elementary neuroanatomic and biochemical bases for drug therapy will not find his or her knowledge so readily superseded. The therapist need know only the class to which an unfamiliar drug belongs, for example, to know something of its actions, applications, appropriateness to a given case, and potential interactions with psychotherapy.

It is possible to read and make use of this book without perusing the material in this section and even giving short shrift to the later chapters on the organization of specific brain systems, but we do not recommend it. Indeed, we see this entire book as background material, one of the steps in the reader's progress toward becoming the new professional that we are calling for.

Neuropharmacology is a derivative science that has only recently come of age as a mature and autonomous branch of science. Its history is therefore, in one sense, less than two decades old. But, in another sense, its history is the combined histories of its forerunners: neurophysiology, neurochemistry, neuroanatomy, and pharmacology. The reader who is interested in a historical perspective should study the following calendar of historical events in neuropharmacology.

Historic dates in four neuroscience disciplines

Pharmacology/Psychopharmacology	Neurochemistry
1856 Bernard localizes site of curare action	1885 Thudichum writes treatise on the chemical constitution of the brain
1868 Crum-Brown and Fraser demonstrate structure-activity relation	1905 Elliott likens epinephrine to sympathetic stimulation
1875 Caton discovers EEG	
1887 Freud studies cocaine	1921 Loewi describes vagusstoff
1892 Kraepelin, the father of psychopharmacology, writes essay on drug effects on psychic processes	1921 Cannon describes SNS secretory substance
	1928 Page heads up first department of brain chemistry in Munich
1899 Dreser introduces aspirin	
1905 Langley develops receptor theory	1929 Dale isolates and identifies ACh
1928 Discovery of monoamine oxidase	1930s Opposing "spark" and "soup" clubs debate nature of transmission
1929 Lucas discovers cyclopropane	
1933 Clark defines the dose-response principle	1949 Bulbring, et al. shows SNS stimulation releases catecholamines
1935 Amphetamines for narcolepsy	1951 Koelle reports CNS distribution of acetylcholinesterase
1937 Marijuana Tax Act	
1938 Merritt and Putman introduce phenytoin	1953 Twarog and Page discover serotonin in the brain
1938 Hofmann isolates LSD	1954 Vogt reports regional brain distribution of norepinephrine
1946 Berger characterizes pharmacology of meprobamate	1954 Eccles identifies ACh as Renshaw cell transmitter
1948 Alquist distinguishes α and β receptors	1956 Von Euler identifies norepinephrine as sympathetic transmitter
1949 Cade reports lithium effectiveness in mania	1957 Brodie and Shore report brain serotonin distribution
1953 Chlorpromazine and reserpine introduced	1957 *Neurochemistry*, (1st ed.)
1954 Bradley et al. ellucidate strychnine mechanism	1958 Curtis and Eccles develop microionophoretic technique
1954 Glutethimide introduced	1961 Elliott identifies factor I as GABA
1957 Monoamine oxidase inhibitor use in depression begins	1962 Gaddum collects CNS secretory substance with a cannula
1957 Kuhn describes antidepressant activity of tricyclics	1962 Falck and Hillarp develop histochemical staining of amines
1960 Randall discovers sedative properties of chlordiazepoxide	1963 Mitchell devices collecting-cup technique
1961 L-dopa therapy introduced	1963 Axelrod reviews elucidation of catecholamine metabolism
1963 Trendelenburg reveals mechanism of amphetamine action	
1965–1966 α-methylparatyrosine and parachlorophenylalanine introduced as tool drugs	

Historic dates in four neuroscience disciplines (continued)

Functional Neuroanatomy	Neurophysiology
1850 Waller describes retrograde degeneration	1840 DuBois Reymond discovers action and resting potentials
1880s Marchi and Algeri devise myelin stain	1902 Bernstein hypothesis relates resting potential to K^+
1885 Golgi develops stain	1937 Cole and Curtis devise giant squid axon preparation
1890s Ramon y Cajal begins mapping	
1897 Sherrington coins term *synapse*	1939 Hodgkin and Huxley begin study of cell potentials culminating in 1963 Nobel prize
1927 Cannon proposes central autonomic centers	
1934 Ramon y Cajal presents neuron doctrine	1940 Harvey and MacIntosh correlate ACh release with extracellular Ca^{++}
1937 Papez circuit described	1941 Dean proposes Na^+ pump
1938 Hess proposes ergotropic and trophotropic centers	1947 Hodgkin, Katz, and Huxley propose Na^+ hypothesis of action potential
1949 Hebb develops cell assembly theory	1951 Keynes measures ion fluxes during action potential
1949 Maruzzi and Magoun discover reticular activating system	1951 Eccles initiates single cell recordings
1950s Beidler develops integrated evoked potential technique	1953 Blaschko and Welch discover granular storage
1951 Eccles postulates synaptic alterations	1956 Euler and Hillarp isolate SNS vesicles
1952 Penfield proposes centrencephalic system	1957 DelCastillo and Katz localize ACh receptors on outer membrane surface
1953 Myers and Sperry discover split brain	1959 Whittaker isolates CNS synaptic vesicles by subcellular fractionation
1954 Olds and Milner devise self-stimulation technique	1963 Lipicky, Hertz, and Shane relate Ca^{++} influx during action potential to ACh release
1958 Dement discovers rapid eye movement sleep	
1962 Holt develops autoradiography	
1963 Carlton proposes limbic-cholinergic system for response inhibition	
1964 Stein describes reward and punishment systems	

Introduction to Functional Neuroanatomy

4

Directions in the central nervous system are designated by terms developed by anatomists. These are illustrated in Figure 4-1. The top of the head is designated *anterior,* or *rostral;* the lower part is designated *posterior* or *caudal.* Toward the back is *dorsal* and toward the front is *ventral. Medial* means toward the middle, while *lateral* means toward the side, left or right. Figure 4-1 will also serve to introduce the major subdivisions of the human brain. With that introduction to the directional terms employed in neuroanatomy, we will consider briefly the anatomy of the nervous system, from a functional point of view.

Peripheral Nervous System

The peripheral nervous system is both the starting point and the end point for an understanding of CNS function, since inputs to the CNS arise from the peripheral nervous system, and outputs are expressed through the peripheral nerves. Moreover, we will need to refer periodically to parts of the peripheral system in our discussions of CNS function. Therefore, a brief review is in order. The peripheral nervous system is divided into two principle parts, the somatic and the autonomic.

The Somatic Division

The somatic division innervates the so-called striated skeletal muscles and carries sensory inputs from receptors in the skin, the muscles, and the joints. Somatic nerves come from the spinal cord at each vertebral level. A spinal nerve consists of a mixed bundle of motor axons heading *away* from the spinal cord (*efferents*) and elongated dendrites of bipolar, sensory cells projecting *toward* the spinal cord (*afferents*). The efferents are of two types: the alpha-(α) motor neurons innervate the skeletal muscle directly while the gamma-(γ) motor neurons control the sensitivity of sensory receptors in the muscles ("spindle organs"). Beside the passage of information to and from the CNS, the spinal cord and peripheral nerves have some limited regulatory capabilities. Relatively simple regulatory mechanisms, of which the knee jerk is a familiar example, require no participation higher than the spinal cord and are referred to as segmental reflexive control. Figure 4-2 shows the entrance and exit of axons from the spinal cord; it also shows a hypothetical monosynaptic reflex.

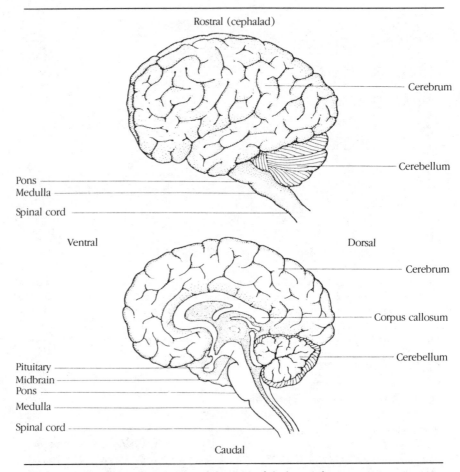

Fig. 4-1. *Lateral (top) and medial (bottom) aspects of the human brain.*

Also part of the peripheral nervous system but having mixed somatic and autonomic functions are the cranial nerves. Some of the principle functions carried by the 12 cranial nerves are olfactory inputs (1st cranial nerve); visual inputs (2nd); muscular and autonomic regulation of the eye (3rd, 4th, and 6th); muscular control and sensations of the face, sinuses, teeth, pharynx, and tongue (including taste) (5th, 7th, and 9th); hearing and sense of balance (8th); parasympathetic regulation of the viscera (10th); and control of the muscles of the neck (11th) and tongue (12th).

The Autonomic Division

The autonomic division innervates the viscera, smooth muscles, cardiac muscles, and glands. The autonomic division is further divided into two subdivisions, the sympathetic and parasympathetic branches.

Sympathetic Branch

The sympathetic nervous system (SNS) controls the mobilization of resources for emergencies. Sympathetic activation leads to increased heart rate and dilatation of

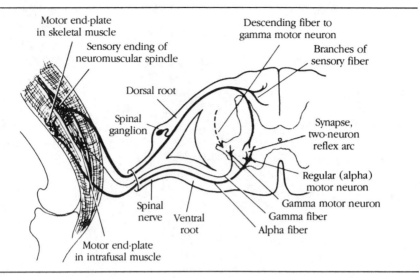

Fig. 4-2. *Skeletal muscle innervation by alpha and gamma motor neurons of the somatic nervous system. Modified from A. J. Gatz.* Clinical Neuroanatomy and Neurophysiology *(4th ed.). Philadelphia: Davis, 1970.*

coronary blood vessels (vasodilatation), dilatation of the pupils, inhibition of gastrointestinal activity and contraction of sphincters, and excitation of sweat glands and the pilomotor (or "hair-raising") apparatus. All these effects are aimed at preparing the subject for "fight or flight."

Unlike the somatic fibers, which do not have synapses until they reach the target muscle, efferent autonomic fibers synapse once outside the spinal cord in addition to the synapse at the target organ (Fig. 4-3). This intermediate synapse is called a ganglion. The axon extending from cord to ganglion is called the preganglionic fiber; the one extending from ganglion to effector organ is called the postganglionic fiber. In the SNS, preganglionic fibers extend a short distance from the cord to one of a chain of ganglia running parallel to the cord referred to as the sympathetic chain. These preganglionic fibers release one transmitter, *acetylcholine*. The postganglionic fibers are relatively long and release *norepinephrine*.

The Parasympathetic Branch

The parasympathetic nervous system (PNS) is complementary in function to the SNS. Its role is to conserve and store bodily resources. Activation of the PNS leads to inhibition of cardiac activity and coronary vasoconstriction, increased digestive and secretory activity, and pupillary constriction. In contrast to the SNS, parasympathetic ganglia lie near the target organ, far from the cord. Therefore, preganglionic fibers are long and postganglionic fibers are short. Like the SNS, preganglionic fibers release acetylcholine, but, unlike the SNS postganglionic fibers of the PNS, they also release acetylcholine.

There are drugs, many of great therapeutic value, that interact more or less specifically at each of the types of synaptic sites of the peripheral nervous system, but discussion of these drugs is beyond the scope of this book. The reader is directed to any standard pharmacology text for detailed information on this topic.

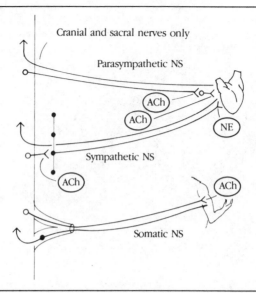

Fig. 4-3. *Somatic and autonomic (sympathetic and parasympathetic) components of the peripheral nervous system showing transmitters released at each type of synapse. ACh, acetylcholine; NE, norepinephrine.*

The Central Nervous System

To understand how drugs may alter mood, arousal state, muscle tone, the relay of sensory information to consciousness, or such complex functions as memory, learning, or motor coordination, we need first to understand the rudiments of normal processes by which the brain performs these functions. In subsequent chapters, we will consider in detail the higher, integrative systems of the brain. In this chapter, we will explore the CNS with the intention of gaining an overview of its function.

The processes of the CNS can be divided for convenience into three categories (Fig. 4-4): (1) the flow of sensory information into appropriate centers; (2) the control of muscles, organs, and glands; and (3) higher processes that involve complex elaborations of sensory inputs, resulting in subtle, purposive patterns of behavior—in other words, inputs, outputs, and processing. Of the three, the inputs are least susceptible to drug modification and therefore have the least claim to our attention for the present purposes. The inputs and outputs can each be further divided into two categories on the same basis: those that provide for interaction of the organism with the environment (sensory and motor systems) and those that provide for maintenance of the internal fluid environment and organ functions (physiochemical and autonomic inputs, autonomic and endocrine regulatory outputs).

Inputs: The Sensory Systems

Sensory information originates in the response of specialized receptors to discrete physical stimuli. These receptors include the rods and cones in the retina of the eye; the hair cells of the ears; taste buds on the tongue; dendrites of the olfactory neurons; somatosensory receptors in the skin for discriminative touch pressure, pain, and temperature; spindle organs of striated muscles; Golgi organs in tendons; and the hair

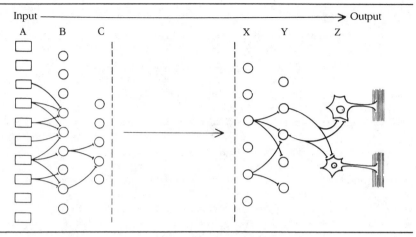

Fig. 4-4. *Overall organization of the brain is indicated in a rough caricature that suggests the flow of information from the input of sensory signals by receptor cells (A) to the eventual output by motor neurons (Z) terminating on muscle cells. The outputs of receptors and neurons usually branch to send diverging signals to the next stage. Most neurons receive converging inputs, both excitatory and inhibitory, from earlier stages. Something is known about the significance of the connections near the input end of the brain (B, C) and near the output end (X, Y). Far less is known about the workings of regions in between, which make up most of the brain. From D. H. Hubel. The brain.* Sci. Am. *241:51, 1979.* © *1979 by Scientific American, Inc. All rights reserved.*

cells of the vestibular system. From the point of view of the psychopharmacologist, the functioning of these specialized receptors is not of particular interest because the development of the "generator potentials" and nerve impulses at these receptors is a process not particularly susceptible to drug influences.

The nerve impulses generated by the interaction of these receptors with an appropriate stimulus travel along somatic afferent fibers. In the case of the cranial sensory nerves, afferent nerve fibers contribute to cranial nerves and synapse at cranial nerve nuclei, which are located throughout the lower region of the brain (the pons, medulla, and midbrain). In the case of afferents from receptors in the trunk, the cell bodies lie in the spinal cord and the axons synapse sometimes on motor neurons at the same level but sometimes not until they reach the brainstem or thalamus. In the spinal cord, sensory fibers travel in tracts grouped according to function.

The somatosensory system consists of two subsystems, the epicritic and the protopathic. The epicritic system has receptors sensitive to light touch, deep pressure, and joint movement. The protopathic system carries the following senses: pain, cold, warmth, and crude touch. Inputs from the head enter the brain via the 5th, 7th, and 10th cranial nerves. All these inputs project to the somatosensory cortex.

The visual system is perhaps the most elaborate of the sensory systems. Most of what we call the eye makes up the accessory structures of the visual system. The cornea produces a rough focusing of light, while the lens produces a fine focusing of light on the retina. The iris controls the quantity of light entering the eye. The retina itself is a screen of neural elements extending about 100 degrees and backed by the choroid, which absorbs light so as to reduce reflection and scattering. The retina contains the receptor cells called rods and cones.

One million fibers project from the eye along the optic nerves. At the optic chiasm, half of these fibers cross over. The net effect of this is that the right visual field is represented in the left hemisphere, while the left visual field is represented in the right hemisphere.

Like the visual system, the auditory system has highly developed accessory structures. The receptor cells of the auditory system are hair cells on the basilar membrane of the cochlea, which are stimulated by movement of the fluid (in the cochlea) produced by sound waves, which cause the basilar membrane to vibrate. Inputs of the auditory system project to the auditory cortex in the temporal lobe.

The receptors for taste are taste buds, found primarily on the tongue, of which there are four types, sweet, bitter, sour, and salty. Impulses originating from these receptors travel by the 7th, 9th, and 10th cranial nerves, terminating in the portion of the somatosensory cortex corresponding to the tongue.

The receptors of the olfactory system are hair-like endings in the nasal mucosa that are actually dendrites of the primary sensory neurons lying in the olfactory bulbs. Factor analysis of human judgments has suggested six categories of receptors: fragrant, ethereal, resinous, spicy, putrid, and burnt. The olfactory inputs project from the olfactory bulbs to the amygdaloid complex and the uncus, the latter being a basal region of the temporal lobe.

The vestibular system is considered part of the extrapyramidal system because of its profound influence on posture and reflexes. The receptors are hair cells (cristae) located in the three semicircular canals of the inner ear and in the utricle, which lies between the three. The hair cells of the semicircular canals are activated by calcium carbonate granules that depress the hairs during movement. Inputs from these cells indicate the position of the head. Inputs from the utricle respond to static position and indicate acceleration and centrifugal and gravitational force.

Inputs: Physiochemical

The brain receives information regarding the status of the internal environment and organ functions in the form of physiochemical inputs. These inputs may be relayed to the brain from peripherally lying receptors or may derive from receptors within the brain itself. Peripherally lying receptors include the baroreceptors that monitor blood pressure and the carotid bodies that monitor oxygenation of the blood. Brain receptors (in the hypothalamus) monitor the state of hydration, core temperature, and glucose levels. The brain is also sensitive to carbon dioxide levels in the blood through activity of specialized receptors on the surface of the medulla. Many endocrine substances exert feedback and perhaps additional regulatory and developmental influences on the brain.

Outputs: The Motor Pathways

Reference has already been made to the efferents of the somatic and autonomic nervous system as well as the efferent component of the cranial nerves. All consequences of CNS activity must ultimately be expressed through these pathways or through the endocrine system. Within the CNS, motor control is divided into two systems: the pyramidal and the extrapyramidal.

The pyramidal system is a well-defined tract arising in the motor cortex. Axons of the pyramidal system are the longest axons known, and they extend without synapses through the internal capsule in the region of the basal ganglia, through the pyramids overlying the brainstem, and thence via the corticospinal tracts of the spinal cord to the motoneurons of the cord. Thus a minimum of only two neurons can be involved in cortically initiated muscular activity. Because of the small number of synaptic delays, and since these fibers are well myelinated, the delay between cortical activity and muscular response is very short. The small number of synapses within the pyramidal system also means that this system is rather insensitive to drug disruption, because drugs usually produce their effects through modulation of synaptic mechanisms.

The extrapyramidal system (Chap. 20) is not so much a system as a conceptual lumping together of all motor influences other than pyramidal. Included in the extrapyramidal system are the cerebellum, the vestibular system, the corpus striatum, and a number of pontine and mesencephalic nuclei, including the red nucleus, subthalamic nucleus, substantia nigra, and zona incerta. Influences from each of these areas converge on the descending reticular formation, which acts as a common discharge pathway for extrapyramidal regulation. The descending reticular axons impinge primarily on gamma motor neurons of the somatic nervous system.

Outputs: Autonomic and Endocrine

The outputs that provide for regulation of internal processes are conveyed by the autonomic and endocrine systems. The activity of these systems is influenced by many categories of drugs, and the physiology of the autonomic and endocrine systems is therefore of vital importance to pharmacology and clinical medicine. However, these are matters beyond the scope of our present undertaking.

Processing: Special Functions of the Various Brain Regions and Systems

The Brainstem

In its ascending projection, the spinal cord gives way to the *medulla oblongata,* the lowest portion of the brain (Fig. 4-5). Not surprisingly, the medulla resembles the cord in shape and organization. A substantial portion of the medulla, as might be expected from its anatomic position, is composed of fibers in transit from higher to lower centers, and vice versa (Fig. 4-6A). Nevertheless, the medulla provides some rather impressive

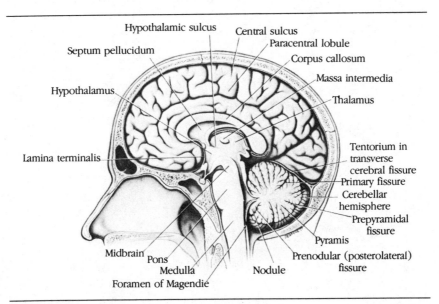

Fig. 4-5. *Medial aspect of the brain. From S. R. Noback.* The Human Nervous System. © *1974 by McGraw-Hill Book Company, New York. Used with permission.*

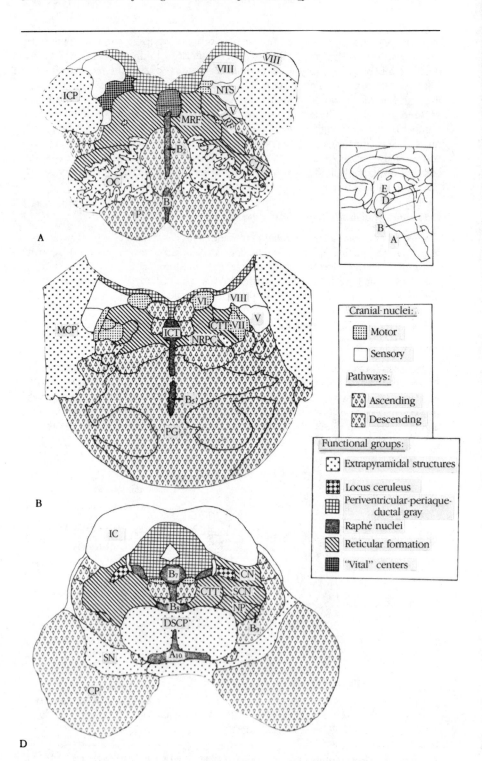

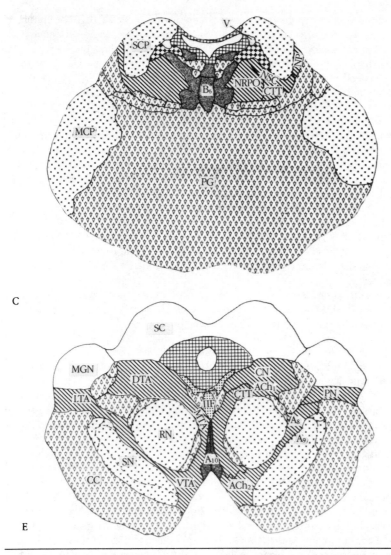

Fig. 4-6. *Cross sections of the brainstem at the levels indicated in the insert. A, B, and C, Medulla. B and C, Pons. D and E, Midbrain. All structures are bilateral, though some are illustrated, for simplicity, on one side only. Nuclei labeled A, B, or ACh with a subscript indicate locations of cell clusters containing specific transmitters: A, norepinephrine or dopamine; B, serotonin; ACh, acetylcholine (see Chap. 6 for details concerning these nuclei). Roman numerals identify cranial nerve nuclei. CC, crus cerebri; CN, cuneiform nucleus; CP, cerebral peduncles; CTT, central tegmental tract; DSCP, decussation of the superior cerebellar peduncle; DTA, dorsal tegmental area; IC, inferior colliculi; ICP, inferior cerebellar peduncle; LRF, lateral reticular formation; LTA, lateral tegmental area; MCP, middle cerebellar peduncle; MGN, medial geniculate nucleus (of thalamus); MRF, medial reticular formation; MTA, medial tegmental area; NP, nucleus pedunculoponticus; NRPC, nucleus reticularis pontis caudalis; NRPO, nucleus reticularis pontis oralis; NSC, nucleus subceruleus; OC, olivary complex; P, pyramids; PG, pontine gray; PN, peripeduncular nucleus; PT, pyramidal tracts; RN, red nucleus; SC, superior colliculi; SCN, subcuneiform nucleus; SCP, superior cerebellar peduncle; SN, substantia nigra; VTA, ventral tegmental area.*

processing capabilities. In the medulla are a number of centers that regulate important bodily functions, the so-called vital functions. The final motor outflow for central influence over respiration, blood vessel tone, heart rate and contractile strength, and gastrointestinal function arises from a dorsal zone in the medulla (Fig. 4-6A) that includes several cranial nerve nuclei (the dorsal motor nucleus of the vagus, the nucleus and tractus solitarius, the hypoglossal and certain parahypoglossal nuclei). This is not to say that higher centers do not influence these same vital processes, but rather that the principal responsibility for their central regulation resides in the medulla. The cyclic operation of respiration arises in cells of the so-called respiratory center in the medullary reticular formation. Two reciprocally inhibitory cell groups are observed, one controlling inspiration and one controlling expiration. Another specialized area of the medulla called the chemoreceptor trigger zone is sensitive to certain noxious chemical substances and elicits vomiting when stimulated.

Several cranial nerve nuclei lie in the medulla (Fig. 4-6A), some, as we have just seen, involved in the regulation of vital functions. Generally, the nuclei for cranial nerves IX, X, XI, and XII and the spinal tract of the 5th cranial nerve reside in the medulla. The afferent nuclei of the cranial nerves provide the first level of processing of cranial nerve inputs, while the efferent cranial nerve nuclei provide the final packaging of efferent signal patterns.

The caudalmost portion (that is, the tail end) of the reticular formation lies in the medulla (Fig. 4-6A). The medial portion of the reticular formation at this level is the common discharge pathway for extrapyramidal influences on motor activity, giving rise to reticulospinal projections. Within the medial reticular formation are numerous especially large cells. The lateral reticular formation is noteworthy for its complement of small cells. In this area there is a somatotopic representation of proprioceptive and tactile afferents that are relayed on to the cerebellum.

Situated dorsally to the reticular formation, beneath the fourth ventricle, is the periventricular gray, which is part of the periventricular punishment system discussed in Chapter 3. Also found in the medulla are a number of extrapyramidal afferent relay nuclei, most notably the olivary complex (Fig. 4-6A).

Many drugs profoundly influence the vital centers of the medulla; for example, sedatives and narcotics depress the respiratory center. Other drugs, such as some of the neuroleptics, exert a depressant influence on the vasomotor center, leading to low blood pressure (hypotension). When depressant drugs are present in doses sufficient to suppress the functioning of the medulla markedly, death is the likely consequence.

The *pons* lies immediately above the medulla; the pons and the medulla together constitute the hindbrain. As in the medulla, many pathways pass through the pons. In fact, they are even more numerous in the pons, since it must provide massive bridgeways connecting the brainstem with the dorsally situated cerebellum. These bridgeways are the superior, middle, and inferior cerebellar peduncles (Fig. 4-6A–D). The ventral, bulbous portion of the pons is a major point of interconnection between the pyramidal system and the cerebellum (Fig. 4-6B and C). Signals reaching the ventral pontine gray are relayed to the cerebellum via the middle cerebellar peduncle. The reticular formation continues to be present in the pons, although somewhat constricted in its contours (Fig. 4-6B and C). One pontine reticular nucleus (nucleus reticularis pontis caudalis [Fig. 4-6B]) is believed to be responsible for stimulating dreaming during the dream phase of sleep.

Cranial nerve nuclei lying in the pons include those for cranial nerves V through VIII (Fig. 4-6B), which serve the muscles and sensory receptors of the face, jaw, and sinuses, as well as innervating the salivatory glands, taste receptors on the front of the tongue, and auditory and vestibular systems.

The *midbrain* overlies the hindbrain and interconnects it with the higher brain centers. The midbrain is one of the chief areas of integration within the brain. The reticular formation continues in its course from pons to thalamus throughout the ventral midbrain. There are highly complex and diffuse interconnections between the reticular formation and limbic system in this area. Indeed, it is primarily in the midbrain that the limbic system expresses its influence on behavior. The ventrolateral portion of the midbrain reticular formation (Fig. 4-6E) serves as the bed nucleus of the ascending reticular activating system, exerting widespread influences on the activity level of the cerebral cortex (see Chap. 10). The reticular formation taken in toto plays a profound role in regulating the flow of afferent and efferent traffic through the brainstem. One portion of the midbrain reticular formation, the cuneiform nucleus (Fig. 4-6D and E), is the likely anatomic site for the formation of the neural interconnections underlying respondent (or Pavlovian) conditioning. Dorsal to the reticular formation is the periaqueductal gray, the rostral continuation of the periventricular gray, and, like it, part of the punishment, or response suppression, system.

The red nucleus and substantia nigra of the extrapyramidal system reside in the midbrain, by and large (Fig. 4-6E). The red nucleus is a center integrating cerebellar and striatal signals, while the substantia nigra projects in the ascending direction and helps to regulate activity of the corpus striatum.

Located on the dorsal surface of the midbrain (the tectum) are two pairs of nuclei, the inferior (Fig. 4-6D) and the superior (Fig. 4-6E) colliculi. The nuclei act as integrative and relay stations for afferent impulses of the auditory and visual systems respectively. In the ventral midbrain (the tegmentum), along with the reticular formation, lie several cranial nerve nuclei (the oculomotor, accessory oculomotor, and trochlear nuclei) that control eye movements via the 3rd and 4th cranial nerves (Fig. 4-6D and E).

Scattered throughout the medulla, pons, and midbrain are nuclei belonging to particular neurotransmitter systems. Two epinephrine-containing nuclei are found in the medulla and are involved in sympathetic regulation. Seven norepinephrine nuclei are found in the brainstem, three in the medulla, and four in the pons. Most of these are involved in sympathetic regulation or response facilitation. One norepinephrine-containing nucleus, the locus ceruleus (Fig. 4-6C and D), is the bed nucleus of the reward system (Chap. 3). Three nuclei containing dopaminergic cell bodies (A_8, A_9, A_{10}) all lie in the midbrain (Fig. 4-6E). These nuclei provide ascending pathways that relate to motor tone, arousal, and aggression, among other functions. These dopaminergic pathways have been implicated in schizophrenia and extrapyramidal disorders. Nine clusters containing serotonergic cell bodies are found in the brainstem: four in the medulla, two in the pons (Fig. 4-6B and C), and three in the midbrain (Fig. 4-6D). Seven of these nine clusters are found in a group of nuclei called the raphé nuclei (the Greek *raphé* means a "ridge" or "surface mark"), and these nuclei appear as features along the midline of the brainstem. One dopamine nucleus (nucleus linearis) is an eighth raphé nucleus, since it, too, appears at the midline. The serotonergic raphé nuclei are involved in gating mechanisms, habituation, and sleep-cycle regulation.

Looking at the brainstem as a whole, the following classes of nuclei are noted: (1) aminergic nuclei, including adrenergic, noradrenergic, dopaminergic, and serotonergic; (2) cranial nerve nuclei, both motor and sensory; (3) extrapyramidal relay nuclei; and (4) nuclei of the reticular formation and central gray. The functions intrinsic to the brainstem (Table 4-1) include regulation of vital functions, response facilitation, response suppression, gating of afferents, motor relay and integration, activation of higher centers in relation to afferents, and regulation of the sleep-wake cycle. While this list of functional capabilities may appear limited in view of the full gamut of potentials in human behavior, it constitutes a truly remarkable set of functions when contrasted

Table 4-1. *Functions of the brainstem*

Regulation of vital functions: dorsal visceral gray
Response facilitation: lateral reticular gray
Response suppression: periaqueductal, periventricular, and subependymal gray
Gating of afferents: raphé nuclei, periaqueductal gray
Motor relay and integration: reticular, tegmental, and ventral pontine gray; extrapyramidal nuclei
Ascending activation: reticular and tegmental gray
Sleep-wake cycle: raphé nuclei, pontine reticular gray

with the very narrow range of processing capabilities intrinsic to the spinal cord. In any case, the rich diversity of behaviors organized by higher centers are realized largely through molding and manipulating the more primitive mechanisms of the brainstem, not through wholly independent processes.

The Diencephalon

The diencephalon includes four areas: the dorsal thalamus (or thalamus), epithalamus, subthalamus, and hypothalamus, structures that participate in a wide variety of regulatory activities.

1. The *dorsal thalamus* is a centrally lying, egg-shaped collection of nuclei that act as relay stations between the cortex and lower brain. Some of the nuclei are relay stations for sensory inputs in the visual, auditory, and somatosensory systems. Another group of nuclei called associative nuclei belong to the diffuse thalamic projection system (Chap. 10) and control the waves of consciousness of the cortex. A third category of nuclei called intrinsic nuclei interconnect other thalamic nuclei and help integrate the flow of discharges. The functions of some nuclei are unknown.
2. The *epithalamus* comprises a few disparate structures that lie on the dorsal boundary of the brainstem. The striae medullaris thalami look like threads overlying the thalamus and are involved in olfaction. The habenulae are nuclei also involved in olfaction. The pineal gland, which, strictly speaking, is a gland attached to, but distinct from, the brain, is involved with biochemical responsiveness to light, diurnal cycles, and possibly gonadotropic control of sexual development.
3. The *subthalamus* is a zone of transition between the tegmentum of the mesencephalon and the thalamus. The anterior portions of the red nucleus and substantia nigra extend into the subthalamus. Pathways interconnecting the corpus striatum with the thalamus, hypothalamus, and extrapyramidal nuclei of the brainstem disseminate throughout the subthalamus (see Chap. 20). In addition, some extrapyramidal integrative function occurs associated with two nuclei of the subthalamus—the subthalamic nucleus (of Luys) and the nucleus of Forel's field.
4. The *hypothalamus,* which lies on the ventral surface of the brain just above the pituitary gland, is a tightly packed cluster of nuclei. It serves as the principle discharge center for the entire limbic system, as well as bearing primary responsibility for a number of regulatory processes. With exceptions, the general direction of flow through the hypothalamus is from higher to lower centers. A full discussion of the hypothalamus is found in Chapter 15.

Various homeostatic (state-maintaining) processes come under the domain of the hypothalamus, including water balance, energy balance, temperature regulation, and sexual function. The hypothalamus has been considered the highest level of integration of the autonomic nervous system. Probably a more accurate view is that the hypothalamus in its various homeostatic functions has regulatory access to the autonomic nervous system.

The hypothalamus elicits integrated motor patterns related to emotional expression. Limbic system–regulated emotional behaviors are directed through the hypothalamus, which acts as the limbic output center.

The hypothalamus is also the communication center between the nervous system and the endocrine system, effecting neural regulation of the pituitary gland, which in turn is the "master" gland of the endocrine system. Reciprocal feedback regulation is exerted over the hypothalamus by the endocrine glands that it controls.

This important area is also involved in arousal regulation insofar as it trasmits limbic system influences to the diffuse thalamic projection system of the thalamus via a tract called the mamillothalamic tract. Lesions of the mamillary bodies of the hypothalamus result in coma.

The Telencephalon

The telencephalon is the dorsalmost extent of the brainstem and therefore immediately underlies the cerebral cortices. The telencephalon includes the basal ganglia and internal, external, and extreme capsules. The last three are fiber tracts passing from cortex to midbrain. The basal ganglia consists of four nuclei. Three of these—the putamen, globus pallidus, and caudate—together form the corpus striatum. The fourth nucleus is the amygdala, which is a part of the limbic system. However, the term *basal ganglia* is often used loosely as a synonym for *corpus striatum*.

The corpus striatum is the highest regulatory center for the extrapyramidal system (Chap. 20), and its three nuclei function together in aspects of involuntary motor control, including coordinated movement and postural tone. They discharge to the extrapyramidal nuclei of the subthalamus and mesencephalon, thence to the descending reticular formation.

The amygdala (Chap. 15) is believed to be involved closely in the regulation of aggressive and rage behavior. Another part of the amygdala is interconnected with the olfactory system. Connections with other limbic structures such as the hypothalamus and hippocampus are extensive.

The Limbic System

The limbic system (Chap. 15) includes, in addition to the amygdala, certain basal cortical regions: the septum, hippocampus, and cingulate gyrus. In addition to these, a number of prominent fiber bundles interrelating these primary areas are properly included in the limbic system.

The limbic system is closely related to the olfactory sense. This area is also critical in the regulation of emotional behavior and much of all learning that occurs. Selective inhibition of subcortical nuclei resulting from limbic system influence makes possible selection of appropriate responses from the behavioral repertoire. And finally, the hippocampus in particular is instrumental in short-term memory and consolidation of learning into retained experience.

The Cerebral Cortex

The seat of consciousness, conscious sensation, and voluntary control of behavior is the cerebral cortex (Chap. 26). The cortex is divided by anatomists into four lobes: frontal, parietal, occipital, and temporal. The frontal lobe regulates delayed responding, response extinction, abstract thought, and motor regulation (pyramidal). The parietal lobe is involved in language, spatial and temporal orientation, bodily sensations, and body image. The occipital lobe is devoted entirely to the visual system, while the temporal lobe is related to the auditory system and limbic system.

Selected References and Further Readings

1. Angevine, J. R., Jr., and Cotman, C. W. *Principles of Neuroanatomy.* New York: Oxford University Press, 1981.
2. Carpenter, M. B. *Human Neuroanatomy* (7th ed.). Baltimore: Williams & Wilkins, 1976.
3. Gatz, A. J. *Clinical Neuroanatomy and Neurophysiology* (4th ed.). Philadelphia: Davis, 1970.

The Physiology
of Nerve Cells

5

R̸

Cytology

Cytology is the study of cells. The nervous system is made up of hundreds of billions of nerve cells, called neurons, and their associated neuroglia, or supporting cells. The neuron is the essential functional subunit in the nervous system, and an understanding of its characteristics and properties contributes substantially to a comprehension of CNS function and the effects of drugs on the CNS. We particularly wish to consider the aspects of nerve cell structure that are referred to in subsequent chapters.

In many ways, nerve cells bear considerable resemblance to other cells. They vary substantially with respect to size and shape, however. Each neuron contains a single nucleus, somewhat larger in relation to the size of the cell than is the case in most non-neural cells. The nuclei contain one or more nucleoli. The nerve cell, like other cells, contains free ribosomes and rough endoplasmic reticulum (both associated with protein synthesis) and a Golgi apparatus (involved in the packaging of secretory products). Like other cells, neurons contain mitochondria (the "powerhouse" of the cell), which are specialized for oxidative phosphorylation, and microtubules.

The cytology of nerve cells is, however, characterized by a number of special properties. Nerve cells are capable of conduction of bioelectric impulses over long distances without loss of signal strength. Nerve cells are highly specific in their interconnections, both with other nerve cells and with innervated tissues (muscles, organs, glands, and sensory receptors).

Connections are almost always synaptic in nature. A synapse is a very small space, usually about 200 Å (about 1/1,270,000 of an inch) in width, separating two nerve cells or a nerve cell and an effector system such as a muscle. Nerve cells do not directly contact one another, and therefore an electrical impulse cannot be passed directly from one cell to another. Rather, communication between neurons is mediated by their sensitivity to chemicals (neurotransmitters, or neuroregulators) released by other nerve cells. It is this intercellular chemical process, called transmission, not the intracellular processes, which is most readily susceptible to the modifying influence of drugs.

The synaptic nature of CNS interconnections was much more difficult to establish than that of the peripheral nervous system. At the end of the nineteenth century, the widely held view among neuroanatomists was that the cells of the brain were anatomically linked together into a syncytium, i.e., a network acting like a single large cell. Even after Ramon y Cajal established in the 1890s the presence of anatomic separations

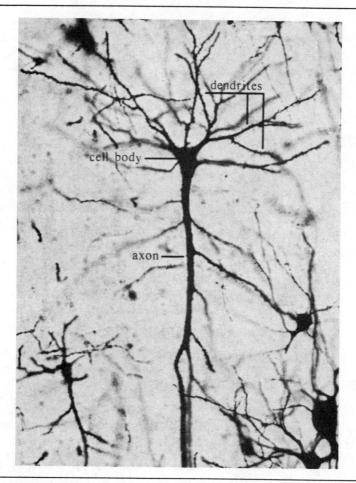

Fig. 5-1. *A neuron of the visual cortex of a cat (× 375). Modified from R. Lewin.* The Nervous System. *New York: Anchor Press/Doubleday, 1974.*

between cells, and pharmacologists demonstrated parallels between central and peripheral drug effects, the controversy between direct electrical and indirect, neuro-chemical interconnectiveness persisted until the 1930s and even beyond.

Closely related to the transmission functions are the specialized "cytoplasmic processes" that characterize nerve cells. A given nerve cell has one or more of these processes extending from its body, or soma. A monopolar cell has just one such process, an axon. An axon is highly specialized for rapid conduction and acts as the output side in the nerve cell's function. In addition to the axon, a bipolar cell possesses a single large dendritic trunk. A dendrite is specialized for receiving and integrating inputs from other nerve cells or sensory receptors. Dendrites are the input side of the nerve cell. Multipolar cells (Fig. 5-1) possess multiple dendritic processes, collateral axonal branches, or both.

Nerve cells are frequently distinguished in terms of their axonal characteristics. Some axons are covered by an insulating fatty sheath (a type of neuroglia) called myelin.

Myelination increases conduction velocity. Fibers vary widely in diameter. Velocity of conduction increases with the diameter of the axon.

In addition to nerve cells, the brain contains neuroglial (or glial) cells. These are of two principal varieties. Those that compose the myelin sheath are called oligodendroglia, satellite cells, or Schwann's cells. Star-like fibrous neuroglia, called astrocytes, surround the surfaces of blood vessels in the vicinity of axons and dendrites and probably function as insulation and structural framework for nerve cells.

The Cell Membrane: A Fluid Mosaic

Crucial to the development of an understanding of nerve cell function is an appreciation of the characteristics of the cell membrane. Nerve cells are in the business of communication and "talk" to each other through the special communication mechanisms inherent in the membrane. But communication is but one of the functions of the membrane, not the most important. The basic role of the membrane, fundamental to life itself, is to maintain the integrity of the cell within a range of external environmental conditions. In the words of Lewis Thomas, "To stay alive, you have to be able to hold out against equilibrium, maintain imbalance, bank against entropy, and you can only transact this business with membranes in our kind of world" [4]. The communication function is carried on cautiously by the cell, in a manner aimed at minimizing the risk of exposing the cell to a challenge that cannot be adequately met.

The messages received by nerve cells are in the form of molecules, some large, some small. The message may be received in either of two ways. Some small molecular messengers may be granted entry into the cell interior. These messengers will then have access to the inner workings of the cell, perhaps influencing enzyme activity, perhaps modifying genetically regulated cell expression, or possibly modulating energy conversions within the cell. Larger messengers and small but suspect messengers will be denied access to the cell but will nevertheless exert minor or major influences by stimulation of specialized receptive sites located in the membrane itself. These receptive sites are commonly termed *receptors*. Stimulation of a membrane receptor sets into motion a cascade of chemical reactions whose character is defined by the identity of the messenger, receptor type, and subsequent effector mechanisms in the cascade.

The cell membrane is viewed as consisting of a fluid mosaic, an ocean of phospholipids on which floats a flotilla of membrane proteins. The phospholipids are organized in a bilayer (Fig. 5-2), each phospholipid molecule oriented so that its polar head faces outward against the aqueous extracellular or intracellular fluid, while its long lipid hydrophobic tail points to the middle of the membrane, abutting the other half of the bilayer. The lipid membrane is largely impermeable to water-soluble molecules.

Three main phospholipids constitute the cell membrane. The inner surface of the membrane consists mostly of phosphatidylethanolamine, and the outer side of the membrane consists largely of phosphatidylcholine. Sandwiched between these two, deep in the membrane, is phosphatidyl-*N*-monomethylethanolamine. Two methyltransferase enzymes control the interconversions of the three phospholipids. Methyltransferase I converts phosphatidylethanolamine into phosphatidyl-*N*-monomethylethanolamine, while methyltransferase II converts the latter into phosphatidylcholine. The activity of these enzymes regulates membrane viscosity because phosphatidyl-*N*-monomethylethanolamine promotes increased membrane fluidity, while phosphatidylcholine causes increased viscosity. Membrane viscosity plays an important role in determining the function of the various membrane proteins (e.g., ion channels, recognition proteins, effector proteins).

The flotilla of proteins, adrift in the membrane, vary in size, location, and function. Some float on the inner surface, some on the outer surface, and some transverse the

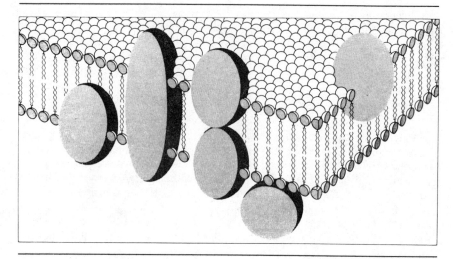

Fig. 5-2. *Structure of the cell membrane is shown schematically according to current conceptions. The basic structure is a double layer of lipid (fat) molecules with their hydrophilic heads pointing outward and their hydrophobic tails pointing inward. Also associated with the membrane are protein molecules, seen here as larger bodies some of which penetrate the membrane and others of which are embedded in one side or the other. Most of the movement of ions into and out of the membrane is by way of channels in the various proteins. From D. C. Tosteson. Lithium and mania.* Sci. Am. *244:166, 1981.* © *1981 by Scientific American, Inc. All rights reserved.*

width of the membrane, extending outward from it on both sides. Some of these proteins serve as carriers, providing transport of needed chemicals into the cell and escorting unwanted molecules to the exterior. Some proteins serve as ion channels, allowing a limited flow of water and small particles across the lipid barrier. Some are catalytic enzymes that regulate important cellular metabolic activities. Some serve as receptor sites, prepared to receive regulatory messages. And some modulate and couple together the activities of the others. Collectively, these membrane proteins, in conjunction with the cytoplasmic constituents and organelles, enable the cell to conduct its functions.

Function: Conduction and Transmission

Many, indeed most, drugs that influence behavior alter the functioning of individual neurons. One can hardly overstate the extent to which a grasp of the electrophysiologic and neurochemical aspects of neuronal function contributes to an understanding of psychotropic drug effects. Our discussion will examine the state of a hypothetical neuron just prior to and during a sequence of events commencing with the excitation of that neuron and ending with the transmission of that signal to the next nerve cell down the line.

The Resting State

An unexcited neuron is said to be in a resting state. In the resting state, a nerve cell (indeed any cell) possesses a resting electrical potential; this means that there is a small difference between the electrical potential on the inside as compared with that on the outside of the cell (about 70 millivolts). The inside of the cell is negative with respect to the outside. This charge separation (or polarization) is related to the cell's ability to control the distribution of certain charged chemical substances, or ions. The cell is able to control the distribution of small ions because (1) its "semipermeable" membrane, the cell wall, limits passage of substances to and fro and (2) carrier proteins, powered by cellular energy, actively "pump" sodium out of cells in exchange for potassium. The activity of this sodium-potassium exchange pump leads to a net charge separation, because a portion of the potassium leaks back out of the cell, along its concentration gradient. Sodium cannot as easily leak back into the cell along its combined concentration and electrical gradient because it has a larger hydrated radius than does potassium. Because any substance seeks to equalize its distribution across the membrane, there is an immediate passive flow of ions and consequent polarity changes if anything occurs to increase the permeability of the cellular membrane.

The Postsynaptic Potential

Certain neurotransmitters increase membrane permeability. The extent of increased permeability is directly related to how much neurotransmitter contacts the receptors of the cell membrane. Excitatory transmitters produce a decrease in the degree of polarization (partial depolarization) in the part of the nerve cell where the membrane has been "attacked" by neurotransmitter substance. Because this partial depolarization tends to "excite" the nerve cell, it is called an excitatory postsynaptic potential (EPSP). An EPSP can occur only in a dendrite or cell body, not in an axon, since the membrane of an axon is insensitive to neurotransmitter substances.

Other chemical substances, inhibitory neurotransmitters, produce an increase in the degree of polarization (hyperpolarization) of a postsynaptic membrane. In this case the *increase* in polarization is referred to as an inhibitory postsynaptic potential (IPSP) because it *stabilizes* the nerve cell. At any given time, a particular area of membrane on a nerve cell may be bombarded by more than one neurotransmitter, perhaps one capable of eliciting an EPSP, another capable of eliciting an IPSP. The net result in such situations is determined by the relative concentrations of the various substances influencing the membrane. Moreover, the concentrations of chemical substances tend not to be fixed, but rather ebb and flow. The postsynaptic membrane acts as a temporal and spatial integrator and responds with great sensitivity to the balance of influences from various sources as they occur from moment to moment.

The Action Potential

If the net change in polarization produced by neurotransmitters at the dendrites and cell body is sufficiently *excitatory,* a chain reaction is set off in the axon of the cell. In the first step, the impermeable state of that part of the axonal membrane adjacent to the cell suddenly breaks down; this is accompanied by a complete loss and even reversal of polarization for a split second. Almost as quickly, the membrane regains its semipermeability and reestablishes the resting potential. This entire sequence of changes, termed the *action potential* (Fig. 5-3), occupies but a fraction of a second at any given point.

At the same time, however, the occurrence of an action potential at a particular point along the axon triggers a similar sequence of events in the adjacent axonal membrane; and as the sequence is replicated there, a similar sequence arises in the next axonal

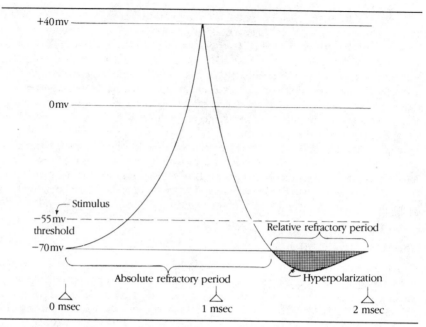

Fig. 5-3. *Hypothetical schema of an action potential indicating refractory periods.*

segment, and so on, on down the line. In this manner, the action potential is propagated like a wave down the length of the axon. This capacity of propagation is critical to the functioning of nerve cells.

Unlike the postsynaptic potential, which is continuously variable or analog and chemically initiated, the action potential is all-or-nothing or digital and electrically initiated (i.e., by the EPSP). During the passage of an action potential, the axon is completely refractory, that is, insensitive, to further initiation of an action potential. Immediately following the action potential, the axon is relatively refractory to initiation of a new action potential (Fig. 5-3).

Chemical Transmission

The last step in the cycle of events occurs at the end of the nerve axon, called the bouton. The bouton is a terminal swelling in the axon that contains large numbers of dense granules or vesicles storing the neurotransmitter substance. The bouton also contains catalytic proteins called enzymes, some (called catabolic or degradative enzymes) capable of destroying the neurotransmitter substance and others collectively capable of manufacturing the neurotransmitter. Neurotransmitter stored in the vesicles is protected from destruction by the catabolic enzymes.

Until recently, it was thought that each nerve cell contains and releases one—and only one—transmitter. This view has been called the Dale hypothesis ever since it first appeared in the literature in 1935. However, it is actually Eccles's corollary statement. Dale asserted only that all the axonal branches of a given neuron could be presumed to release the same transmitter(s). Eccles's later statement, which he misnamed "The Dale hypothesis," asserted that each neuron releases but one transmitter. There is no current experimental evidence to refute Dale's actual statement, but there is now considerable evidence indicating that the Eccles version does not hold for all neurons. Some neurons release both a "classical" neurotransmitter and a peptide neuromodulator.

When an action potential arrives at the bouton, the increased permeability of the membrane permits the ejection or extrusion of neurotransmitter from the nerve cell into the synaptic cleft adjacent to the bouton. The mechanism by which this occurs has not yet been elucidated except that it is apparent that the influx of calcium ions accompanying the arrival of the action potential plays a crucial role.

Once the neurotransmitter has been released, it diffuses freely in all directions. Some of it crosses the synaptic space and contacts receptor sites on the postsynaptic membrane of another nerve cell or effector system (organ, muscle, etc.), thus completing the cycle where we took it up and initiating a new and comparable cycle of events. At the same time, the transmitter begins to be inactivated. This serves to limit the duration of its action. Three processes contribute to inactivation of transmitter: (1) simple diffusion, which progressively dilutes its concentration; (2) the action of enzymes, which degrade or break down the transmitter and are located in the synapse; and (3) the reuptake of neurotransmitter by the presynaptic neuron, that is, the neuron that released the transmitter.

Since the vast majority of drugs of interest in psychopharmacology modify chemical transmission between nerve cells, this process will be considered in Chapter 6 in considerable detail.

Selected References and Further Readings

1. Capaldi, R. A. A dynamic model of cell membranes. *Sci. Am.* 230:27–33, 1974.
2. Guyton, A. C. *Textbook of Medical Physiology* (6th ed.). Philadelphia: Saunders, 1981.
3. Lewin, R. *The Nervous System.* New York: Anchor Press/Doubleday, 1974.
4. Thomas, L. *The Lives of a Cell.* New York: Bantam, 1975.

Neurotransmission
6

In this chapter we will consider some aspects of neurochemistry that bear a close relationship to the overall task of elucidating the brain functions and actions of psychotropic drugs. We will focus our attention on substances believed to be neurotransmitters in the CNS or believed to mediate the effects of transmitters. The neurochemicals selected for discussion are those that have been the best studied so far. Before examining the characteristics of specific transmitters, we will first examine the general case with an eye to three issues: (1) the mechanisms of synaptic transmission, (2) acute drug interactions with synaptic transmission, and (3) adaptive changes in synaptic mechanisms.

Mechanisms of Synaptic Transmission

Fortunately for the student of transmitter neurochemistry, the similarities in the transmission mechanisms of the various neurotransmitters are greater than the dissimilarities. As a consequence, it is useful to study transmission mechanisms in the general case. Exceptional features in the transmission mechanisms of particular transmitters can be noted as deviations from the usual situation. We will therefore examine neurotransmission in considerable detail for a hypothetical typical transmitter. The reader is urged to examine Figure 6-1 carefully while studying the text description of transmission mechanisms.

Synaptic transmission is a communicative event. The message sender is called the presynaptic neuron, and the recipient is designated the postsynaptic neuron. The sending of a message is a function that is largely intrinsic to the axonal ending, or nerve terminal, of the presynaptic neuron. Before a given instance of transmission can occur, the presynaptic nerve terminal must be readied through carrying out a number of preparatory steps. These preparatory steps include the maintenance of a resting potential (as described in Chap. 5), synthesis and storage of neurotransmitter, and the movement of filled vesicles into position on the interior face of the presynaptic cell membrane. The maintenance of the resting potential derives from the semipermeable quality of the fluid mosaic membrane, together with the electrogenic capacity of the sodium-potassium exchange pump.

Synthesis of neurotransmitter occurs in one or more steps regulated by synthetic enzymes. A precursor substance is made available to the cell by active transport of the

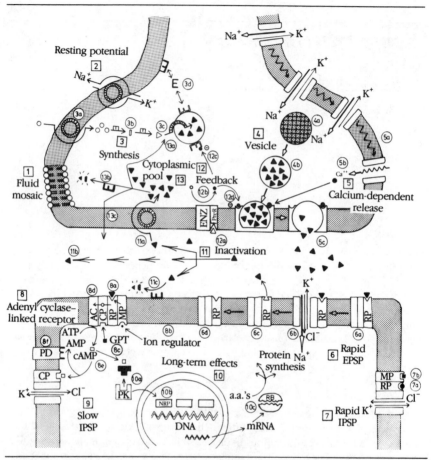

Fig. 6-1. *Neurotransmission mechanisms. a.a.'s, amino acids; AC, adenyl cyclase; AMP, adenosine monophosphate; ATP, adenosine triphosphate; cAMP, cyclic adenosine monophosphate; CP, coupling protein; DNA, deoxyribonucleic acid; EPSP, excitatory postsynaptic potential; ENZ, enzyme; IPSP, inhibitory postsynaptic potential; MP, modulatory protein; mRNA, messenger ribonucleic acid; PD, phosphodiesterase; PK, protein kinase; NRP, nuclear regulatory proteins; RB, ribosome; RP, recognition protein. (1) the fluid mosaic membrane; (2) Na^+-K^+ exchange pump; (3a) precursor uptake; (3b) transmitter synthesis; (3c) vesicular uptake (storage); (3d) enzyme pool shifts; (4a) vesicle (protein mesh and gangliosides); (4b) movement and recognition of full vesicle; (5a) arrival of propagated action potential; (5b) influx of calcium through divalent ion channel; (5c) release; (6a) binding; (6b) activation; (6c) dissociation; (6d) regeneration; (7a) binding of an inhibitory transmitter; (7b) regulation of transmitter affinity by a modulatory protein; (8a) activation of adenyl cyclase–linked receptor; (8b) modulation of transmitter affinity; (8c) guanididine triphosphate regulation of coupling protein; (8d) adenyl cyclase stimulation; (8e) increased cAMP; (8f) phosphodiesterase metabolism of cAMP; (9) cAMP-mediated slow IPSP; (10a) cAMP activation of soluble protein-kinase; (10b) protein-kinase derepression of DNA via nuclear regulatory protein; (10c) mRNA activation of protein synthesis; (11) inactivation of transmitter by: (11a) reuptake; (11b) diffusion; (11c) enzymatic degradation; (12a) binding to presynaptic receptor; (12b) enzymatic formation of inhibitor (or suppression of cofactor synthesis); (12c) inhibition of synthesis; (12d) inhibition of release; (13a) uptake from cytoplasmic pool into vesicle; (13b) intracellular enzymatic degradation; (13c) low-level spontaneous release.*

substance from the extracellular fluid into the cell interior. The initial precursor accumulated by the cell is a molecule widely available in the body, such as an amino acid or metabolic intermediary of glucose metabolism. Rarely, the substance may be an essential dietary constituent.

Often, one step in the synthetic sequence is slower than the others and is therefore rate-limiting in the overall rate of transmitter synthesis. Fractional inhibition of the rate-limiting enzyme has a more significant effect on the production of transmitter than a similar fractional inhibition of any other step. Total inhibition of any step of course stops transmitter synthesis entirely. The synthetic enzymes may be free-floating in the cytoplasm (soluble) or membrane-bound. The membrane-bound fraction may be associated with vesicular membranes or the cellular membrane. Thus, there may be three distinct enzyme pools. Activity of the enzyme will change as it shifts among the pools. Generally, vesicular membrane–bound enzyme is most active, and enzyme bound to the cell membrane is least active.

Often, the final step in synthesis is linked with vesicular membrane uptake and storage of the transmitter. In any case, much of the newly synthesized transmitter is incorporated into storage vesicles, or granules, that are abundant in axonal endings. Storage serves two purposes: It protects the transmitter from enzymatic degradation by cytoplasmic enzymes, and it packages the transmitter in uniform amounts for quantal release.

The synaptic vesicles are believed to consist of a protein mesh with gaps occluded by a kind of lipid called a ganglioside. A fully packed vesicle is identified by a recognition protein in the presynaptic cell membrane. At this point the presynaptic neuron is prepared for a transmission event.

Transmission begins with the arrival of an action potential at the nerve terminal. Since an action potential results from the conduction process, the initial sequence of events that follows its arrival at the nerve terminal is referred to as conduction-transmission coupling. Arrival of the action potential is accompanied by a sharp increase in the permeability of the cell membrane as ion channels momentarily open. The increase in permeability leads to an influx of calcium (among other ions), because active calcium secretion from the cell during the resting state generates a substantial concentration gradient. The calcium ion that flows into the cell binds in part to vesicles. The filled vesicles attached to the presynaptic membrane are stimulated by calcium, triggering apposition and fusion of the vesicle with the cell membrane. The gangliosides of the vesicle wall dissolve in the lipid bilayer of the cell membrane, vesicular pores are exposed, and the transmitter escapes into the synaptic cleft. This is *release* of the neurotransmitter or, more specifically, calcium-dependent release. A small amount of calcium-independent, spontaneous release occurs continuously.

The neurotransmitter released into the synapse begins to flow outward, diffusing in every direction. Because the synaptic cleft is tiny, a substantial portion of the released transmitter contacts the postsynaptic cell membrane. Some of the transmitter comes into contact with recognition proteins (receptor sites) on the postsynaptic membrane. Recognition proteins are often coupled with an effector protein and associated with one or more modulatory proteins to form a receptor complex. Figure 6-1 illustrates the effect of transmitter at three types of receptor complexes. One type of receptor complex generates rapidly developing excitatory postsynaptic potentials. The nicotinic, cholinergic receptor is an example of this type of receptor complex. The transmitter receptor interaction involves four steps: binding, receptor activation, dissociation, and regeneration of activatable receptor. Receptor activation leads to increased effector activity to the extent that the receptor is coupled to an effector protein. The effector for this type of complex is a large ion channel. Influx of sodium ions through the opened channels generates the excitatory postsynaptic potential. These receptor mechanisms will be discussed in more detail in Chapter 7.

Another type of receptor complex, exemplified by the gamma-aminobutyric acid (GABA) receptor, generates rapid inhibitory postsynaptic potentials by activating effector proteins associated with chloride channels. The activated effector protein undergoes a change in conformation that opens up the chloride channel. Sometimes, this type of effector protein is referred to (somewhat inaccurately) as a chloride *ionophore*. The result of chloride influx into the cell is a hyperpolarization, which makes the postsynaptic cell less excitable.

A third type of receptor complex is one in which the effector protein is the enzyme adenyl cyclase. The receptor sites of this type are said to be adenyl cyclase–linked. Norepinephrine receptors of the beta type and most dopamine receptors are of this type. The enzyme adenyl cyclase catalyzes the formation of cyclic adenosine monophosphate (cAMP) from adenosine triphosphate (ATP). Cyclic AMP is said to be a "second messenger," relaying the message signaled by the transmitter through regulation of intracellular and membrane mechanisms. Generally, effects mediated by adenyl cyclase–linked receptors are slower in onset but longer lasting than effects produced by receptors of the ion channel type. Figure 6-1 shows cAMP producing a slow inhibitory potential through its effect on a small ion channel, and also generating long-term modifications by regulation of genetic expression through protein synthesis. The cellular levels of cAMP are controlled in part by the enzyme phosphodiesterase, which degrades cAMP.

Another type of receptor is found on the presynaptic cell membrane and has been dubbed the *presynaptic receptor*.* The presynaptic receptor exerts a feedback effect on the neurotransmission process. Activation of the presynaptic receptor causes an inhibition of synthesis and release of transmitter. The mechanism for presynaptic receptor–mediated inhibition of synthesis is not established but could involve synthesis of an inhibitory substance or suppression of synthesis of a necessary cofactor. Synthesis inhibition might involve enzyme pool shifts. Two mechanisms have been postulated for the inhibition of release mediated by presynaptic receptors: (1) stimulation of a presynaptic receptor–linked cyclic guanosine monophosphate–generating enzyme in the presynaptic membrane, and (2) activation of the Na^+-K^+ exchange pump to produce hyperpolarization. The presynaptic receptor helps to prevent an excess accumulation of transmitter in the synapse.

Presynaptic receptors have been noted in noradrenergic, adrenergic, dopaminergic, and serotonergic nerve terminals of the CNS. In the case of peripheral norepinephrine terminals, calcium-dependent, action potential–evoked release of norepinephrine is modulated not only by norepinephrine itself, but also by acetylcholine, dopamine, opiate peptides, cyclic nucleotides, and prostaglandins. Angiotensin II can increase norepinephrine release. In the brain, release of norepinephrine from terminals is facilitated by GABA and inhibition by opiates. Thus, there appears to be a real mosaic of presynaptic receptors capable of influencing transmitter release.

---

*By common practice, the terms *presynaptic receptor* and *autoreceptor* are used interchangeably to refer to three distinct receptor types: (1) receptors located on a bouton membrane that respond to the transmitter released by that bouton, to provide feedback regulation of turnover rate (the kind under discussion in the text above); (2) receptors located on cell dendrites or soma that respond to the same transmitter released by that cell to provide feedback regulation of firing rate; and (3) postsynaptic receptors associated with axoaxonal synapses, located on boutons, that respond to the transmitter released by the presynaptic cell, to control release of transmitter from the postsynaptic bouton. In this book, we have adopted the convention of designating the first type presynaptic receptors, the second type, autoreceptors, and the third type, axoaxonal postsynaptic receptors.

Even as the transmitter is acting on the various receptor sites, it is also undergoing inactivation. Inactivation provides a means of shutting off a given instance of transmission, so that it does not continue to exert its influence indefinitely. Inactivation involves three distinct mechanisms: (1) reuptake by the presynaptic nerve terminal by a high-affinity, energy-dependent transport process; (2) diffusion out of the synapse; and (3) enzymatic breakdown by degratory enzymes. Degratory enzymes may be free-floating in the extracellular fluid or membrane bound. They may be extracellular or intracellular. The reuptake mechanism is in two stages, in the sense that the transport mechanism in the cell membrane carries the transmitter from the synapse to the cytoplasm, and then the vesicular uptake mechanism transports the transmitter into a vesicle.

Acute Drug Interactions with Synaptic Transmission

The "business end" of the transmission process is the extent to which an effect is generated in the postsynaptic cell. Therefore, it is useful, when given the mechanism of any drug, to make a practice of analyzing the impact of that particular mechanism on the activity of effector proteins in the target cell. Several different drugs each of which cause an increase in the activity of a particular effector protein in a group of postsynaptic cells, regardless of the specific means by which that end is accomplished, will produce effects that are at least superficially similar, especially in the span of acute effects. But these effects will be dramatically different and generally the opposite of effects produced by drugs that decrease activity of the same effector proteins in the same group of cells.

Before going on to the following section, the reader is urged to take a few minutes to compile as complete a list as possible of mechanisms for modifying synaptic transmission. Start with two headings: (1) drug effects that increase postsynaptic effector activity and (2) drug effects that decrease postsynaptic effector activity. After you finish, check your list against the established drug mechanisms listed in Table 6-1.

Acute Drug Effects That Increase Postsynaptic Effector Activity

A systematic approach might be to review each of the steps in the transmission process for possible points of intervention. As we proceed, we will observe that some possibilities correspond to known drug mechanisms, while certain other hypothetical possibilities are either not feasible in practice or of heuristic interest only.

Interference with maintenance of the resting potential of the presynaptic cell (e.g., by elevation of extracellular potassium) will cause release of transmitter. This technique is useful to laboratory scientists and even has clinical application in cardiology. This intervention is not of value as a clinical manipulation of CNS synapses, because it dissociates transmission from conduction.

The availability of precursors for transmitter synthesis can be increased by *administration of precursor,* provided the substance is one that is able to cross the blood-brain barrier. An example of this technique is the use of levodopa, a precursor of dopamine. Recent experimental work indicates that dietary manipulations can significantly alter availability of precursors for certain of the transmitters, most notably serotonin. Both carbohydrates and proteins contain significant amounts of tryptophan, the precursor of serotonin, but protein-rich foods do not elevate brain serotonin. The tryptophan in protein must compete with other amino acids of protein for uptake into the brain, and this competition is not favorable to uptake of tryptophan. Carbohydrates and tryptophan itself have been found effective in promoting sleepiness in babies and adults when

Table 6-1. *Acute drug interactions with synaptic transmission*

Ultimate effect on postsynaptic effector activity	
Increase activity	Decrease activity
Administer precursor	Inhibit synthesis
Diet enriched with precursor	Diet deficient in precursor
Block storage (initial response)	Block storage (main response)
Decrease firing rate of presynaptic cell	Increase firing rate of presynaptic cell
Increase Ca^{2+} influx per action potential	Decrease Ca^{2+} influx per action potential
Release transmitter (uncouple transmission from conduction)	Block release
Increase affinity of postsynaptic receptor for transmitter (via modulatory protein)	Decrease affinity of postsynaptic receptor for transmitter (via modulatory protein)
Increase receptor-effector coupling (via coupling protein)	Uncouple receptor from effector
Inhibit degradation of second messenger	Inhibit effector protein
Administer postsynaptic receptor agonist	Administer postsynaptic receptor antagonist
Block reuptake	Stimulate reuptake
Inhibit transmitter degradation	Activate degratory enzymes
Administer presynaptic receptor antagonist	Administer presynaptic receptor agonist

these substances are ingested in the evening (a finding that is at odds with the conventional wisdom that sugar makes children hyperactive and convicts aggressive). Brain levels of catecholamines are not so readily influenced by diet, but these transmitters can be elevated by precursor loading with tyrosine.

Another hypothetical means of increasing synthesis is to increase the amounts of synthetic enzymes. It is not generally feasible to administer enzymes for purposes of influencing body activities, because enzymes are too large to enter or leave the circulatory system intact. This limitation is not a factor when the desired locus of action is within the gastrointestinal tract or on the surface of the skin, but it precludes manipulation of enzyme levels in the brain. The amount and activity of enzymes may be altered as an adaptive mechanism when a synapse is subjected to a prolonged challenge, as will be discussed subsequently.

Storage of transmitter in synaptic vesicles may be inhibited by certain drugs. Such drugs are called *depletors*—reserpine is an example. Depletors cause a prolonged decrease in transmission, but this decrease may be preceded by a transient stimulation as newly formed and stored transmitter spills out into the cytoplasm and synapses.

The number of action potentials reaching the nerve terminal may be increased if the *firing rate* of the presynaptic cell is enhanced by activation of the neuron at the level of its dendrites or cell body. This possibility somewhat begs the question at hand, since it invokes an intervention at a different synapse. Elevations in extracellular calcium will increase the amount of transmitter released per action potential, but it is generally impractical to change calcium levels systemically, because the body very carefully guards the level of this important cation through the action of thyrocalcitonin and parathyroid hormone. There is some indication that *calcium influx* per action potential may be regulatable. Stimulation of norepinephrine receptors of the α-1 type is thought to elevate calcium influx.

Release is generally tightly coupled to conduction, but certain drugs, called *releasers,* may stimulate release even in the absence of an action potential. A prominent example of this type of drug is amphetamine, which releases norepinephrine and dopamine.

The binding of a transmitter to a postsynaptic receptor site is subject to modulation by modulatory proteins associated with the receptor site. Some drugs can *increase binding* of a transmitter by exerting an influence on a modulatory protein adjacent to the transmitter receptor site. Benzodiazepines produce this effect on GABA-binding. *Coupling* proteins are also subject to regulation by endogenous peptides and nucleotides. It is likely that in the coming years a new generation of drugs will become available, some of which will be able to increase receptor-effector coupling. In the case of receptors linked to adenyl cyclase, receptor-mediated effects may be increased by *inhibitors of phosphodiesterase.*

Another approach to increasing receptor activation is the administration of a transmitter *mimic,* a drug that is an agonist at the postsynaptic receptor. An agonist binds to the receptor and activates it in the same manner as the transmitter itself. Some are many times more potent than the natural transmitter.

Still another means of increasing postsynaptic effector activity is to prolong the presence of the transmitter in the synapse. This can be accomplished by interfering with the inactivation mechanisms. Drugs such as imipramine *block reuptake* of norepinephrine and serotonin, while another class of antidepressants *inhibit the degratory enzyme* monoamine oxidase, which acts on several transmitters. Diffusion is not susceptible to drug or experimental manipulation, short of freezing the brain in liquid nitrogen, a technique of limited clinical value.

Synaptic transmission can also be enhanced by preventing the feedback regulation exerted through the presynaptic receptor. Thus, a drug that is a selective *antagonist at presynaptic receptors* will free the presynaptic cell from feedback inhibition. Yohimbine has this effect on noradrenergic neurons. An antagonist is a drug that binds to a receptor but does not activate it. Its action is related to its ability to deny the transmitter access to the receptor.

Acute Drug Effects That Decrease Postsynaptic Effector Activity

One approach to decreasing transmission is by *inhibition of synthesis.* Inhibition of the rate-limiting step is most effective. Inactivation of enzyme may be accomplished through pool shifts as well. If the precursor happens to be an essential dietary constituent, synthesis inhibition can be accomplished by *dietary restrictions* that eliminate sources for the precursor. *Depletion* of stored transmitter also renders transmission ineffective.

Some of the most potent toxins known act by *preventing release* of transmitter. For example, release of acetylcholine is prevented by *Clostridium botulinum* toxins.

A very commonly encountered mechanism in pharmacology is the use of a *postsynaptic receptor antagonist.* Neuroleptics are antagonists at dopamine receptor sites, preventing dopamine's access to the receptor sites.

The affinity of transmitter for postsynaptic receptor sites may be decreased by modulatory proteins associated with the receptor. Certain cholinergic receptors (the nicotinic type) exhibit *decreased affinity* for acetylcholine in the presence of peptide modulators. *Uncoupling* of the dopamine receptor sites from the adenyl cyclase effector protein can be brought about by drugs that stimulate formation of guanidine nucleotides. Narcotics have this effect and are said to produce a "functional blockade" of dopamine receptors.

Stimulation of presynaptic receptors by a *selective presynaptic receptor agonist* will diminish synthesis and turnover rates of the corresponding transmitter. The drug clonidine has this effect on presynaptic receptors of norepinephrine neurons. Turnover rate can also be decreased by drugs that *slow the firing rate* of the presynaptic neuron.

Adaptive Changes in Synaptic Mechanisms

Long-term drug effects often cannot be adequately explained solely on the basis of acute interactions with synaptic processes. Even with acute administration, the total drug effect is substantially more (and in a way less) than just the primary effect, because the body's compensatory mechanisms play a significant role in determining the total effect of a drug. This becomes ever more apparent as the duration of treatment is increased, as compensatory mechanisms become stabilized as adaptations, or, contrariwise, undergo tolerance. The therapeutic effects of antidepressants and antipsychotic drugs, which occur in each case only after 2 weeks or more of treatment, can be understood only through an appreciation of adaptive mechanisms. Pharmacodynamic tolerance and the related physical dependence that accompanies the chronic use of narcotics and sedative-hypnotics likewise find explication in adaptive mechanisms. Although each example of an adaptive mechanism develops at a unique and characteristic pace, it is convenient for didactic purposes to view these compensatory and adaptive events as occurring within two general time frames: (1) short-term compensatory mechanisms occurring in minutes to hours; and, (2) long-term adaptations developing in approximately 6 days to 3 weeks of chronic drug administration.

Short-Term Compensatory Mechanisms

Short-term compensatory changes are feedback processes, apparently not dependent on synthesis of new protein. Five examples of short-term compensatory mechanisms are shown in Figure 6-2A. Since the activity of some synthetic enzymes is dependent on concentrations of one or more common ions, marked changes in the distribution of ion species because of an altered firing rate over a period of time may cause positive or negative influences on rates of transmitter synthesis. Synthesis rate as well as the rate of release may also be suppressed by chronic activation of the presynaptic receptor on the nerve terminal.

The firing rate of the presynaptic cell—and hence transmitter release—is subject to autoregulation through the action of the same or different transmitters on the cell body or dendrites of the neuron. Autoregulatory influences involve multineuronal feedback loops in some instances; in others, the influence may result from the action of transmitter released by the cell's own feedback collateral axons. In some cases, the autoreceptors may respond to changes in overall brain level of the transmitter that it binds.

Two other short-term compensatory mechanisms relate to receptor sensitivity. Postsynaptic receptors exhibit multiple affinity and excitability states. A decrease in affinity or excitability state (or both) that develops and disappears with particular rapidity as a result of maximal stimulation of a receptor population is called tachyphylaxis. It probably occurs because a large proportion of the receptors have shifted to the activated state. Changes in affinity or excitability states, or both, over a longer time period may result from activation or inhibition of modulatory proteins and coupling proteins associated with a receptor-effector complex. This mechanism is implicated in short-term

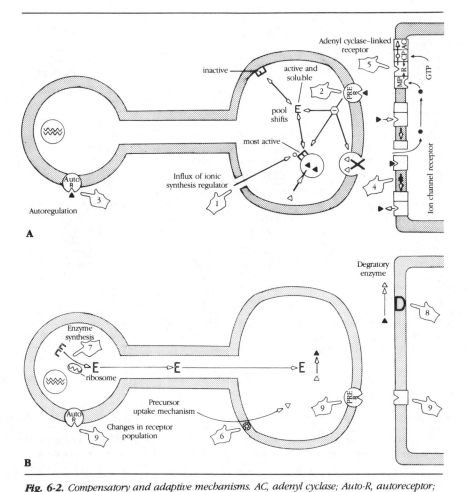

Fig. 6-2. *Compensatory and adaptive mechanisms. AC, adenyl cyclase; Auto-R, autoreceptor; CP, coupling protein; D, degratory enzyme; E, synthetic enzyme; GTP, guanidine triphosphate; MP, modulatory protein; Pre-R, presynaptic receptor; R, receptor. A. Compensatory mechanisms. (1) Influx of an ionic regulator may stimulate or inhibit activity of enzymes involved in transmitter synthesis; (2) activation of presynaptic receptors by free transmitter or agonist in the synapse leads to inhibition of release and inhibition of synthesis (possible mechanisms for the latter include enzyme pool shifts, production of an inhibitory substance, or suppression of cofactor production); (3) autoregulation of firing rate of the presynaptic cell is mediated by action of free transmitter or agonist on autoreceptors located on cell bodies or dendrites of the presynaptic cell; (4) the affinity and/or excitability state of most postsynaptic receptors diminishes during maximal stimulation because a higher proportion of the receptors are in the modified state (this is called tachyphylaxis); (5) postsynaptic receptors (whether associated with ion channels or linked to adenyl cyclase) are subject to changes in affinity state and receptor-effector coupling. The illustration depicts the likely case for opiate receptors: an ion-sensitive modulatory protein alters affinity states for agonists and antagonists (possibly by regulating the rate of regeneration of receptor to the ground state); a guanidine nucleotide–sensitive coupling protein alters affinity states (for agonists but not antagonists) and alters receptor-effector coupling. B. Adaptive mechanisms. (6) A prolonged increase in synthesis demand may induce the precursor uptake mechanism; (7) similarly, the production of the synthetic enzymes may be induced or repressed in relation to changing rates of synthesis; (8) degratory enzyme production may be induced or repressed in relation to degratory rates; (9) prolonged elevation of the levels of transmitter or appropriate agonists may lead to a decrease in receptor population (binding capacity). Chronic receptor blockade, denervation, and diminished turnover may stimulate an increase in receptor populations. Receptor types vary in their capacity for this type of adaptation. Receptor adaptations of this type are implicated in drug dependence and in the mechanisms of tricyclic antidepressants and neuroleptics.*

pharmacodynamic tolerance to narcotics, as well as in down-regulation of noradrenergic receptors of the α-1 type in response to chronic antidepressant therapy.

Long-Term Adaptive Mechanisms

When a change in neuronal function in response to chronic contact with a drug depends on altering the pattern of protein synthesis of the neuron, the time frame over which the change occurs is extended, and it is called an adaptation rather than a compensatory mechanism. As long-term adaptations develop, the compensatory mechanisms may be replaced. On the other hand, the long-term adaptation may involve the development of tolerance to the primary drug effect, the compensatory mechanisms, or both. The synthesis of a given protein may be induced (increased) or repressed (diminished). Adaptations involving induction or repression of protein synthesis have been noted with respect to synthetic enzymes, degratory enzymes, precursor transport proteins, and transmitter recognition proteins (receptor sites). Changes in the number of receptor sites have been noted in the down-regulation of β-adrenergic receptors by chronic antidepressant administration and in the up-regulation of dopamine receptors following long-term neuroleptic administration. Precursor availability has been shown to be a significant factor in controlling brain levels of serotonin, catecholamines, and acetylcholine, so that it is to be expected that induction of the precursor transport mechanism could have an impact on rate of transmitter synthesis.

Acetylcholine

Historical Highlights

The growth in understanding of the role of acetylcholine (ACh) actually predates its structural identification. As indicated in the discussion of the peripheral nervous system, acetylcholine is the transmitter substance throughout the parasympathetic and somatic nervous systems and at the preganglionic nerve terminals of the sympathetic nervous system. Indeed, only the postganglionic fibers of the sympathetic nervous system release any other transmitter. The earliest knowledge of acetylcholine comes from its role in the peripheral, not the central, nervous system.

In 1921, Loewi described a substance of unknown structure that was released by stimulation of the vagus (10th cranial) nerve. Loewi named this substance *Vagusstoff*. It was capable of producing all the effects on the heart normally associated with vagal stimulation. Eight years later, Dale isolated and identified *Vagusstoff* as acetylcholine. Progress in ACh research, however, was hindered by the lack of a simple chemical assay for ACh, and investigators were forced to turn their attention to a search for the presence of the enzyme that breaks down ACh rather than the transmitter itself. In 1951, Koelle reported the histochemical distribution of this enzyme, acetylcholinesterase, in the CNS. Then, in 1954, Eccles identified ACh as the transmitter that acts on the Renshaw cell of the spinal cord. This was the first—and to date the only—definitive establishment of the identity of a CNS transmitter.

Synthesis

Acetylcholine is synthesized in the body in a one-step reaction requiring acetylcoenzyme A and choline as substrates. Acetylcoenzyme A is an intermediate in the

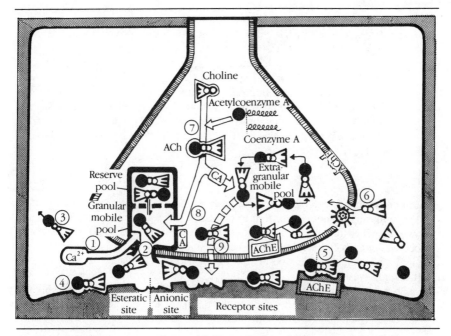

Fig. 6-3. Cholinergic synapse. ACh, acetylcholine; AChE, acetylcholinesterase; CA, choline acetylase. (1) Influx of extracellular calcium (Ca^{2+}); (2) release of ACh from granules attached to presynaptic nerve ending; (3) ACh diffusion; (4) receptor activation; (5) AChE hydrolysis of ACh; (6) choline uptake; (7) synthesis of ACh; (8) movement of newly synthesized ACh into empty granules to replace the released material; (9) continuous release of cytoplasmic ACh independent of extracellular Ca^{2+}. Modified from A. K. Swonger. Nursing Pharmacology. Boston: Little, Brown, 1978.

metabolism of glucose and is therefore in abundant supply. The simple reaction is catalyzed by the enzyme cholinecetylase, which is found in nerve terminals of cholinergic (which means acetylcholine-containing) neurons. Because the enzyme is located within the cell, only choline within the cell can be utilized to make ACh. Therefore, the cholinergic nerve terminal has a mechanism (an uptake pump) for accumulating choline from the synapse (Fig. 6-3). Much of the choline in the synapse derives from the breakdown of already released acetylcholine.

Degradation

Enzymatic destruction of ACh is carried out by a class of enzymes called cholinesterases. Cholinesterases hydrolyze acetylcholine, producing acetate and choline. There are two broad categories of cholinesterases: *Acetylcholinesterase* (AChE) (also called *true* or *specific* cholinesterase) has a high degree of preference for ACh over other substrates and is found in neural tissue and in erythrocytes. *Pseudocholinesterase* (or *nonspecific* cholinesterase) metabolizes ACh only slowly and is prevalent in plasma and nonneural tissue.

Acetylcholinesterase is of particular interest to pharmacologists, since a number of drugs increase ACh levels by inhibiting AChE. AChE is a large protein molecule with a high molecular weight (about 260,000). There are two sites on this long molecule involved in the interaction with ACh. One site (called the anionic site) binds the ACh, while the other (called the esteratic site) donates electrons and thus cleaves the ACh. Inhibitors of AChE bind at one or both sites and prevent ACh's access to AChE. The inhibitor may or may not itself be broken down. So-called reversible inhibitors, such as physostigmine, attach at both sites and are themselves slowly hydrolyzed. Irreversible inhibitors, such as organophosphates, attach at both sites, are cleaved, but fail to dissociate completely from the AChE.

Release

Within the axon terminal of the neuron, much of the ACh is sequestered into storage vesicles, although some remains in the cytoplasm. When an action potential (a nerve impulse) reaches the nerve terminal, these vesicles approach the cell membrane and eject their contents into the synaptic space. The release of ACh is largely dependent on the influx of calcium ion that occurs during the action potential.

The storage vesicles provide quantification to the release process. It has been shown that ACh is released in quanta, or approximately equal, discrete packets. The number of packets released presumably depends on the timing of action potentials and the concentration of calcium surrounding the cell.

The Acetylcholine Receptor

Once the ACh has been released, it diffuses freely in all directions. A portion of it finds its way across the synapse and there attaches to receptors of the postsynaptic cell membrane. After activation, the receptor assumes a refractory state for a brief period during which it is not susceptible to further activation. Thus, termination of the effect does not necessarily await the removal of ACh from the synapse. A subsequent regenerative process then reactivates the receptor. In the meantime, the already released ACh is undergoing inactivation. This is accomplished by metabolic degradation and diffusion.

Cholinergic receptors are of two general types: muscarinic and nicotinic. The terms derived from the fact that although acetylcholine itself activates both types, the drug muscarine stimulates only the muscarinic type, while the drug nicotine is selective for the nicotinic type. The nicotinic type is associated with large ion channels, and thus the receptor complex produces short-latency, excitatory postsynaptic potentials when activated (Table 6-2). The muscarinic type is not as well understood. Activation leads to a decrease in adenyl cyclase activity, perhaps through the exigency of elevating levels of guanidine nucleotides.

Role in the Central Nervous System

Acetylcholine is a ubiquitously distributed neurotransmitter, and its functional significance is correspondingly diverse and multifaceted.

Brainstem

Many cells in the brainstem are responsive to ACh application, notably cells of the respiratory center and cochlear nuclei. Many cranial nerve efferent nuclei contain

Table 6-2. *Cholinergic receptor-complex characteristics*

	Muscarinic	Nicotinic
Receptor types[a]	Muscarinic	Nicotinic
Affinity states[b]	SH, H, L	Packing of subunits modifies affinities and effect (Na^+ conductance)
Chemical constituents		
Receptor	Recognition protein	Circular clusters of proteinous subunits
Effector	Guanidyl cyclase (?)	Sodium channel
Other	Guanosine triphosphate–sensitive coupling protein	Substance P and enkephalin-sensitive modulatory protein (?)
Selective agonist	Muscarine	Nicotine
Selective antagonist	Atropine	Hexamethonium
Regional distribution	Diffuse: cerebrum, especially lower strata, caudate nucleus, hippocampus, hypothalamus, thalamus, cerebellum	Ascending reticular activating system, lateral geniculate nucleus, supraoptic nucleus, cingulate gyrus
Effect of activation	Inhibition of adenyl cyclase	Rapid excitatory postsynaptic potential
Adaptability	High	?

SH, superhigh affinity; H, high affinity; L, low affinity.

[a]Noninterconverting.

[b]Rapidly interconverting states regulated by modulatory and coupling protein activity.

cholinergic cell bodies. Approximately one-third of the cells of the reticular formation are excited by ACh; approximately 10 percent are depressed. There appear to be two subcortical cholinoceptive sites where ACh can alter arousal level: one in the subthalamus, where ACh depresses the ascending reticular activating system but enhances spinal reflexes, and a second in the lateral reticular formation, where ACh enhances arousal.

There are two reticular nuclei of the midbrain that are cholinergic, each the bed nucleus for a major system of ascending projections to diffuse targets (Fig. 6-4). One of these nuclei, called the cuneiform nucleus (see Fig. 4-6), receives inputs from every sensory system and interconnects with extrapyramidal and autonomic output centers. It is a likely site for the development of conditional linkages subserving Pavlovian-type (respondent) conditioning. It discharges to various brainstem nuclei (which accounts for the cholinoceptive neurons of the lateral reticular formation) and sends ascending projections to the thalamus via the dorsal tegmental pathway.

The other cholinergic cell group of the midbrain reticulum is in the ventral tegmentum (see Fig. 4-6). It sends ascending projections via the ventral tegmental tract to join the medial forebrain bundle (Fig. 6-4). These fibers reach the septal region of the limbic system and portions of the hypothalamus and corpus striatum. From these relay points, signals are passed on to the cortex. This cholinergic system is considered to be part of the ascending reticular activating system and helps to produce externalization of attention.

A third brainstem cholinergic fiber system interconnects the pons and medulla with the cerebellum (Fig. 6-5).

Corpus Striatum

The caudate nucleus of the corpus striatum has particularly high rates of formation and breakdown of ACh because of the presence of intrinsic cholinergic neurons. Many cells in the caudate nucleus are excited by ACh application, while a few are depressed. Certain anticholinergic substances are effective antiparkinsonian agents; parkinsonism is believed to involve the corpus striatum.

A nucleus called substantia innominata, lying just beneath the globus pallidus of the corpus striatum, is both a recipient and a point of origin of cholinergic projections (Fig. 6-4). This nucleus receives inputs from the ventral tegmental cholinergic system and sends widespread cholinergic projections to most regions of the cerebral cortex. Apparently, this nucleus serves as a relay station in the ascending reticular activating system. About 50 percent of the ACh in the cortex disappears when the axons to the cortex from the substantia innominata are severed.

A descending cholinergic system arises from the globus pallidus of the corpus striatum and projects to the subthalamic nucleus, the hypothalamus, and thalamus (Fig. 6-5). It is an extrapyramidal discharge pathway.

Limbic System

The hippocampus receives cholinergic fibers from the septal region, and many hippocampal neurons are cholinoceptive (Fig. 6-6). There are numerous similarities between hippocampal lesions and the pharmacologic actions of cholinergic blockers. In the hypothalamus, several important functions are influenced by ACh. It appears to bring about release of antidiuretic hormone and adrenocorticotropic hormone (ACTH)

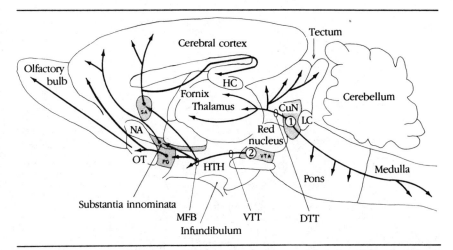

Fig. 6-4. *Ascending cholinergic systems. (1) Projections from the cuneiform nucleus (CuN) of the midbrain reticular formation to the brainstem, thalamus, and tectum. (2) Projections from the ventral tegmental area (VTA) of the midbrain reticular formation to the limbic system, hypothalamus (HTH), corpus striatum, and substantia innominata and from these relay points to the cerebral cortex. DTT, dorsal tegmental tract; HC, hippocampus; LC, locus ceruleus; MFB, medial forebrain bundle; NA, nucleus accumbens; OT, olfactory tubercle; PO, preoptic area; SA, septal area; VTT, ventral tegmental bundle.*

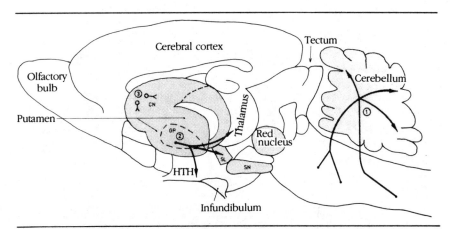

Fig. 6-5. *Extrapyramidal cholinergic pathways. Extrapyramidal brain regions are shaded. (1) Cholinergic connections between the brainstem and cerebellum; (2) striatal discharge system from the globus pallidus (GP) to the subthalamic nucleus (SN), hypothalamus (HTH), and thalamus; (3) intrinsic cholinergic neurons of the striatum. CN, caudate nucleus; SL, subthalamic nucleus (of Luys).*

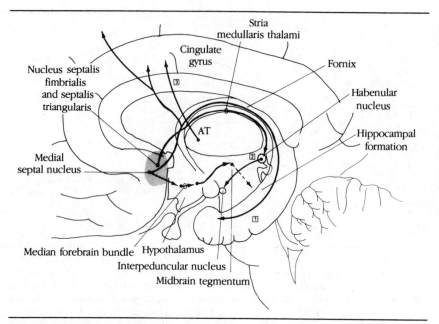

Fig. 6-6. *Cholinergic pathways of the limbic system. (1) Septal-hippocampal projections of the fornix; (2) septal-habenular projections of the stria medularis thalami, and habenulointerpeduncular projections of the fasciculus retroflexus; (3) anterior thalamic radiations.*

from the pituitary by stimulation of regulating hypothalamic nuclei. Cholinergic stimulation of the hypothalamus can elicit hypothermia, i.e., subnormal body temperature. The medial and lateral septal areas are cholinoceptive. The preoptic area of the hypothalamus receives cholinergic inputs from the ventral tegmental area of the midbrain. Cholinergic neurons in the preoptic area project to the prefrontal cortex. Two cholinergic pathways of the limbic system are the fasciculus retroflexus, which connects the habenula nucleus to the interpeduncular nucleus, and the anterior thalamic radiations to the cingulate gyrus.

Thalamus

Many cells of the thalamus respond to ACh, particularly units in nuclei connected with the diffuse thalamic system (Chap. 10) and sensory relay nuclei. Cholinergic inputs reach these thalamic nuclei from the cuneiform nucleus of the midbrain. The thalamus also receives cholinergic projections from the cerebellum.

Cerebrum

The final link of the ascending arousal system, the pallidocortical tract, is cholinergic. Cholinergic blockers produce slow-wave activity in the EEG. Acetylcholine is released profusely by the cortex, and this release is elevated by electrical stimulation of the cortex or reticular formation or by convulsants. Atropine, a cholinergic blocker, raises the threshold for EEG activation by reticular stimulation.

Behavioral Effects

Cholinergic blockers produce a characteristic anticholinergic syndrome marked by memory impairment, slurred speech, drowsiness, ataxia, confusion, disorientation, and hallucinations. In behavioral tests, cholinergic blockers seem to impair especially those behaviors requiring suppression of a response. In humans, anticholinergics impair short-term memory and attention.

Norepinephrine

Historical Highlights

Like ACh, norepinephrine (NE) is a peripheral transmitter substance, and, as with ACh, understanding of adrenergic (meaning NE-containing) nerve function grew out of study of peripheral synapses. In 1931, Cannon reported on an epinephrine-like substance released during sympathetic stimulation. The nature of this substance was not firmly established until 1956, when Von Euler identified it as NE. The development of histochemical staining techniques in 1962 by Falck et al. provided a means for subsequent "mapping" of CNS adrenergic pathways by Dahlstrom et al. In 1965, the introduction of a α-methylparatyrosine, a specific depletor of NE, by Spector et al. provided new ways of determining the role of NE. Alquist made the distinction between α- and β-receptors in 1948, and Lands added the further specification of β-1 and β-2 receptors in 1967.

Synthesis

The synthesis of NE is a three-reaction sequence that begins with the amino acid L-tyrosine (Fig. 6-7). L-tyrosine can be converted by the enzyme tyrosine hydroxylase to dihydroxyphenylalanine (dopa). Tyrosine hydroxylase can be inhibited by several drugs, including, notably, α-methylparatyrosine. When tyrosine hydroxylase is inhibited, the content of NE in the brain begins to decline because of the inability to replenish the supply by synthesis of new NE. This is referred to as depletion. Tyrosine hydroxylase is subject to feedback inhibition, which means that the end product of the pathway, NE, can competitively inhibit tyrosine hydroxylase. This prevents excess buildup of NE levels.

The second step in the synthesis of NE is the conversion of dopa to dopamine. Dopamine is important in its own right as a neurotransmitter. This reaction is regulated by the enzyme l-aromatic amino acid decarboxylase, which incidentally is also involved in the synthesis of serotonin.

The third step in the synthesis of NE is the oxidation of dopamine to NE. The enzyme for this step is thought to be located in the membrane of the vesicles that store NE in adrenergic synaptosomes. Some drugs, such as FLA63, inhibit this step.

Degradation

Two enzymes are capable of destroying NE. One of these, monoamine oxidase (MAO), is associated with mitochondrial membranes. This is a highly nonspecific enzyme that

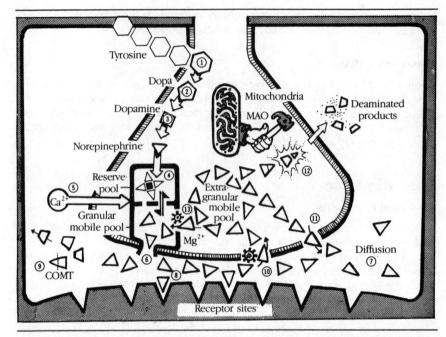

Fig. 6-7. *Noradrenergic synapse. Δ, norepinephrine; MAO, monoamine oxidase; COMT, catechol-O-methyltransferase. (1) Conversion of tyrosine to dihydroxyphenylalanine (dopa) (blockade by alpha-methylparatyrosine); (2) conversion of dopa to dopamine (competitively inhibited by methyldopa); (3) conversion of dopamine to norepinephrine (NE) (inhibited by disulfiram); (4) storage of NE in granules (inhibited by reserpine and guanethidine); (5) influx of calcium (Ca²⁺) during action potential; (6) release of NE from granular mobile pool by an action potential (blocked by bretylium, guanethidine, and MAO inhibitors); (7) diffusion of NE; (8) receptor-binding and activation by NE (mimicked by sympathomimetics, blocked by adrenergic-blocking drugs); (9) metabolism of NE by COMT (blocked by glucocorticoids); (10) cellular reuptake of NE (blocked by tricyclic antidepressants, cocaine, and ouabain); (11) drug-induced release of NE from extragranular mobile pool (induced by amphetamine or tyramine); (12) metabolism of NE by MAO to form deaminated products (inhibited by MAO inhibitors); (13) granular reuptake of NE (inhibited by reserpine). Modified from A. K. Swonger. Nursing Pharmacology. Boston: Little, Brown, 1978.*

metabolizes a large variety of substances. Inhibitors of MAO, such as tranylcypromine and isocarboxazid, have been used as antidepressants (Chap. 18). The other enzyme capable of breaking down NE is catechol-O-methyltransferase (COMT). This enzyme is found outside of the nerve cells in the surrounding milieu and can be inhibited by a drug called tropolone. Norepinephrine can be acted on by either or both of these enzymes, so there is a total of three possible products of NE breakdown.

Release

Release of NE is believed to be effected by the influx of calcium ions accompanying the arrival of an action potential, just as occurs with ACh. Release of stored NE may also be facilitated by various drugs, notably amphetamine. Guanethidine, an antihypertensive agent, has the opposite effect, preventing neuronal release of NE even in the presence of an action potential. Storage of NE by the vesicles can be impaired by drugs such as reserpine. This leads to a depletion of stored NE. Guanethidine also produces a reserpine-like depletion.

Adrenergic Receptors

Once NE is released into a synapse, it is free to act on receptors on the postsynaptic membrane. Adrenergic receptors are classified into four subgroups (called α-1, α-2, β-1, and β-2), based on differential susceptibility to various blocking and stimulating drugs (Table 6-3). Many drugs, called sympathomimetics, imitate the action of NE. Phenylephrine, a commonly used decongestant found in cold remedies, stimulates peripheral α-adrenergic receptors, for example. The β-receptors and some of the α-2 receptors are linked to adenyl cyclase, but α-1 receptors are not, and they are largely or entirely presynaptic receptors.

Inactivation

Released NE can be inactivated by any of three mechanisms: enzymatic breakdown, diffusion (and thus dilution), and reuptake by the presynaptic neuron. This last process is an energy-utilizing process quantitatively of great importance in inactivating NE. The high affinity carrier protein that carries out this reuptake of norepinephrine can also take up dopamine, serotonin, and a number of substances structurally similar to NE. The tricyclic antidepressants, such as imipramine, inhibit the activity of this neuronal re-uptake pump and thus prolong the presence of NE in the synapse.

The neuronal uptake mechanism is distinct from the granular storage mechanism. The latter is unaffected by imipramine but is inhibited by reserpine.

Role in the Central Nervous System

Noradrenergic pathways are more limited in number and noradrenergic nuclei are more discretely localized than was the case for cholinergic systems. Figure 6-8 portrays the major noradrenergic pathways of the CNS. The ascending noradrenergic pathways arise in nuclei of the pons and medulla and extend without synapsing to areas of the hypothalamus, limbic system, and cerebral cortex. The distribution of projections is very diffuse indeed. For example, a given nerve cell in one of these pontine nuclei, the locus ceruleus, may send axon collaterals to both the cerebellum and cerebrum. Because of the diffuseness of these pathways, as well as pharmacologic evidence implicating NE, it is believed that these pathways control generalized CNS functions, including mood, motor activity level, and reward mechanisms.

The ascending NE fibers are divisible into three groups. A dorsal tegmental bundle carries axons mainly from locus ceruleus (group A_6 in Fig. 6-8) and projects to the thalamus, corpus striatum, hypothalamus, cerebral cortex, limbic system, and colliculi (sensory relay nuclei in the midbrain). A ventral tegmental bundle carries axons originating in other noradrenergic nuclei (A_1, A_2, A_5, and A_7) and projects to the periventricular gray of the rostral pons and midbrain, including the locus ceruleus itself and the dorsal raphé nucleus. The dorsal and ventral tegmental bundles both travel through the pons and medulla in the central tegmental tract and ascend in the medial forebrain bundle at the level of the subthalamus. The third noradrenergic tract carries fibers from various noradrenergic nuclei (A_2, A_5, A_6, and A_7) to periventricular areas of the hypothalamus. These target areas belong to the punishment system.

Table 6-3. *Noradrenergic receptor-complex characteristics*

	Alpha-1 (α-1)	Alpha-2 (α-2)	Beta-1 (β-1)	Beta-2 (β-2)
Receptor types[a]				
Affinity states[b]	Ca^{2+}-dependent	α-2, high; α-2, low		
Chemical constituents				
Receptor	Recognition protein	Recognition protein	Recognition protein	Recognition protein
Effector	Unknown	Unknown	Adenyl cyclase	Adenyl cyclase
Other	Ca^{2+}-sensitive coupling protein	GTP-sensitive coupling protein	Calmodulin-sensitive coupling protein; GTP-sensitive modulatory protein	Calmodulin-sensitive coupling protein; phospholipid methyltransferase; GTP-sensitive modulatory protein
Selective agonist	Phenylephrine	Clonidine	Dobutamine	Salbutimol
Selective antagonist	Prazosin	Yohimbine	Practolol	Butoxamine
Regional and synaptic distribution	Throughout CNS; post-ganglionic SNS; post-synaptic; conc. in HTH, CS, cerebrum	Presynaptic	Throughout CNS; post-ganglionic SNS; post-synaptic; conc. in cerebrum	Throughout CNS; post-ganglionic SNS; post-synaptic; conc. in cerebellum
Effect of activation	↑ Ca^{2+} flux; ↓ cGMP (secondary ?)	↓ NE synthesis and release	↑ cAMP; slow PSPs	↑ cAMP; slow PSPs
Adaptability	Poor vis-à-vis number of receptors, but coupling can increase	High	High (either number or coupling can be involved)	Poor

GTP, guanosine triphosphate; HTH, hypothalamus; CS, corpus striatum; cAMP, cyclic adenosine monophosphate; PSP, postsynaptic potentials.
[a] Alpha-1, beta-1, and beta-2 can slowly interconvert by recoupling with different effector proteins. Alpha-2 is noninterconverting with others.
[b] Rapidly interconverting states regulated by modulatory and coupling proteins.

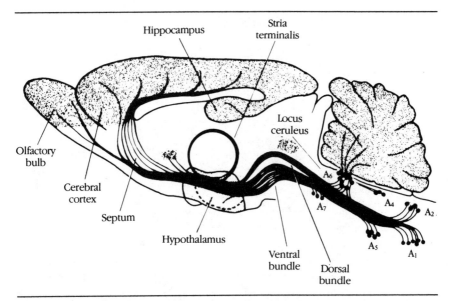

Fig. 6-8. *Ascending norepinephrine pathways. The strippled regions indicate the major nerve terminal areas. A_1-A_3 are in the medulla; A_1 lies in the lateral reticular formation; A_2 lies in the dorsal visceral gray; A_3 is the dorsal accessory olive. A_4-A_7 are in the pons: A_4 is the facial nucleus (motor nucleus of the 7th cranial nerve); A_5 is the motor nucleus of the trigeminal nerve; A_6 is the locus ceruleus (bed nucleus of the reward system); A_7 is part of the subceruleus nucleus.* Modified from J. R. Cooper et al. The Biochemical Basis of Neuropharmacology (3rd ed.). New York: Oxford University Press, 1978.

In addition to these elongated pathways, there are adrenergic cells with short axons in and around the reticular formation. Many cells in the reticular formation respond to local application of NE or amphetamine, which causes NE to be released.

There is considerable evidence implicating NE in affective disorders, especially endogenous depression. This hypothesis is discussed fully in Chapter 18, in which it is shown that many psychoactive drugs alter noradrenergic function.

Dopamine

Historical Highlights

The importance of dopamine (DA) as a neurotransmitter was first postulated by Blaschko in 1959. Until then, it was considered to be important only as the precursor of NE. The mapping of DA pathways in the brain and the discovery that certain behaviors are specifically related to dopaminergic stimulation have spurred progress in this field.

Metabolism

The metabolism of DA is closely related to that of NE. In dopaminergic neurons, the pathway originating with tyrosine simply stops with the formation of DA (Fig. 6-9). The same two enzymes that act on NE destroy DA.

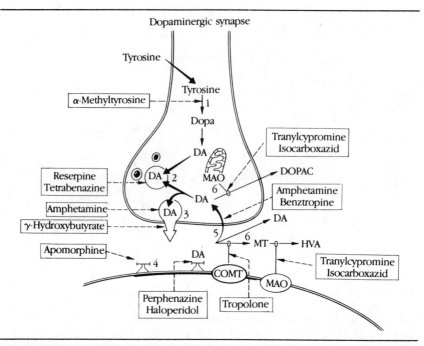

Fig. 6-9. *Dopaminergic synapse.* Solid arrows *depict normal cellular processes.* Dashed arrows *indicate points in the sequence where specified drugs intervene, either to facilitate or to inhibit normal activities. DA, dopamine; MAO, monoamine oxidase; COMT, catechol-O-methyltransferase; DOPAC, 3,4-dihydroxyphenylacetic acid; MT, 3-methoxytyramine; HVA, homovanillic acid. (1) Synthesis; (2) storage by vesicles; (3) release; (4) receptor stimulation; (5) cellular reuptake; (6) degradation. Modified from J. R. Cooper et al.* The Biochemical Basis of Neuropharmacology *(3rd ed.). New York: Oxford University Press, 1978.*

Release

Release of DA is similar to that of NE. Amphetamine is a potent releaser of DA. Gamma-hydroxybutyrate is believed to prevent normal release of DA, just as guanethidine blocks NE release. Storage of DA, like that of NE, is prevented by reserpine.

Dopaminergic Receptors

Despite the similarity in structure between DA and NE, there is a high degree of specificity in their actions, each on its own receptor. Dopaminergic receptors are found peripherally in the renal and mesenteric vascular beds, where DA produces vasodilatation. It is interesting that this effect of DA is not blocked by either α- or β-adrenergic blockers but is readily blocked by a specific dopaminergic-blocking drug, haloperidol. Similarly, the contrast between the effects of centrally acting dopaminergic and noradrenergic stimulants indicates a specificity in central dopaminergic and noradrenergic receptors. Apomorphine is a potent dopaminergic stimulant having about twice the potency of DA itself. Central dopaminergic receptors exhibit an increased sensitivity (or supersensitivity) when chemically deprived of activation. Supersensitivity is a long-term adaptive mechanism aimed at ensuring a set level of dopaminergic activation of receptors over the long run.

Dopaminergic receptors are divided into two types, D_1 and D_2 (Table 6-4). The D_1-receptor is linked to adenyl cyclase, but the D_2 is not. Some D_2-receptors are presynaptic. Additional binding sites with distinctive ligand affinities have been observed, but it remains a matter of contention as to whether these are alternative affinity states of the two fundamental receptor types or distinctly different receptor populations. We suspect the former.

Inactivation

Dopamine is inactivated in the same manner as NE: by enzymatic degradation, by reuptake, and by diffusion. The dopaminergic reuptake mechanism has a higher affinity for DA than NE and is inhibited by amphetamine and benztropine but not by the tricyclic antidepressants.

Feedback Regulation of Dopaminergic Pathways

Drugs that block dopaminergic postsynaptic receptors (chlorpromazine, haloperidol) produce an increase in the firing rate of the dopamine-containing (presynaptic) neuron and consequently an increased release of dopamine. Conversely, drugs that stimulate dopaminergic receptors (apomorphine, D-amphetamine) decrease the firing rate of DA pathways and the release of DA. In other words, dopaminergic neurons, through compensatory and adaptive mechanisms, tend to overcome the effects of any drug that modifies the activity of dopaminergic receptors. Alterations in turnover are short-term compensatory mechanisms that, in the longer run, are supplanted by the adaptive supersensitivity or hyposensitivity of receptors. There is considerable evidence that dopaminergic compensatory and adaptive mechanisms are involved in the development of pharmacodynamic tolerance of, and physical dependence on, narcotics, as well as tardive dyskinesias produced by neuroleptics.

Role in the Central Nervous System

There are five dopaminergic pathways in the CNS (Fig. 6-10). The best studied of these (the nigrostriatal pathway) arises in the substantia nigra (pars compacta, A_9) of the midbrain and extends to the corpus striatum and amygdala. This pathway is involved in modulation of extrapyramidal motor control and perhaps in aggression. The second dopaminergic pathway arises in the tegmentum of the midbrain (A_8 and A_{10}) and runs to the nucleus accumbens of the septal area and the olfactory tubercles. A third pathway, also arising in the midbrain tegmentum, projects to the frontal cortex. A fourth, short dopaminergic pathway arises in the arcuate nucleus of the hypothalamus and innervates the infundibular region of the hypothalamus. A fifth pathway is the short-axon incertohypothalamic system carrying signals from the zona incerta of the subthalamus, as well as from the dorsomedial and periventricular nuclei of the hypothalamus, to anterior and preoptic hypothalamic areas and the lateral septal nucleus. The last two pathways are involved in neuroendocrine regulation.

Behavioral Effects

Aggression is a complex behavior involving many brain regions, so it is likely that many transmitters contribute to its regulation; one of these is DA. Exaggerated dopaminergic

Table 6-4. Dopaminergic receptor-complex characteristics

	D_1	D_2
Receptor types[a]	D_1	D_2
Affinity states[b]	Type 1, type 2 (GTP-determined)	D_2, D_3, D_4
Chemical constituents		
Receptors	Recognition protein	Recognition protein
Effectors	Adenyl cyclase	? (not adenyl cyclase)
Other	Calmodulin-sensitive coupling protein; GTP-sensitive modulatory protein	
Selective agonist	Apomorphine	Apomorphine
Selective antagonist	Sulpiride	Clopramide
Neuroleptic affinities	Phenothiazines > butyrophenones	Butyrophenones > phenothiazines
Regional and synaptic distribution	CNS (especially corpus striatum, frontal lobe, amygdala); small, intensely fluorescent cells of sympathetic ganglia	Presynaptic receptors in corpus striatum and nucleus accumbens; hypothalamic receptors regulating prolactin
Effect of activation	↑ cAMP	↓ Prolactin release; ↓ dopamine release and synthesis
Adaptability	High	Yes

GTP, guanosine triphosphate; cAMP, cyclic adenosine monophosphate.

[a]Noninterconverting.

[b]Type 1 and type 2 are rapidly interconvertible affinity states; D_2, D_3, and D_4 may be interconverting affinity states or distinct receptor types.

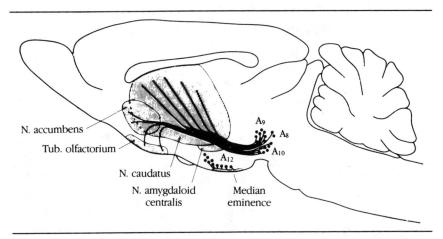

Fig. 6-10. *Ascending dopaminergic pathways. The stippled regions indicate the major nerve terminal areas. A_8–A_{10} are in the midbrain: A_8, in the lateral tegmental field; A_9 is the pars compacta of the substantia nigra; A_{10} is the nucleus linearis intermedius (nucleus parabranchialis pigmentosis). A_{11}–A_{14} are in the diencephalon. A_{12} is the arcuate nucleus in the infundibular region of the hypothalamus. A_{11}, A_{13}, and A_{14} (not shown) are located in the hypothalamus. Modified from K. E. Moore and P. H. Kelly. Biochemical Pharmacology of Mesolimbic and Mesocortical Dopamine Neurons. In M. A. Lipton et al. (Eds.), Psychopharmacology: A Generation of Progress. © 1978 by Raven Press, Publishers/New York.*

stimulation, particularly in animals withdrawn from morphine, elicits fierce aggression. Stereotypy is another effect of overstimulation of dopaminergic receptors. Stereotypy is a pattern of repetitive acts, such as gnawing, head-swinging, and biting. Locomotor activity is greatly reduced, but the subject remains obviously awake. This pattern requires an intact corpus striatum and so presumably is related to dopaminergic receptors innervated by the nigrostriatal pathway. The mesocortical dopamine pathway is involved in arousal, and the mesolimbic dopamine pathway is implicated in schizophrenia.

Epinephrine

Epinephrine is a third catecholamine transmitter. Abundant in the periphery because of its production and release by the adrenal medulla, it has limited distribution in the brain. Two epinephrine nuclei have been identified in the brain, both in the medulla oblongata. At least one of these nuclei is involved in sympathetic regulation.

Serotonin (5-Hydroxytryptamine)

Historical Highlights

The discovery of serotonin in the mammalian CNS by Twarog and Page dates back about thirty years to 1953. Four years later, Brodie and Shore reported its regional distribution in the CNS. Serotonin pathways were mapped by fluorescent techniques in the 1960s, along with the catecholamine (DA and NE) pathways. The identification of the raphé system as the principal serotonin-containing pathway, along with the introduction in

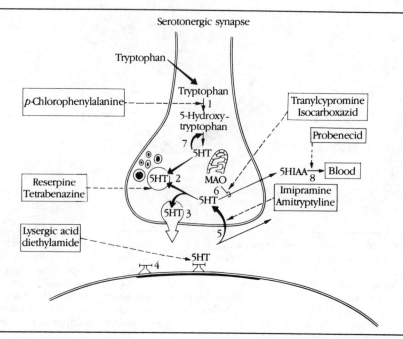

Fig. 6-11. *Serotonergic synapse.* Solid arrows *depict normal cellular processes.* Dashed arrows *indicate points in the sequence where specified drugs intervene either to facilitate or inhibit normal activities. 5-HT, 5-hydroxytryptamine (serotonin); MAO, monoamine oxidase; 5-HIAA, 5-hydroxyindole acetic acid. (1) Synthesis; (2) uptake by vesicles; (3) release; (4) receptor stimulation; (5) cellular reuptake; (6) degradation; (7) feedback regulation of synthesis; (8) transport of metabolite into blood. Modified from R. H. Rech and K. E. Moore.* An Introduction to Psychopharmacology. © *1971 by Raven Press, Publishers/New York.*

1966 of parachlorophenylalanine as a selective serotonin depletor, has aided the elucidation of serotonin's role in behavior.

Synthesis

The synthesis of 5-hydroxytryptamine (5-HT) is a two-step process beginning with the amino acid tryptophan (Fig. 6-11). Tryptophan is distributed ubiquitously in mammalian organisms. It cannot be synthesized by mammalian cells and is thus an essential dietary constituent. Tryptophan is rapidly taken up into the brain and is actively transported into synaptosomes. There it is converted by the enzyme tryptophan-5-hydroxylase to 5-hydroxytryptophan. It is this step that limits the rate of formation of serotonin. Parachlorophenylalanine is a selective inhibitor of tryptophan-5-hydroxylase and causes a depletion of brain serotonin.

The second step in the synthesis pathway for serotonin, and the one leading directly to serotonin, is the decarboxylation of 5-hydroxytryptophan to serotonin (or 5-HT) by l-aromatic amino acid decarboxylase, the same enzyme that converts dopa to dopamine. This reaction is subject to feedback inhibition by the product, serotonin.

Degradation

Like NE and DA, serotonin is broken down by MAO. Inhibitors of MAO protect all three transmitters, although a given inhibitor may protect more with respect to one substrate than another. The oxidative product of the action of MAO on 5-HT is unstable and is further acted on by either of two common enzymes, aldehyde dehydrogenase or alcohol dehydrogenase. The most common product (the one arising from aldehyde dehydrogenase) is 5-hydroxyindoleacetic acid. This substance is actively transported out of the brain into the blood by a carrier mechanism that can be blocked by probenecid.

Release

Serotonin is localized in nerve terminals in discrete storage granules, along with enzymes for its synthesis and degradation. Electrical stimulation of cell bodies corresponding to these terminals causes release of serotonin into the adjacent synaptic cleft. Storage of serotonin, like that of DA and NE, is blocked by reserpine, so that reserpine treatment leads to depletion of serotonin. Unlike the other neurotransmitters, 5-HT release is not calcium-dependent.

Serotonin Receptors

Serotonin receptors are found in the periphery as well as the brain. Peripheral serotonin receptors in the smooth muscle of the gut are of two types: M- receptors and D-receptors, differentiated on the basis of blocker susceptibility. In the CNS, serotonin receptors can be differentiated into at least three categories (Table 6-5). Most postsynaptic serotonin receptors are of the type designated 5-HT$_1$. This type is not linked to adenyl cyclase. It is present in three distinct affinity states. The hallucinogen lysergic acid diethylamide (LSD) is an antagonist at 5-HT$_1$ receptors. Receptors of the 5-HT$_2$ variety are linked to adenyl cyclase. Serotonin autoreceptors located on the cell bodies of serotonin neurons are of a third type; LSD is an agonist at these receptors.

Inactivation

Released serotonin, like DA and NE, is inactivated in three ways: by degradation, by reuptake into the releasing neuron, and by diffusion. The 5-HT reuptake pump is inhibited by the same substances that inhibit NE reuptake, but often with differential potency. The degradation of 5-HT involves the enzyme MAO.

Feedback Regulation of Serotonergic Pathways

Serotonergic pathways are subject to feedback regulation in much the same way as dopaminergic pathways. Monoamine oxidase inhibitors and certain tricyclic antidepressants, which elevate 5-HT levels in the synapse, decrease the firing rate of raphé cell bodies. The 5-HT$_1$ type of receptor is highly adaptable, exhibiting both down-regulation and up-regulation under appropriate circumstances.

Role in the Central Nervous System

Like the catecholamines, serotonin is largely contained in a limited number of pathways. Ascending pathways arise from the raphé nuclei of the caudal midbrain and pons

Table 6-5. Serotonergic receptor-complex characteristics

	5-HT$_1$	5-HT$_2$	Autoreceptors
Receptor types[a]			
Affinity states[b]	Type 1a, 1b, 2		
Chemical constituents			
Receptor	Recognition protein	Recognition protein	?
Effector	? (not adenyl cyclase)	Adenyl cyclase	?
Other	GTP-sensitive coupling protein; modulatory protein	?	?
Selective agonist	5-HT	5-HT	5-HT or LSD
Selective antagonist	LSD, methysergide, cinanserin		
Regional and synaptic distribution	Postsynaptic; forebrain, corpus striatum, thalamus, etc.	Postsynaptic; forebrain, etc.	Raphé cell bodies
Effect of activation	EPSPs; IPSPs (?)	↑ cAMP	↓ Raphé firing rate
Adaptability	High	?	Poor

EPSP, excitatory postsynaptic potentials; IPSP, inhibitory postsynaptic potentials.

[a]Nonintercoverting.

[b]Type 1a, 1b, and 2 are rapidly interconverting affinity states of the 5-HT$_1$ receptor regulated by the modulatory and coupling protein activities. Type 2 favors antagonist (spiroperidol) binding, type 1 favors agonist (5-HT or metergoline) binding and is GTP-dependent (thus the 1a and 1b states). Types 1 and 2 are equally abundant in the forebrain; type 1 predominates in other brain regions.

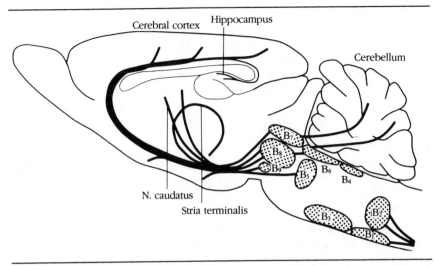

Fig. 6-12. *Serotonergic pathways of the raphé system. B_1–B_4 are in the medulla: B_1 is the raphé pallidus; B_2 is the raphé obscurus; B_3 is the raphé magnus; B_4 is in the chemical trigger zone. B_5–B_6 are in the pons: B_5 is the raphé pontis; B_6 is the superior central tegmental nucleus. B_7–B_9 are in the midbrain: B_7 is the raphé dorsalis; B_8 is the raphé medianus; B_9 is a small cluster dorsal to the medial lemniscus. Modified from K. Fuxe and G. Jonsson. Further mapping of central 5-hydroxytryptamine neurons.* Adv. Biochem. Psychopharmacol. *10:2, 1974.* © *1974 by Raven Press, Publishers/New York.*

and project to the hypothalamus, septum, amygdala, cingulum, cortex, hippocampus, and corpus striatum (Fig. 6-12). Descending pathways originate in the medulla and project into the cord.

Many individual cells in the regions innervated by the raphé system respond to local application of serotonin, either with increased or decreased firing rates. Low doses of 5-hydroxytryptophan, which is converted in the brain to 5-HT, produce sedation and EEG synchronization. Larger doses produce excitation, or convulsions, or both, but this is an artifact related to displacement of NE from its storage sites.

Jouvet and others have implicated serotonin in control of slow-wave sleep (see Chap. 10). Sleep deprivation increases 5-HT synthesis. Administration of 5-hydroxytryptophan increases slow-wave sleep. Destruction of the dorsal raphé nucleus (B_7 in Fig. 6-12) or depletion of serotonin by parachlorophenylalanine causes a marked decrease in slow-wave sleep.

The raphé nuclei are also involved in sensory gating mechanisms. Serotonergic projections (mainly from B_9) to the thalamus regulate the flow of visual, auditory, tactile, and pain sensations to the cortex. Nucleus raphé magnus (B_3) is involved in regulating transmission of pain sensations at the level of the spinal cord (Chap. 22).

Ascending serotonergic projections form four pathways. A lateral mesencephalocortical pathway carries fibers from B_7, B_8, and B_9 via the median forebrain bundle to the limbic system (cingulum, septal region, amygdala, and hippocampus) and cerebral cortex. A medial mesencephalosubcortical pathway carries fibers from B_7 (and perhaps B_5 and B_6) to the hypothalamus and preoptic area. A far-lateral pathway reaches the striatum from B_7. The fourth pathway carries projections from B_5, B_6, and B_7 to the cerebellum.

Behavioral Effects

Increases in brain serotonin produce sedation, lethargy, depressed operant responding, and visual discrimination defects. Lesions of the dorsal raphé nucleus (B_7) produce
insomnia. Depletion of serotonin produces insomnia, enhanced brightness discrimination, habituation defects, hyperreactivity, increased startle responses, and persevera-
tion. These behavioral changes also occur with lesions of the median raphé nucleus
(B_8).

Gamma-Aminobutyric Acid

Gamma-aminobutyric acid (GABA) was identified as a constituent of the CNS in 1950.
In 1961, Elliott identified inhibitory factor I, found in brain perfusate as GABA.

Synthesis

The metabolic pathway involving GABA is known as the GABA shunt because it occurs
as a "side trip" off the Krebs' cycle, a major metabolic pathway in the metabolism of
glucose. The GABA shunt begins and ends with intermediates of the Krebs' cycle (Fig.
6-13). The precursor of GABA, glutamic acid, is formed from α-ketoglutarate, a Krebs'
cycle intermediate; GABA is formed from glutamic acid by the enzyme glutamic acid
decarboxylase (GAD), which is found only in the mammalian CNS, is localized in
synaptosomes, and is of primary importance in regulating GABA levels.

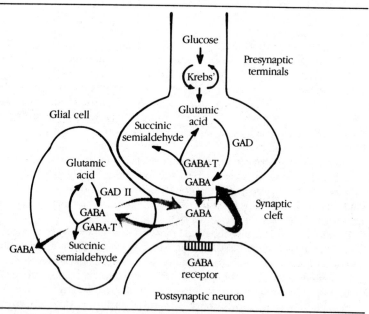

Fig. 6-13. A gabaminergic synapse. GABA, gamma-aminobutyric acid; GABA-T, GABA-trans-
aminase; GAD, glutamic acid decarboxylase. Modified from C. C. Mao and E. Costa, Biochemical
Pharmacology of GABA Transmission. In M. A. Lipton et al. (Eds.). Psychopharmacology: A
Generation of Progress. © 1978 by Raven Press, Publishers/New York.

Degradation

Gamma-aminobutyric acid is metabolized by GABA-transaminase (GABA-T) into succinic semialdehyde, which can in turn be converted into succinic acid, a Krebs' cycle intermediate. Both GABA-T and GAD require a coenzyme, pyridoxal phosphate, for maximal activity, but drugs that decrease the availability of pyridoxal phosphate decrease the activity of GAD more than that of GABA-T and hence decrease GABA levels. Glial cells play an important role in the metabolism of GABA.

Gamma-Aminobutyric Acid Receptors

Three types of GABA receptors have been reported in the literature. The classic GABA receptor, or G_1 type, apparently exists in three affinity states in relation to the influence of associated coupling and modulatory proteins (Table 6-6). The G_1-receptor complex includes at least five constituents: a recognition protein for the transmitter, two modulatory proteins, a coupling protein, and an effector protein, which is a chloride channel. Binding of GABA to the recognition protein can be influenced by either modulatory protein or the coupling protein. One modulatory protein is the receptor site for drugs of the benzodiazepine class. This modulatory protein is sensitive to an endogenous peptide called GABA-modulin (and possibly endogenous inosine and hypoxanthine nucleotides as well). Under the influence of GABA-modulin, GABA-binding to its recognition protein is diminished, but this action can be inhibited by benzodiazepines.

The second modulatory protein is a receptor site for barbiturates, which increase GABA-binding, and certain convulsant drugs, which decrease GABA-binding. The coupling protein is sensitive to sodium ion. Activation of the effector protein opens a chloride channel, which leads to a rapidly developing inhibitory postsynaptic potential. These G_1-receptors have been shown to exhibit adaptability.

The other two types of GABA receptors are poorly understood. One is found in axoaxonal synapses where GABA is released presynaptically, and it serves to decrease release of the transmitter contained in the target bouton. The third type of GABA receptor is located intracellularly. Its function is unknown.

Role in the Central Nervous System

Gamma-aminobutyric acid is an exclusively inhibitory transmitter substance. It is released by the cerebral cortex. In cats, this release is three times faster during sleep than during the waking state. The turnover of GABA in the cerebral cortex derives from intrinsic (or local-circuit) neurons of the stellate type (Chap. 27). These stellate cells play an important role in cortical function, contributing to the processing of afferents and the generation of transcortical inhibition (Fig. 6-14).

The cerebellum likewise contains a vast number of gabaminergic intrinsic neurons. Of the five major types of intrinsic neurons of the cerebellum, four (the Purkinje's, basket, Golgi, and stellate cells) are gabaminergic. Recent estimations of the number of gabaminergic neurons in the cerebellum alone exceed by a factor of 10 what until recently passed as the total number of neurons in the entire brain!

Other locations of intrinsic neurons containing GABA include the hippocampus, the corpus striatum, the habenular nuclei, and the pons.

A few extended gabaminergic pathways have been identified. Efferents from the cerebellar cortex are carried by gabaminergic Purkinje cells to the deep-lying cerebellar nuclei or to the brainstem. Similarly, a portion of descending efferent projections from

Table 6-6. *Gamma-aminobutyric acid receptor-complex characteristics*

	G_1	G_2	G_3
Receptor types[a]			
Affinity states[b]	Type 1a, 1b, 2		
Chemical constituents			
Receptor	Recognition protein	Recognition protein	?
Effector	Chloride channel	Chloride channel	?
Other	Na⁺-sensitive coupling protein; Barbiturate and analeptic-sensitive modulatory protein; Benzodiazepine and GABA-modulin-sensitive modulatory protein	Na⁺-sensitive coupling protein; no benzodiazepine receptor	?
Selective agonist	Muscimol	Muscimol	Muscimol-insensitive
Selective antagonist	Bicuculline	Bicuculline-insensitive	
Regional and synaptic distribution	Cerebrum, striatum, cerebellum, etc.; postsynaptic and presynaptic; type 2 more abundant in cerebellum	Axoaxonal	Intracellular
Effect of activation	Rapid IPSP	↓ Release of NE, DA, ACh, etc.	?
Adaptability	Yes	?	?

[a]Noninterconverting

[b]Type 1a, 1b, and 2 are rapidly interconverting affinity states regulated by modulatory and coupling protein activity.

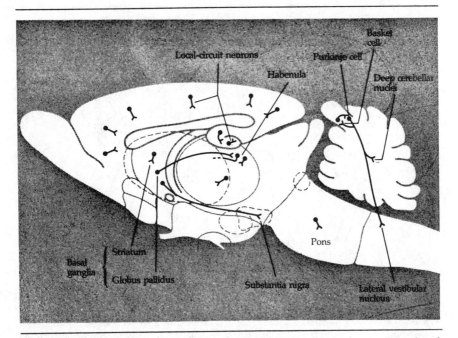

Fig. 6-14. *GABA systems in the brain. From J. B. Angevine, Jr., and C. W. Cotman,* Principles of Neuroanatomy. *New York: Oxford University Press, 1981.*

the corpus striatum release GABA, namely the striatonigral pathway, the pallidosub-thalamic pathway, and a striatal discharge pathway to the entopeduncular nucleus. An afferent GABA pathway reaches the globus pallidus and the related substantia innominata from the septal nucleus.

Glycine

Glycine is a second inhibitory amino acid transmitter (Fig. 6-15). It is found mainly in the spinal cord, where it has an inhibitory effect on reflex circuits. The highly poisonous strychnine is a glycine antagonist. Strychnine causes death from convulsions.

Glutamate and Aspartate

Glutamate and aspartate are also amino acid transmitters, but excitatory in their action. These two transmitters have overlapping specificities, each activating the other's receptor sites to some extent. To date, glutamate has been studied more extensively, but presumably the two exhibit similar synaptic mechanisms. A glutamate-releasing neural process is illustrated in Figure 6-16. As in the case of GABA, glial cells contribute to the metabolism of these excitatory amino acids.

Glutamate is the transmitter of the pyramidal cells of the cerebral cortex. Most outputs from the cerebral cortex are conveyed by pyramidal cell axons. These cortical outputs (Fig. 6-17) reach the corpus striatum, brainstem, hippocampus, and other neo-

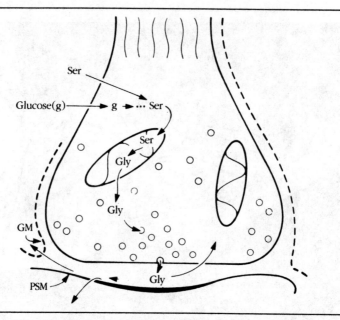

Fig. 6-15. *A glycine synapse. Gly, glycine; GM, glia membrane; PSM, postsynaptic membrane; SER, serine. Modified from M. H. Aprison et al. Neurochemical Evidence for Glycine as a Transmitter and a Model for Its Intrasynaptosomal Compartmentation. In S. Berl et al. (Eds.).* Metabolic Compartmentation and Neurotransmission. *New York: Plenum, 1976.*

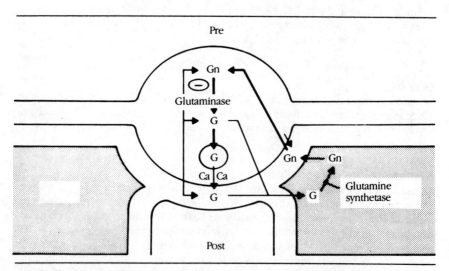

Fig. 6-16. *A glutaminergic synapse. G, glutamate; Gn, glutamine. Modified from C. W. Cotman et al. An overview of glutamate as a neurotransmitter.* Adv. Biochem. Psychopharmacol. *27:10, 1981.* © *1981 by Raven Press, Publishers/New York.*

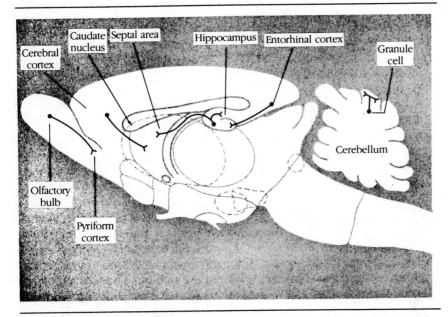

Fig. 6-17. *Glutamate systems in the brain. From J. B. Angevine, Jr., and C. W. Cotman,* Principles of Neuroanatomy. New York: Oxford University Press, 1981.

cortical regions (via transcortical projections). Another important glutamate pathway connects the hippocampus to the septal region. Granule cells, one type of intrinsic neuron of the cerebellum, release glutamate. The lateral olfactory stria from the olfactory bulb to the amygdala and surrounding temporal cortex also release glutamate. Aspartate is found in the cortex and cerebellum, in the latter case associated with a type of afferent projection to the cerebellum called the climbing fibers.

Three types of receptors for excitatory amino acids have thus far been identified (Table 6-7). It is uncertain whether or not these represent three distinct, noninterconvertible receptor types or three affinity states of one receptor protein. Activation of receptors for excitatory amino acids leads to excitatory postsynaptic potentials (EPSPs) and an increase in cyclic guanidine monophosphate (which may be secondary to influx of ions during the EPSPs).

Histamine

Histamine is a putative CNS transmitter and another amino acid (Fig. 6-18). It is especially concentrated in the hypothalamus. There is evidence that, in the hippocampus and cerebral cortex, activity of the histamine-synthesizing enzyme histadine decarboxylase is associated with afferent nerve terminals. Two types of histamine receptors, one linked to adenyl cyclase, one not, are known to exist in the periphery. The CNS histamine-binding sites are largely of the H_2 type, being linked to adenyl cyclase. Diphenhydramine is a selective H_1 blocker; 2-methylhistamine is an H_1 agonist. Cimetidine, on the other hand, selectively blocks H_2-receptors while dimaprit stimulates them. H_2-receptors exhibit adaptability.

Table 6-7. *Characteristics of receptor-complexes for excitatory amino acid transmitters*

Receptor types or affinity states	Type 1	Type 2	Type 3
Chemical constituents			
Receptor	Recognition protein	Recognition protein	Recognition protein
Effector	Sodium channel	Sodium channel	Sodium channel
Other	Ca^{2+}- and leupeptin-sensitive modulatory protein	Ca^{2+}-sensitive modulatory protein	—
Selective agonist	Quisqualic acid	N-methyl-D-aspartic acid	Kainate
Selective antagonist	l-Glutamate diethylester	D-α-Aminoadipic acids	—
Transmitter affinities	Glutamate > aspartate	Aspartate > glutamate	?
Effect of activation	Rapid EPSP; ↑ cGMP (secondary ?)	Rapid EPSP; ↑ cGMP (secondary ?)	?

EPSP, excitatory postsynaptic potential; cGMP, cyclic guanosine monophosphate.

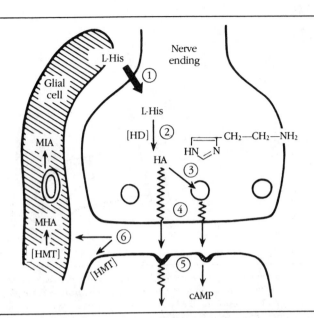

Fig. 6-18. *A histaminergic synapse. cAMP, cyclic adenosine monophosphate; HA, histamine; HD, histadine decarboxylase; HMT, histamine-N-methyltransferase; L-His, L-histadine; MHA, methylhistamine; MIA, methylimidazoleacetic acid. (1) Uptake of L-histadine; (2) synthesis by the action of HD; (3) storage in vesicles; (4) release; (5) stimulation of postsynaptic receptors (most are adenyl cyclase-linked in the CNS); (6) transformation by HMT into MHA, which is then deaminated into MIA. Modified from J. C. Schwartz et al. Neurochemical evidence for histamine acting as a transmitter in mammalian brain.* Adv. Biochem. Psychopharmacol. *15:112, 1976.* © *1976 by Raven Press, Publishers/New York.*

Peptide Neuroregulators

Another class of neuroregulators is the peptides. The number of putative peptides involved in neuroregulation is rapidly increasing at the present time. It is possible that some peptides are transmitters, but most probably serve as neuroregulators or cotransmitters. The implication of the term *neuroregulator* relates to the time course over which effects occur, suggesting slowly developing and long-lasting influences on metabolic processes rather than polarity states. The term *cotransmitter* has been coined to describe the ability of certain peptides (e.g., GABA-modulin) to modulate binding of a primary transmitter.

A hypothetical peptide-releasing neuron is illustrated in Figure 6-19. The major point of distinction in the peptide-releasing neuron is the role of the Golgi body and associated rough endoplasmic reticulum in the packaging of the peptide.

Foremost among the peptides, in terms of present experimental and clinical interest, are the endorphins. The endorphins include β-endorphin and two pentapeptides, met-enkephalin and leu-enkephalin. These substances are the endogenous ligands for the receptors acted on by narcotic analgesics. Thus, narcotics may be viewed as agonists at endorphin receptors. The endorphins are important in gating of pain sensations and inhibition of the punishment system. The role and distribution of the endorphins will be discussed more thoroughly in Chapter 22.

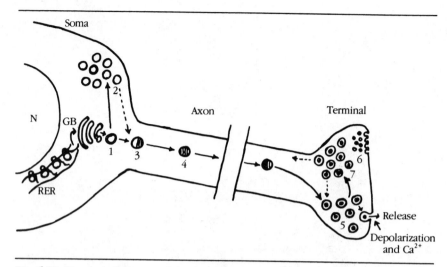

Fig. 6-19. *Hypothetical diagram of the intracellular processes of synthesis, storage, processing, transport, and release of peptides (or proteins) in a peptidergic neuron. RER, rough endoplasmic reticulum; GB, Golgi body; N, nucleus. (1) Newly formed granule; (2) granule pool (in soma) available for axoplasmic transport; (3 and 4) various stages of maturation of granules during transport; (5) granule pool in the axon terminal containing fully processed proteins ready for release; (6) recycled granule membranes in form of small vesicles; (7) pool of stored granules in terminal in nonreleasable form. Modified from H. Gainer. Peptides and neuronal function. Adv. Biochem. Psychopharmacol. 15:202, 1976. © 1976 by Raven Press, Publishers/New York.*

Substance P is a peptide that is involved in conveying pain sensations. The bipolar cells of the dorsal root ganglia of the spinal cord release substance P. These cells carry signals arising from peripheral pain receptors into the spinal cord. Substance P is also found in the striatonigral tract of the extrapyramidal system and in a limbic system pathway connecting the habenular nuclei and interpeduncular nucleus. This transmitter produces long-lasting inhibitory effects on postsynaptic cells.

Other peptides currently under investigation as brain neuroregulators are growth-hormone inhibitory factor, vasoactive intestinal polypeptide, cholecystokinin, adrenocorticotropic hormone, thyrotropin-releasing factor, luteinizing hormone releasing factor, melanocyte stimulating hormone, neurotensin, angiotensin II, antidiuretic hormone, and oxytocin.

Cyclic Nucleotides

Adenosine 3′:5′-monophosphate (cyclic AMP [cAMP]) mediates many hormonal effects in peripheral tissues. Many of the actions of epinephrine are related to cAMP, including insulin release and sugar and fat utilization. Cyclic AMP has been designated a "second messenger" because of this role of translating the presence of various hormones into specific cellular effects. Cyclic AMP is found in high concentration in the brain and plays a role in the CNS similar to its role in the endocrine system.

Metabolism

Cyclic AMP is formed from adenosine triphosphate, a universal cellular constituent, by the enzyme adenyl cyclase (Fig. 6-20). Adenyl cyclase is the effector protein for many of

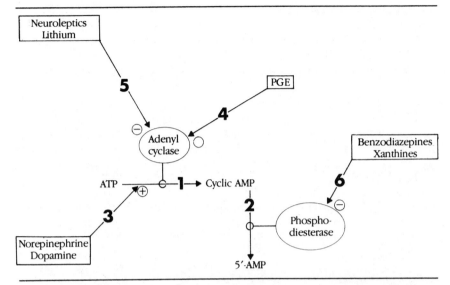

Fig. 6-20. *Metabolism of cyclic AMP (cAMP) indicating known and postulated drug modifications. AMP, adenosine monophosphate; ATP, adenosine triphosphate; PgE, prostaglandin E. (1) Synthesis of cAMP by adenyl cyclase; (2) degradation of cAMP by phosphodiesterase; (3) mediation of NE and DA effects by cAMP; (4) PgE inhibition of adenyl cyclase; (5) inhibition of adenyl cyclase as proposed mechanism for lithium and neuroleptics; (6) inhibition of phosphodiesterase by xanthines and as proposed mechanism of anxiolytics.*

the CNS receptor complexes. Adenyl cyclase activity is stimulated by a number of neurotransmitters, including NE, DA, serotonin, and histamine. Increased adenyl cyclase activity leads to an elevation in cAMP levels.

Destruction of cAMP is catalyzed by the enzyme phosphodiesterase. A group of drugs called xanthines, including theophylline and caffeine, are effective inhibitors of phosphodiesterase. These inhibitors of phosphodiesterase potentiate the effects of cAMP.

Role in the Superior Cervical Ganglion

Greengard has studied the role of cAMP in sympathetic ganglia of the rabbit. Electrical stimulation of the preganglionic cells causes an increase in levels of cAMP, an increase that is related to the intensity of stimulation. Stimulation of the postganglionic cells has no effect. Local application of DA produces a hyperpolarization of postganglionic cells, and this hyperpolarization is enhanced by theophylline. Since theophylline is a phosphodiesterase inhibitor, it appears that preganglionic fibers containing DA are responsible for the hyperpolarization as well as the increased cAMP levels and that the two are related. Dopamine effects are also blocked by prostaglandin E (PgE), a drug known to reduce levels of cAMP.

Role in the Cerebellum

A similar set of studies has indicated that effects of β-adrenergic receptors of the cerebellum are imitated by stimulators of nerve cells lying in the locus ceruleus of the brainstem. The fibers from the locus ceruleus release NE. If NE is depleted, no inhibition of Purkinje's cells can take place. Moreover, direct application of NE to Purkinje's cells produces an effect identical to stimulation of the cells in the locus ceruleus.

The inhibitory action of Purkinje's cells produced by NE or by stimulation of the locus ceruleus is reproduced exactly by direct application of cAMP. All three effects can be potentiated by phosphodiesterase inhibitors or blocked by prostaglandin E.

Role in the Cerebral Cortex

Norepinephrine, DA, serotonin, and histamine all elevate cAMP levels. Acetylcholine has no direct effect on cerebral cAMP levels, but it does elevate levels of another cyclic nucleotide, cyclic guanosine monophosphate (cGMP). This elevation of cGMP induced by ACh is blocked by atropine, a cholinergic blocker.

The role of cGMP has been less well studied than that of cAMP. In the perfused rat heart, however, it has been reported that the antagonistic physiologic actions of isoproterenol (a β-adrenergic stimulant) and ACh are mediated by cAMP and cGMP respectively. A theory that has evolved from that work is that it is the ratio of the two cyclic nucleotides that is the crucial relationship, not either alone (the so-called yin-yang hypothesis).

Effects Mediated by Cyclic Nucleotides

As illustrated in Figure 6-1, cAMP exerts a modulatory effect on membrane and soluble enzymes in the cell interior. The best-understood mechanism is the activation of soluble protein kinase. The cAMP-dependent protein kinase exists as a holoenzyme composed of two subunits. A regulatory subunit exerts an inhibitory effect on the catalytic subunit. When cAMP contacts the holoenzyme, it splits the enzyme and binds to the regulatory subunit, freeing the catalytic subunit to produce its cellular actions, for example, modulation of nuclear regulatory proteins.

The levels and activity of cyclic nucleotides are subject to regulation by cellular proteins. A protein called phosphodiesterase enzyme activator (PDEA) is stored in vesicles of nerve terminals and released by a cAMP-dependent process. This protein increases the activity of phosphodiesterase, the degratory enzyme of cAMP. Another cellular constituent, protein kinase modulator (PKM), can regulate the activity of cAMP and cGMP. Protein kinase modulator consists of two subunits: (1) an inhibitory component that turns off cAMP-dependent protein kinase and (2) an excitatory component that stimulates cGMP-dependent protein kinase. Thus, PKM may play a role in controlling the balance of activity of the two opposing cyclic nucleotides.

Psychotropic Drugs and Cyclic Adenosine Monophosphate

A number of neuroleptic drugs prevent the rise in cAMP produced by NE in brain slices. Moreover, there is a good correlation in a series of phenothiazines between their efficacy in preventing the NE-induced increase in cAMP and their potency as antipsychotic agents. Lithium has also been reported to inhibit adenyl cyclase activity.

Conversely, a group of psychedelic drugs, including LSD, has been reported to elevate levels of cAMP. A congenor of LSD, bromo-LSD, does not raise cAMP levels and does not have the hallucinatory effects of LSD.

Last, the action of anxiolytics has been postulated to be related to cAMP. Diazepam and chlordiazepoxide are potent inhibitors of phosphodiesterase. A significant correlation is found between antianxiety potency and degree of inhibition of phosphodiesterase. And antianxiety potency has been reported for xanthines that inhibit phosphodiesterase as well as a derivative of cAMP itself, dibutyryl cAMP.

Selected References and Further Readings

General

1. Angevine, J. B., Jr., and Cotman, C. W. The Chemical Coding of Neural Circuits. In *Principles of Neuroanatomy*. New York: Oxford University Press, 1981. Chap. 14.
2. Cooper, J. R., Bloom, F. E., and Roth, R. H. *The Biochemical Basis of Neuropharmacology* (3rd ed.). New York: Oxford University Press, 1978.
3. Creese, I., and Sibley, D. R. Receptor adaptations to centrally acting drugs. *Annu. Rev. Pharmacol. Toxicol.* 21:357–391, 1981.
4. Kelly, R. B., Deutsch, J. W., Carlson, S. S., and Wagner, J. A. Biochemistry of neurotransmitter release. *Annu. Rev. Neurosci.* 2:399–446, 1979.

Acetylcholine

5. Cheney, D. L., and Costa, E. Biochemical Pharmacology of Cholinergic Neurons. In M. A. Lipton et al. (Eds.), *Psychopharmacology: A Generation of Progress*. New York: Raven, 1978.
6. Kuhar, M. J. Central Cholinergic Pathways: Physiological and Pharmacological Aspects. In M. A. Lipton et al. (Eds.), *Psychopharmacology: A Generation of Progress*. New York: Raven, 1978.
7. Lewis, P. R., and Shute, C. C. D. Cholinergic Pathways in CNS. In L. L. Iversen et al. (Eds.), *Handbook of Psychopharmacology*. New York: Plenum, 1978. Vol. 9.

Cyclic Nucleotides

8. Bloom, F. E. The Role of Cyclic Nucleotides in Central Synaptic Function. In E. Costa et al. (Eds.), *First and Second Messengers: New Vistas, (Advances in Biochemical Psychopharmacology,* Vol. 15). New York: Raven, 1976.
9. Daly, J. Role of Cyclic Nucleotides in the Nervous System. In L. L. Iversen et al. (Eds.), *Handbook of Psychopharmacology*. New York: Plenum, 1975. Vol. 5.
10. Kuo, J. F., Kuo, W.-N, and Shoji, M. Regulation by Cyclic GMP and Stimulatory Protein Kinase Modulation of Cyclic GMP-dependent Protein Kinase from Brain and Other Tissue. In E. Costa et al. (Eds.), *First and Second Messengers: New Vistas, (Advances in Biochemical Psychopharmacology,* Vol. 15). New York: Raven, 1976.
11. Nathanson, J. A., and Greengard, P. "Second messengers" in the brain. *Sci. Am.* 237:108–119, 1977.

Dopamine

12. Bunney, B. S., and Aghajanian, G. K. Mesolimbic and Mesocortical Dopaminergic Systems: Physiology and Pharmacology. In M. A. Lipton et al. (Eds.), *Psychopharmacology: A Generation of Progress*. New York: Raven, 1978.
13. Costa, E., and Gessa, G. L. (Eds.). *Nonstriatal Dopaminergic Neurons, (Advances in Biochemical Psychopharmacology,* Vol. 16). New York: Raven, 1977.
14. Moore, R. Y., and Bloom, F. E. Central catecholamine neuron systems: Anatomy and physiology of the dopamine systems. *Annu. Rev. Neurosci.* 1:129–169, 1978.
15. Roberts, P. J., Woodruff, G. N., and Iversen, L. L. (Eds.). *Dopamine, (Advances in Biochemical Psychopharmacology,* Vol. 19). New York: Raven, 1978.

Epinephrine

16. Goldstein, M., Lew, J. Y., Matsumoto, Y., Hökfelt, T., and Fuxe, K. Localization and Function of PNMT in the Central Nervous System. In M. A. Lipton et al. (Eds.), *Psychopharmacology: A Generation of Progress*. New York: Raven, 1978.

Gamma-Aminobutyric Acid

17. DeFeudis, F. V., and Mandel, P. (Eds.). *Amino Acid Neurotransmitters, (Advances in Biochemical Psychopharmacology*, Vol. 29). New York: Raven, 1981.
18. DiChiara, G., and Gessa, G. L. (Eds.). *GABA and the Basal Ganglia, (Advances in Biochemical Psychopharmacology*, Vol. 30). New York: Raven, 1981.
19. Fonnum, F., and Strom-Mathisen, J. (Eds.). Localization of GABA-ergic Neurons in the CNS. In L. L. Iversen et al. (Eds.), *Handbook of Psychopharmacology.* New York: Plenum, 1978. Vol. 9.
20. Iversen, L. L. Biochemical Psychopharmacology of GABA. In M. A. Lipton et al. (Eds.), *Psychopharmacology: A Generation of Progress.* New York: Raven, 1978.
21. Johnston, G. A. R. Neuropharmacology of amino acid inhibitory transmitters. *Annu. Rev. Pharmacol. Toxicol.* 18:269–289, 1978.

Glutamate and Aspartate

22. DeFeudis, F. V., and Mandel, P. (Eds.). *Amino Acid Neurotransmitters, (Advances in Biochemical Psychopharmacology*, Vol. 29). New York: Raven, 1981.
23. DiChiara, G., and Gessa, G. L. (Eds.). *Glutamate as a Neurotransmitter, (Advances in Biochemical Psychopharmacology*, Vol. 27). New York: Raven, 1981.
24. Evans, R. H. Excitatory amino acid transmitters. *Annu. Rev. Pharmacol. Toxicol.* 21:165–204, 1981.
25. Johnston, G. A. R. Biochemistry of Glycine, Taurine, Glutamate and Aspartate. In L. L. Iversen et al. (Eds.), *Handbook of Psychopharmacology.* New York: Plenum, 1975. Vol. 4.

Glycine

26. Aprison, M. H. Glycine as a Neurotransmitter. In M. A. Lipton et al. (Eds.), *Psychopharmacology: A Generation of Progress.* New York: Raven, 1978.
27. Johnston, G. A. R. Biochemistry of Glycine, Taurine, Glutamate and Aspartate. In L. L. Iversen et al. (Eds.), *Handbook of Psychopharmacology.* New York: Plenum, 1975. Vol. 4.

Histamine

28. Green, J. P., Johnson, C. L., and Weinstein, H. Histamine As a Neurotransmitter. In M. A. Lipton et al. (Eds.), *Psychopharmacology: A Generation of Progress.* New York: Raven, 1978.
29. Schwartz, J.-C. Histaminergic mechanisms in the brain. *Annu. Rev. Pharmacol. Toxicol.* 17: 325–339, 1977.
30. Schwartz, J.-C., Barbin, G., Garbarg, M., Pollard, H., Rose, C., and Verdiere, M. Neurochemical Evidence for Histamine Acting as a Transmitter in Mammalian Brain. In E. Costa et al. (Eds.), *First and Second Messengers: New Vistas, (Advances in Biochemical Psychopharmacology*, Vol. 15). New York: Raven, 1976.
31. Taylor, K. M. Brain Histamine. In L. L. Iversen et al. (Eds.), *Handbook of Psychopharmacology.* New York: Plenum, 1975. Vol. 3.

Norepinephrine

32. Lindvall, O., and Bjorklund, A. Organization of Catecholamine Neurons in the Rat Central Nervous System. In L. L. Iversen et al. (Eds.), *Handbook of Psychopharmacology.* New York: Plenum, 1978. Vol. 9.
33. Moore, R. Y., and Bloom, F. E. Central catecholamine neuron systems: Anatomy and physiology of the norepinephrine and epinephrine systems. *Annu. Rev. Neurosci.* 2:113–168, 1979.

Peptides

34. Loh, H. H., and Ross, D. H. (Eds.). *Neurochemical Mechanisms of Opiates and Endorphins, (Advances in Biochemical Psychopharmacology,* Vol. 20). New York: Plenum, 1979.
35. Martin, J. B., Reichlin, S., and Bick, K. L. (Eds.). *Neurosecretion and Brain Peptides, (Advanced Biochemical Psychopharmacology,* Vol. 28). New York: Plenum, 1981.
36. Nicoll, R. A., Schenker, C., and Leeman, S. E. Substance P as a transmitter candidate. *Annu. Rev. Neurosci.* 3:227–268, 1980.
37. Snyder, S. H., and Childers, S. R. Opiate receptors and opiate peptides. *Annu. Rev. Neurosci.* 2:35–64, 1979.
38. Snyder, S. H., Pasternak, G. W., and Pert, C. B. Opiate Receptor Mechanisms. In L. L. Iversen et al. (Eds.), *Handbook of Psychopharmacology.* New York: Plenum, 1975. Vol. 5.

Serotonin

39. Aghajanian, G. W., and Wang, R. Y. Physiology and Pharmacology of Central Serotonin Neurons. In M. A. Lipton et al. (Eds.), *Psychopharmacology: A Generation of Progress.* New York: Raven, 1978.
40. Azmitia, E. C. The Serotonergic-Producing Neurons of the Midbrain Median and Dorsal Raphé Nuclei. In L. L. Iversen et al. (Eds.), *Handbook of Psychopharmacology.* New York: Plenum, 1978. Vol. 9.
41. Fuller, R. W. Pharmacology of central serotonergic neurons. *Annu. Rev. Pharmacol. Toxicol.* 20:111–127, 1980.

Principles of
Pharmacology
7

Receptors

The effects produced by a drug (or for that matter by an endogenous hormone) on a living system are the physiologic consequence of an interaction between the drug and some locus in or on the target cells. It is presumed that in most cases these loci are macromolecular components of the postsynaptic cell membrane. Pharmacologists refer to these loci as receptors. Most receptors are proteins, but some drugs interact with the lipid membrane.

A given receptor population bears a specificity for certain chemical substances, usually a group of structurally similar substances, but is not acted on by all pharmacologically active substances. An effector cell possesses a multitude of identical receptors for each receptor type found associated with that cell. Drugs may interact with receptor proteins in either of two fundamental ways (Fig. 7-1): (1) as *agonists*, or stimulants, and (2) as *antagonists*, or blockers. An agonist binds with the receptor and activates it by producing some physiochemical alteration. An antagonist binds to the receptor but does not activate it. In occupying the receptor, the antagonist prevents access of the agonist to the receptor or, in other words, affords "protection" to the receptor. The action of an antagonist, therefore, is not direct, but related to the prevention of the normal agonistic action of an endogenous or exogenous agonist. It is presumed, perhaps without basis, that for every receptor there is an endogenous substance capable of activating it.

With respect to neurotransmitters and their receptors, it should be kept in mind that receptor activation does not necessarily lead to electrical excitation of the target neuron. The activated receptor may mediate hyperpolarization of the target neuron or activate an enzyme in the target neuron.

Theoretically, four steps are involved in the drug-receptor interaction (Fig. 7-2): (1) Attracted by electrostatic forces, the drug and receptor associate are reversibly bound by some combination of various kinds of chemical bonds; (2) the receptor is modified or "activated" if the drug has agonistic properties; (3) the drug dissociates from the receptor, leaving a still modified and unexcitable receptor; (4) a "ground-state," or excitable, receptor is regenerated. Steps 1 and 3 are governed by dissociation constants; step 4 may be regulated enzymatically by a modulatory protein, while step 2 occurs at a rate determined by the "efficacy" of the drug. Normally, the "affinity" of a

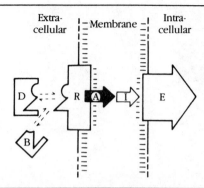

Fig. 7-1. *Drug-receptor interactions. D, agonist drug; B, blocking (antagonist) drug; R, receptor; A, signal from activated receptor; I, intermediate steps; E, effector mechanism constituting the response. Modified from R. H. Rech and K. E. Moore (Eds.),* An Introduction to Psychopharmacology. © *1971 by Raven Press, Publishers/New York.*

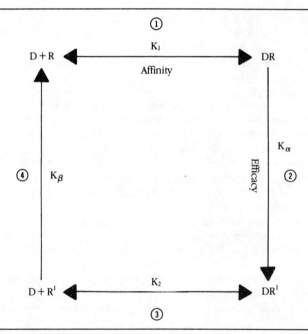

Fig. 7-2. *The interactions of a drug and receptor. D, drug; R, receptor in the ground state; R', receptor in the modified or activated state.* K_1 *and* K_2 *are dissociation constants for the binding of drug to the receptor.* K_α *is the rate constant for activation of the receptor and is a reflection of the efficacy of the drug.* K_β *is the rate constant for regeneration of ground state receptor. (1) Binding; (2) activation; (3) dissociation; (4) regeneration of activable receptor.*

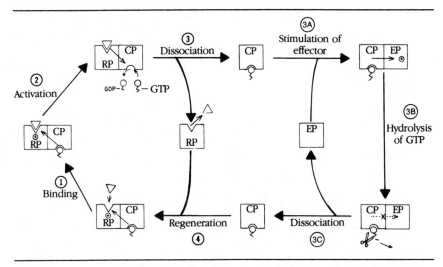

Fig. 7-3. *Receptor mechanisms. (1) The ground state receptor consists of two subunits: the recognition protein (RP) and the coupling protein (CP). The latter has a molecule of guanydyl diphosphate (GDP) attached that promotes binding of the two subunits as well as having a positive influence on affinity of the recognition protein for the transmitter molecule. This high affinity state promotes binding. (2) As a result of transmitter-binding, guanydyl triphosphate (GTP) replaces GDP at the nucleotide binding site on CP, which constitutes receptor "activation." (3) This leads to dissociation of the transmitter from RP and dissociation of the two subunits (CP and RP). (3A) CP with GTP attached is capable of binding to the effector protein (EP) and enhances its activity. (3B) This persists until the GTP undergoes hydrolysis to GDP. (3C) Hydrolysis of the GTP causes CP to dissociate from EP, and EP activity returns to the basal level. (4) CP can now link up with a free RP to regenerate an excitable receptor.*

drug or transmitter for the receptor reflects the dissociation constant for step 1. This is generally the case when all or most of the receptor population is in the "ground state."

The termination of the action of a drug is related not only to the removal of the drug from the vicinity of the receptors but also reciprocally to the rate at which receptors are regenerated to the excitable state. If all or most of the receptors of a given type on a given cell are in the modified form, the drug can no longer exert an influence. The reduction in excitable receptors that sometimes occurs in the presence of high concentrations of an agonist drug is called tachyphylaxis.

Receptor complexes vary in the number of elements involved from transmitter binding to actualization of an effect. The nicotinic receptor (for acetylcholine) is a relatively simple one. The transmitter molecules apparently bind directly to the protein subunits that constitute the effector unit, a large-ion channel. More typically, a receptor complex consists of a recognition protein (or receptor site) for the neurotransmitter (or drug), an effector unit (ion channel or enzyme), a coupling protein that communicates between the recognition protein and effector, and one or more modulatory proteins that control binding of the transmitter to the recognition protein. The interconversions of this typical receptor complex are illustrated in Figure 7-3.

Dose-Response Relationship

The response of a biologic system to a drug is graded such that within a fairly wide range increasing concentrations of a drug produce increasing magnitude of response. This is

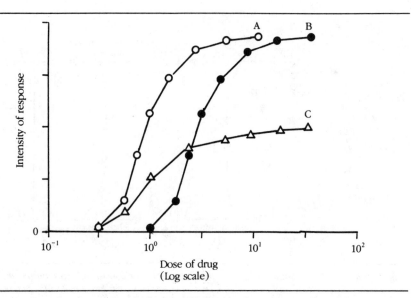

Fig. 7-4. *Intensity of response as a function of dose of a drug. Curve A shows the response to a hypothetical agonist in the absence of an inhibitor. Curve B shows the parallel shift brought about by the presence of a competitive antagonist. Curve C shows the effect of a noncompetitive antagonist. Note that the maximal intensity of response is reduced by the noncompetitive antagonist. Modified from A. K. Swonger.* Nursing Pharmacology. *Boston: Little, Brown, 1978.*

called the dose-response relationship (Fig. 7-4). It is impossible to overstate the importance of a thorough grasp of this principle. Interpretation and judgments regarding the consequences of drug applications are meaningless unless dose is taken into consideration.

It is generally assumed that the response is proportional to the number of receptors in the activated state. This assumption, however, has not yet been proved. An alternative is that response is related to the rate at which the receptor is modified (step 2 in Fig. 7-2). In either case, the rate of activation of the receptor is itself dependent on the concentration of drug in its vicinity, since the greater the concentration of drug, the greater is the likelihood of an effective collision between a drug molecule and a receptor. The presence of an antagonist reduces the effective number of receptors available to any agonist.

Antagonists may be either competitive or noncompetitive. A competitive antagonist has affinity for the same site as the corresponding agonist. The antagonist or agonist can occupy the receptor site, and the total number of sites occupied by each (i.e., the balance of competition) will be determined by the relative concentrations and relative affinities of the two substances. If the concentration of the antagonist is increased, the competitive balance shifts toward blockade of the receptors, but this can be overcome by increases in agonist concentration. A noncompetitive antagonist, on the other hand, interacts with the receptor in a manner that impairs its ability to bind the agonist. Noncompetitive antagonists cannot be reversed by high concentrations of an agonist drug (Fig. 7-4).

Two drugs that act at the same receptor may differ widely in ability to stimulate the receptor. These two drugs are said to differ in potency. Differences in potency may be related to a difference in ability to attach to the receptor (affinity) or a difference in ability to activate the receptor (efficacy). Antagonists may also differ in affinity for the receptor. A partial agonist is a drug with good affinity but low efficacy.

For any given response system, there is a drug dose that elicits the maximal response beyond which additional concentrations of drug have no further effect. This is called the ceiling effect and is an expression of efficacy.

The concentration of drug around the receptor is determined by the dose administered. In addition, many factors may influence the delivery of drug from the site of administration to the receptors in question. One important factor is the route of administration.

Routes of Administration

Drugs may be administered topically to a restricted part of the body or systemically. Therapeutic application of centrally active drugs is invariably systemic. Topical application of drugs to a part of the brain may be employed in experimental work in laboratory animals, but will not be discussed here. There are three categories of systemic administration: oral, rectal, and parenteral.

Oral administration is the most common, usually the least unpleasant, and the easiest. Absorption of the drug can occur at any point along the gastrointestinal tract. The chemical properties of the drug are extremely important here, since they will determine if the drug is to be absorbed from the acid medium in the stomach or from the neutral medium in the intestine. The quantity of material in the gastrointestinal tract will also influence absorption. Greater absorption will occur in an empty stomach.

In rectal administration, a drug is given as an enema or suppository. This is not a commonly employed technique; it is reserved primarily for patients who are not able to take drugs orally.

Parenteral administration means literally not through the gastrointestinal tract. We will discuss briefly six parenteral routes. Intravenous administration is commonly employed and has several advantages, including rapid delivery, controllability of dose, and rate of onset. It is a good route for drugs that are poorly absorbed from or irritate the gastrointestinal tract. Its disadvantages are that rapid injection may lead to embolisms or elevated blood pressure. Hepatitis can result if nonsterile instruments are employed.

Subcutaneous administration is a simple route but with variable results. Absorption is usually slow and dependent on blood flow and the lipid solubility of the drug. Somewhat similar to subcutaneous administration is the intramuscular route. The deltoid muscle is usually employed. Absorption is generally fairly rapid, and large volumes can be administered with little irritation.

Inhalation is a rapid means of administering gases and aerosols. The major application is with the volatile anesthetics, but this may also be a common route of self-administration, as in cannabis, tobacco, or cocaine. Two routes not employed in human subjects are the intraperitoneal and the intraventricular routes. The latter is used as a means of circumventing the blood-brain barrier (see the next section).

Once a drug enters the circulatory system from any of these routes, it is rapidly distributed throughout the body. Distribution is not necessarily uniform, since some drugs have an affinity for lipid tissue, others for aqueous media. Moreover, distribution may be restricted by penetration barriers or altered by active accumulation into particular regions. Drugs that are highly lipid soluble generally exhibit more rapid and more complete transit across the various penetration barriers because the membranes that comprise such barriers are composed largely of phospholipids. Lipid soluble drugs often have a larger apparent volume of distribution than drugs with low lipid solubility.

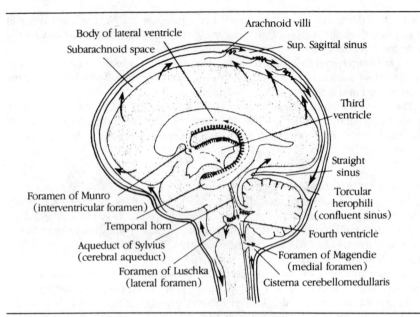

Fig. 7-5. *The circulation of the cerebrospinal fluid. Modified from A. J. Gatz.* Clinical Neuro-anatomy and Neurophysiology *(4th ed.). Philadelphia: Davis, 1970.*

Lipid soluble drugs are usually shorter acting than less lipid soluble congeners because lipid soluble drugs move out more rapidly, through the penetration barriers back into the general circulation, during the drug elimination phase. Ultimately, elimination from the circulatory system is accomplished by metabolism, excretion, and tissue accumulation of the drug.

The Blood-Brain Barrier

The access of drugs to the CNS is governed by an additional and unique consideration. In addition to having a rich vascular supply, the brain is bathed by the cerebrospinal fluid (CSF) flowing throughout the cerebral ventricles and the subarachnoid space, which separates the cortex from its overlying sheaths (Fig. 7-5). The passage of chemical substances from the circulatory system into either the brain or the CSF is highly restricted, and this functional restriction is referred to as the blood-brain barrier. This term does not denote a particular anatomic structure, but rather a functional phenomenon. Many drugs do not cross the blood-brain barrier to any appreciable extent and so have little central effect. These include dopamine, norepinephrine, and serotonin, three endogenous CNS transmitters. The membranes that separate the blood from the CSF and from the brain also possess specialized carrier mechanisms to accumulate or discharge selected materials. The metabolic breakdown products of dopamine and serotonin are actively extruded from the CSF into the blood, for example.

Drug Metabolism and Elimination

The duration of a drug action is determined in part by its metabolism and elimination. The time required for the body to reduce the plasma concentration of a drug by half is called the half-life of a drug, and is a commonly employed convention for quantifying the rate at which the body disposes of a particular drug (Table 7-1). Certain drugs can be metabolized by cells throughout the body but most drugs are metabolized largely by enzymes in the liver that are highly specialized for the degradation of drugs. These drug-metabolizing enzymes play a significant part in the inactivation of many chemical substances. The degradative products from these reactions can be returned to the circulatory system or excreted in the bile.

Elimination of drugs or their metabolites from the body is accomplished chiefly by the kidneys and lungs. Some substances are actively secreted by the kidneys, while others are simply filtered along with the plasma and not reabsorbed. In either case, the substance is then excreted in the urine. Volatile substances may be eliminated from the body by exhalation from the lungs.

Drug Interactions

One drug can alter the effect of another in three basic ways: (1) by altering its availability, (2) by a physiologic interaction, or (3) by a pharmacologic interaction. An interaction affecting availability (or metabolic interaction) is often related to the liver-metabolizing enzymes discussed in the preceding section. Certain drugs, particularly some sedative-hypnotics and antiepileptics, increase the activity of the liver drug-metabolizing enzymes. This increases the rate of metabolism of all drugs broken down by these enzymes, including many analgesics, anticoagulants, antihistamines, anti-inflammatory agents, antiepileptics, steroids, anxiolytics, and sedative-hypnotics. Another type of metabolic interaction occurs when a drug inhibits an enzyme that degrades another drug. Monoamine oxidase inhibitors prolong the action of all drugs broken down by monoamine oxidase; these include barbiturates, cocaine, and meperidine. A third type of metabolic interaction occurs when one drug displaces another from an inactive binding site. An example of this is the displacement of phenytoin or penicillin from plasma albumin binding sites by aspirin. Aspirin increases the pharmacologic response to a given dose of diphenytoin by decreasing the fraction of it that is inactively bound by the albumin. This type of interaction is significant only for drugs that are very highly bound to plasma proteins, generally in excess of 80 percent (see Table 7-1).

The term *physiologic interaction* denotes the relationship of two drugs that affect the same response system but not at the same receptor site. If the drugs have an effect in the same direction, this is called *additive;* if the net effect is greater than the sum of the individual effects, this is called *synergistic.* If the drugs have opposing actions, this is called a *physiologic* or *functional antagonism.* All CNS depressants (sedatives, tranquilizers, narcotics) have additive depressant actions. The relationship between pentobarbital (a sedative) and strychnine (an analeptic) is one of physiologic antagonism.

Pharmacologic interactions are those that occur at a given receptor. In the discussion of receptors, above, we discussed agonists (receptor stimulators) and antagonists (blockers). The interaction between a receptor stimulator and a blocker is called pharmacologic antagonism. The interaction between morphine and naloxone (Chap. 23) is an example of pharmacologic antagonism. Pharmacologic antagonism is more direct and quantitative than physiologic antagonism.

Multiplicity of Effects

Throughout, we have made an effort to define, where possible, the action of psychotropic drugs in terms of specific brain systems. A severe limitation imposed on this effort

Table 7-1. *Pharmacokinetic parameters for important CNS drugs*

Drug	Route of elimination	Elimination half-life (hr)	Percent bound to plasma proteins
Acetaminophen	Renal	0.9–3.3	15–25
Amitriptyline	Hepatic	41–45	94–97
Amobarbital	Hepatic	14–42	41–60
Amphetamine	Renal	7–34	low
Aspirin	Renal	2.4–19*	40–70
Caffeine	Renal	3.5–6	
Carbamazepine	Renal	20–37	75–82
Chloral hydrate	Renal	1	40
Chlordiazepoxide	Hepatic	6–34	94–98
Chlorpromazine	Hepatic	11–58	95–98
Clonazepam	Hepatic	22–33	45
Codeine	Renal	3–6	
Desmethyldiazepam	Hepatic	15–96	85–98
Diazepam	Hepatic	27–87	80–99
L-dopa	Renal	2.5–3.0	
Ethanol	Hepatic	0.15–0.35	0
Ethchlorvynol	Renal	21–105	
Ethosuximide	Renal	30–56	20–30
Flurazepam	Hepatic	24–100*	low
Glutethimide	Hepatic	5–22	54
Haloperidol	Renal	13–35.5	
Heroin	Renal	1–2	
Ibuprofen	Hepatic	2	99
Imipramine	Renal	3.5	95
Lithium	Renal	7–24	0
Lorazepam	Hepatic	10–20	90–95
LSD	Hepatic	1.7–3.0	
Meperidine	Hepatic	3.2	40–60
Meprobamate	Hepatic	6–16	low
Methadone	Renal	10–25	83–87
Methamphetamine	Renal	12–14	low
Methaqualone	Renal	10–43	70–90
Methylphenidate	Hepatic	1–2	
Morphine	Renal	1.3–3.4	35
Naloxone	Hepatic	1.5	low
Nortriptyline	Hepatic	18–35	94
Oxazepam	Hepatic	3–21	80–95
Pentazocine	Renal	2.5–6.0	
Pentobarbital	Renal	42–50	45
Phenobarbital	Hepatic	53–160	32–36

Table 7-1 (continued)

Drug	Route of elimination	Elimination half-life (hr)	Percent bound to plasma proteins
Phenytoin	Renal	7–42	88–93
Primidone	Hepatic	3–12	19
Propoxyphene	Hepatic	1.6–4.1	
Protriptyline	Hepatic	78	92
Secobarbital	Hepatic	15–40	44
Δ^9-THC	Hepatic	56	
Valproic acid	Renal	6–10	90–95

*Includes half-life of active metabolite.

is that most, if not all, drugs affect many brain systems. There is no such thing as a "clean" drug—one imposing a single, neat, and circumscribed challenge to the CNS. To attribute all the clinical effects of a given drug to a single known pharmacologic action is therefore usually erroneous.

A related rule (which we have designated the principle of *multa loca tenens*) states that if a drug can substitute in some regard for a given endogenous chemical, it can probably substitute in other respects as well, albeit to a greater or lesser extent. If a drug bears sufficient structural similarity to a given CNS transmitter so that it can stimulate its receptors, it may also compete for its reuptake pump and its metabolic enzymes. There are numerous examples of such multiple interactions. One that springs to mind is p-chloroamphetamine, which competes with serotonin both for monoamine oxidase and the vesicular binding sites. Consequently, a known interaction between a drug and some neurochemical system in the brain may or may not be the principal action contributing to its observable effects. Therefore, the reader should view cautiously discussions of the mechanisms of action of a drug, whether here or elsewhere. At best, these are "state-of-the-art" interpretations based on considerable but incomplete knowledge of how drugs work.

Selected References and Further Readings

1. Gatz, A. J. *Clinical Neuroanatomy and Neurophysiology* (4th ed.). Philadelphia: Davis, 1970.
2. Goldstein, A., Aronow, L., and Kalman, S. M. *Principles of Drug Action* (2nd ed.). New York: Harper & Row, 1974.
3. Gilman, A. G., Goodman, L. S., and Gilman, A. *The Pharmacological Basis of Therapeutics* (5th ed.). New York: Macmillan, 1980.
4. Levine, R. R. *Pharmacology: Drug Actions and Reactions* (2nd ed.). Boston: Little, Brown, 1978.
5. Usdin, E., Bunney, W. E., Jr., and Davis, J. M. (Eds.). *Neuroreceptors: Basic and Clinical Aspects.* New York: Wiley, 1981.

Drug Use, Drug Abuse III

We now turn our attention to de facto aspects of drug utilization. Chapters 8 and 9 spotlight respectively the two distinct situations under which psychotropic drugs are widely employed, namely, in the clinic and on the street.

In Chapter 8, technical aspects of the clinical application of psychotropic medication and nonpharmacologic variables influencing drug response are considered in depth. This chapter is furnished principally for the benefit of readers, such as psychiatric nurses or physicians, who may be somewhat more directly involved in the administration of psychotropic drugs, but it is hoped that it will be profitable reading, nevertheless, for others as well.

In Chapter 9, the pharmacologic aspects of drug abuse are more explicitly defined and discussed than was possible in previous chapters dealing with potential drugs of abuse. No attempt is made here to consider the important and multifaceted psychological aspects of drug abuse—a topic that would well extend by itself to book length. This omission should not be taken to indicate that the authors view drug abuse as primarily a pharmacologic issue. On the contrary, we view it as principally a psychological one.

Clinical Psycho-pharmacology* 8

The manner in which the clinician actually prescribes and administers psychotropic drugs reflects much more (and sometimes much less) than the pharmacology of these agents. The pharmacologic mechanisms of most drugs currently in use are not completely understood, and there are inevitable delays in the passage of that knowledge from clinical research and laboratory to clinic. In the meantime, the physician is confronted with patients in genuine distress for which the means of amelioration may be at hand in psychopharmacologic agents. Nonpharmacologic theories, traditions, even hunches and personal preferences, are assembled to fill the void and permit practice to continue in the face of inadequate information. To this must be added the interests of the pharmaceutical industry, their "detail" men, and the specialized media by which drugs are brought to the physician's awareness—all these shape the pattern of a physician's method. Local custom and regional and national differences are also factors. Not surprisingly, then, actual practice in clinical psychopharmacology is every bit as large an area of inquiry, mystery, and partial theory as the underlying chemical, anatomic, and physiologic bases that form the bulk of this book.

As if that were not enough, this already messy area of inquiry must be complicated further by the introduction of patient variables, the personal factors and social circumstances. Finally, doctor and patient form an interactive system which has influences and shows effects of its own on the outcome of drug therapy.

Rational Psychotherapeutics

The component parts of rational clinical utilization of psychotropic drugs are therefore numerous, and their enumeration must, of necessity, be somewhat arbitrary.

To begin with, it needs to be understood that every instance of therapy constitutes a miniature experiment and not simply the application of fixed principles. Although in current medical practice precise data collection is frequently not carried out, failure to do so constitutes a compromise of best medical practice in the name of expediency. The selection of one or more drugs, the determination of dosages, the route and frequency of administration, as well as many decisions regarding nondrug elements of treatment become interventions or manipulated independent variables that may, or

*Portions of this chapter are modified from A. K. Swonger, *Nursing Pharmacology.* Boston: Little, Brown, 1978.

may not, result in beneficial changes in the dependent variables. The dependent variables are, of course, the indicators of the patient's condition, both as regards the disease state and unrelated symptoms (side effects). It is not enough to assume that because a therapeutic intervention has succeeded in other patients it will necessarily benefit the present case, although the accumulated experience of many such cases constitutes the jumping-off point for the initial selection of treatment approaches. The clinical judgment of the medical team must be supported by careful appraisal, involving specific measurements and a well-planned and well-executed treatment protocol that incorporates features of experimental design. Only then will valid assessment of the efficacy of a given approach be possible. So far, only a small minority of patients are receiving treatment based on this experimental model of therapeutics.

Successful application of the experimental model of therapeutics depends on the extent to which three prerequisites are met: (1) accuracy of diagnosis; (2) knowledge and competence in the areas of psychopathology, psychopharmacology, and the psychological aspects of drug therapy; and (3) adequacy of the therapeutic design.

Diagnosis

Early in this book we stressed the importance of diagnosis in identifying the organic base of observed disturbed behavior. Differential diagnosis in psychiatry involves classifying patients into nosologic categories that are assumed to be related to both causes and appropriate cures of the "psychopathology." The differentiation of similar symptomatologies and histories can involve observations and decision procedures of some subtlety. It may be easy to mistake some patterns in the group of schizophrenias for the manic state in a manic-depressive disorder, and vice versa. The question of the general validity of such global classifications aside, the fine partitioning of symptomatology and syndromes is important to clinical psychopharmacology only insofar as there are demonstrable differences in the responses of persons in different diagnostic categories to different specified drugs or to agents of different drug classes.

The state of knowledge and the relative importance attached to particular distinctions are continuously shifting. At one time, clinicians employed neuroleptics with comparatively low sedating effects for "withdrawn schizophrenics" and the more sedating neuroleptics for more "active schizophrenics." The rationale for this has not survived replications of carefully controlled research, though it is probable that individual practices may still reflect this intuitively appealing idea.

The specificity of psychotropic drugs within a given class is low. Pharmaceutical manufacturers, in an effort to achieve product differentiation and capture markets, have frequently emphasized a degree of specificity and special effectiveness that the greater mass of research findings does not support. Furthermore, many drugs have novel, cross-class applications, where demonstrated effectiveness is not readily explainable in terms of the general theories appropriate to the drug class and the type of disorder. Neuroleptics may sometimes be effective in cases of depression. Certain antidepressants (doxepin and amitriptyline) have sometimes been found to be effective for relief of anxiety, as has the antiparkinsonian agent diphenhydramine. Unexpected specificity also occurs, as in the effectiveness of haloperidol in the treatment of the Gilles de la Tourette syndrome, which has led some psychopharmacologists to propose that new drugs be tested on a limited scale across many different applications, including "inappropriate" ones. All too often, screening practices uncover only new agents that greatly resemble established ones and fail to reveal potentially valuable pharmacologic strategies that are truly novel.

Some diagnostic distinctions are important, despite the general imprecision and obscurities we have alluded to. An example of a major differentiation problem is that between schizophrenic and manic-depressive syndromes. Neuroleptics may be effective in the manic phase of manic-depressive disorder. Prior to the advent of lithium therapy, chlorpromazine, haloperidol, and even reserpine were commonly used to treat mania. But lithium therapy does not seem to be useful in schizophrenia, even with a pronounced manic component. Patients with active, extroverted, achievement-oriented personalities, regardless of diagnosis, may do better without drugs than with them. With a person who is more accurately classified as schizophrenic, an antidepressant may actually exacerbate psychotic behavior. Other distinctions may also be important: the relative appropriateness of neuroleptics in chronic as opposed to acute or episodic schizophrenia or the importance of the endogenous-exogenous distinction in depressions.

Rational therapeutics presupposes an accurate diagnosis. Obviously, if the nature of the morbid condition is misunderstood, then much of the treatment effort will be misdirected. Beyond this self-evident observation, it should be realized that even if the diagnosis is accurate within the limitations of current psychiatric nosology, the restraints imposed by that nosology may be a serious handicap to understanding the patient's condition. For one thing, classification of psychiatric conditions is based primarily on presenting symptoms, which, in a sense, are the final or temporary results of the underlying disease. Different disease states may produce similar morbid symptoms, or a given disease state may lead to a variety of behavioral changes in different patients. Current diagnostic procedures tend to overemphasize overt manifestations and to underutilize etiologic distinctions. Another effect of diagnostic labeling is to create the illusion that the disease state is a fixed entity, while in fact it is dynamic over time and highly variable across patients. It is important that the psychotherapist retain an attitude that permits continual reevaluation and therapeutic adjustments.

One approach to diagnosis is the use of a "decision tree" (Fig. 8-1). This provides a systematic consideration of all possibilities through the application of established criteria of evaluation. Diagnosis by exclusion is not appropriate. Psychiatric diagnosis is reached by means of a clinical interview of the patient and supportive laboratory testing.

The major categories in the psychiatric nosology are: (1) organic brain syndrome; (2) psychoses; (3) affective disorders; (4) anxiety states; (5) other neuroses, nonpsychotic disorders, and personality disorders; and (6) disorders usually first noted in infancy, childhood, or adolescence. The usefulness of pharmacotherapy is largely confined to three of the categories: psychoses, affective disorders, and anxiety states (Table 8-1). In Chapter 2, we discussed organic brain syndrome and the limited application of drugs in that condition. Pharmacotherapy for "other nonpsychotic disorders" is largely limited to symptomatic relief of concomitant anxiety, depression, or psychophysiologic reactions (skin reactions, muscle tension or backache, bronchial spasms, migraine, hypertension, ulcers and other gastrointestinal reactions, sleep disturbances, or neurologic symptoms). A specialized drug application in this category is the use of antiandrogens (cyproterone in Europe and medroxyprogesterone in the United States) to suppress libido in paraphilias that are repeatedly expressed in antisocial behavior. The pharmacotherapy of disorders first evident in infancy, childhood, or adolescence is likewise limited to a few specific conditions, such as separation anxiety, Gilles de la Tourette's syndrome, functional enuresis, and attention-deficit disorders. Psychoses will be discussed in detail in Chapter 16, anxiety states in Chapter 17, and affective disorders in Chapters 18 and 19. For the time being, it might be well to clarify a few descriptive terms.

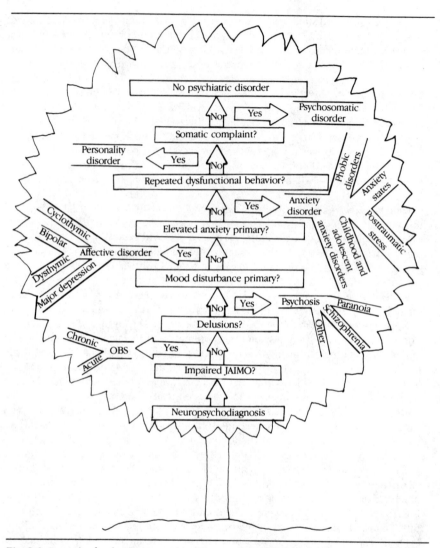

Fig. 8-1. *Example of a decision tree approach to psychiatric diagnosis. JAIMO, judgment, affect, intellect, memory, or orientation impaired; OBS, organic brain syndrome.*

The term *functional* is used to denote conditions for which the etiology is at the psychological level of organization. Historically, the term has been applied to all of the psychiatric disorders except organic brain syndrome. The distinction between *functional* and *organic* is losing a good deal of its value as it becomes apparent that schizophrenia and depression may often arise primarily at the organic level of organization. One could argue that endogenous depression is organic, while reactive depression is functional, but even that assertion may blur when the discussion turns to the possibility of organic predisposition to reactive depression or acute reactive psychoses. The term *reactive* can, however, be useful in specifying those conditions for which the etiology is largely or entirely at the psychological level of organization.

The terms *psychosis* and *neurosis* have narrowed in their application. The latter term has been largely abandoned in favor of *anxiety state* and subdesignations within that group and elsewhere in the nosology (see Table 8-1). The term *psychosis* may still be applied collectively to schizophrenia, paranoid disorders, and other psychotic conditions. But affective disorders are no longer distinguished as psychotic or neurotic in the third edition of the *Diagnostic and Statistical Manual* (DSM-III) of the American Psychiatric Association.

Acute and *chronic* are still useful terms for distinguishing conditions of short and long duration respectively, and they often also carry implications as to prognosis or rapidity of onset. The terms are applied especially to organic brain syndrome, psychoses, and anxiety states.

Knowledge Prerequisites

The second prerequisite for successful therapeutics is adequate knowledge of the psychiatric condition itself, of the drugs used for treatment, and of the psychological aspects of drug therapy, together with the ability to apply this knowledge in the treatment of the patient.

Knowledge of the Psychiatric Problem

A thorough understanding of the pathophysiology of the patient is of great importance to rational therapeutics. Knowledge of the etiology of the disease state is the foundation for developing and comprehending the therapeutic rationale. Often, the relationship between the action of a drug and the biochemical or physiologic deficits associated with the disease is at least tentatively understood and provides the rationale for the use of the drug.

Many psychiatric and neurologic disorders are progressive or pass through predictable stages. Even for diseases that are relatively uniform in a qualitative sense, the condition is dynamic in terms of severity. The psychotherapist who is aware of the dynamic characteristics of the disease in question is cognizant of the need to reevaluate continually the selection of drugs and the dosage regimen.

Another important feature of the interaction between disease state and drugs is the extent to which a given condition can be expected to respond to a given drug. Severe drug reactions often occur when a drug is being used for a condition that is only minimally responsive to that agent. This misuse of drugs can be avoided by adjusting expectations regarding efficacy to a level that is justified by the realities of clinical experience with the agent.

Knowledge of Drugs

The application of drug knowledge to the clinical setting begins with the evolution of the therapeutic rationale. As the plan develops, the physician at some point—and frequently at many points—must make a choice as to whether or not to use a drug and, if so, which one. Frequently, the difficult, but best, choice is to administer no drug or perhaps to give a placebo. Specific expectations as to the benefit to be derived from the drug should be established and criteria formulated for assessing the extent to which those expectations are indeed met. Drug prescriptions that are unnecessary or inappropriate are not merely nonefficacious but may also be responsible for producing toxic side effects or iatrogenic disorders. Moreover, such ill-conceived drug regimens

Table 8-1. Diagnostic categories for mental disorders

Diagnostic category	Type[a]	Incidence[b]	Sex ratio	Drug treatments
Organic mental disorders				
Dementias (includes chronic organic brain syndrome)	P/NP	++	F > M	Cerebral metabolic stimulants; other psychotropics
Delirium and other acute organic brain syndromes	P/NP	++	M = F	Varies with cause
Drug-induced				
Intoxication	NP	++	M > F	Various antagonists and symptomatic treatments
Withdrawal	P	++	M > F	
Toxic psychoses	P	+	M > F	
Psychotic disorders				
Schizophrenia	P	+++	M > F	Neuroleptics
Paranoid disorders	P	R	M > F	Neuroleptics
Other[c]	P	++	?	Neuroleptics
Affective disorders				
Major				
Bipolar	P	+	M = F	Lithium
Major depression	P	+++	F > M	Antidepressants
Other				
Cyclothymic disorder	N	+	F > M	Lithium
Dysthymic disorder	N	++	F > M	Anxiolytics, neuroleptics, antidepressants
Anxiety disorders				
Phobias	N	R/C	F > M	Barbiturates (adjunctive); MAO inhibitors
Panic disorder	N	+	F >> M	Antidepressants
Generalized anxiety disorder	N	++	F > M	Anxiolytics
Obsessive-compulsive disorder	N	R	M = F	Anxiolytics, L-tryptophan, trazodone
Posttraumatic stress disorder	N	Situational	?	Anxiolytics
Other nonpsychotic disorders				
Somatoform disorders[d]	N	+	F > M	None
Dissociative disorders[e]	N	R	F > M	None

Psychosexual disorders				
Gender identity disorders	N	R	?	None
Paraphilias[f]	N	R	M>>F	Antiandrogens
Psychosexual dysfunctions	N	R/C	Varies	None
Substance use disorders[g]	NP	+++	Varies	Rarely (e.g., methadone)
Disorders of impulse control[h]	NP	+	Varies	None
Factitious disorders	NP	R	M>F	None
Adjustment disorders[i]	NP	++	?	None
Psychosomatic disorders[j]	NP	(+++)	Varies	Various
Personality disorders[k]	PD	+++*	Varies	None
V codes[l]	O	+++	Varies	None
Disorders first evident in infancy, childhood, or adolescence				
Major brain dysfunctions				
Mental retardation	NP	++	M>F	No effective treatment; thioridazine and other psychotropics for symptom control
Autism and other pervasive developmental disorders	P	+	M>>F	
Minimal brain dysfunctions				
Attention deficit disorders	NP	++	M>>F	Stimulants
Specific developmental disorders[m]	NP	+++	M>F	None
Anxiety disorders				
Separation anxiety	N	R	M>F	Antidepressants
Overanxious disorder	N	++	M>F	Anxiolytics
Personality disorders				
Avoidant disorder	PD	R	F>M	None
Conduct disorder	PD	+++	M>>F	Phenothiazines
Aggressive, undersocialized				None
Unaggressive, undersocialized				None
Socialized				None
Other[n]	PD	++	Varies	None

Table 8-1 (continued)

Diagnostic category	Type[a]	Incidence[b]	Sex ratio	Drug treatments
Disorders with physical manifestations				
Eating disorders				
Anorexia nervosa	NP	+	F>>M	Cyproheptadine or chlorpromazine
Bulimia	NP	++	F>M	Anorexics
Pica	NP	R	M=F	None
Motor disorders				
Gilles de la Tourette's syndrome	NP	R	M>F	Haloperidol
Tics	NP	R/C	M>F	Diazepam or haloperidol
Speech disorders				
Stuttering	NP	+	M>>F	None
Elective mutism	PD	R	F>M	None
Functional enuresis	NP	+	M>F	Imipramine

[a]Includes psychosis (P); neurosis (N); nonpsychotic disorders not classified as neuroses (NP); personality disorders (PD); conditions not due to a mental disorder (O).

[b]A condition is designated rare (R) when it occurs in <1.5% of the presenting mental health population, adult or minor, as appropriate; + indicates occurrence in 1.5–4%; ++ indicates occurrence in 5–15%; +++ indicates occurrence in >15%; (+++) indicates common occurrence but presentation as a physical disorder; R/C indicates a disorder that is rarely of clinical significance but is probably common in the overall population.

[c]Includes schizophreniform disorder, brief reactive psychosis, and schizoaffective disorder.

[d]Includes somatization and conversion disorders, psychogenic pain, and hypochondriasis.

[e]Includes psychogenic amnesias or fugues, multiple personalities, and depersonalization disorder.

[f]Fetishism, pedophilia, and voyeurism, for example.

[g]Includes abuse or dependence. Men more commonly abuse alcohol and street drugs including heroin/morphine, methadone, PCP, marijuana, methaqualone, and cocaine. Women more often abuse drugs obtained legally, by prescription or over-the-counter, including benzodiazepines, antidepressants, nonnarcotic analgesics, propoxyphen, barbiturates, and meprobamate.

[h]Pathologic gambling (M>F), kleptomania (F>M), and pyromania (M>F), for example.

[i]Maladaptive reactions to identifiable psychosocial stressors.

[j]Tension and migraine headaches, asthma, acne, cardiac arrhythmias, angina, sacroiliac pain, ulcers, and gastrointestinal disturbances, for example.

[k]Includes paranoid, schizoid, schizotypal, histrionic, narcissistic, antisocial, borderline, avoidant, dependent, compulsive, or passive-aggressive personalities.

[l]Conditions not attributable to a mental disorder that are focuses of attention or treatment: malingering; borderline intellectual functioning; adult antisocial behavior; academic or occupational problems; uncomplicated bereavement; noncompliance with medical treatment; phase-of-life problem; marital or parent-child problem; other family or interpersonal problems.

[m]Developmental arithmetic, language, and reading disorders, for example.

[n]Includes reactive attachment disorder, schizoid disorder, oppositional disorder, and identity disorder.

may prolong or worsen certain disease states or result in failure to make use of more effective therapeutic approaches. About 5 percent of hospital admissions may be attributable to hypersensitivity reactions to drugs. Approximately one in four inpatients suffers a hypersensitivity reaction during the hospital stay.

Identification of Psychiatric Side Effects

The vast majority (about 80 percent) of adverse reactions to drugs are predictable, and many of these are also avoidable. The psychotherapist who is aware of the potential adverse reactions to psychotropic drugs will be able to assess the influence of these reactions on the overall clinical picture. For that reason, heavy emphasis is placed on the psychiatric side effects of drugs throughout this book.

Knowledge of Drug Actions and Interactions

General Considerations

When a drug is to be added to a preexisting therapeutic regimen, the requirements for establishing a sound therapeutic rationale must not be relaxed. What is the objective of the addition? How is the efficacy of the new drug to be assessed? What is the rationale for use of the drug for this condition? What are the expected benefits, and how do they compare with the expected risks? As regards the risks of adding a second or third or nth drug, one must consider not only the composite list of adverse drug reactions but also the possibility of drug interactions. The use of drug combinations increases the likelihood of significant adverse reactions and taxes the limits of the therapist's knowledge. The psychotherapist should become familiar not only with multiple lists of possible adverse reactions but also with the known drug interactions involving these substances.

Another sort of interaction is the effect of drugs on coexisting medical conditions. For example, the presence of renal disease is critically important in lithium administration, because lithium is cleared from the body largely by the kidney. On the other hand, neuroleptics, tricyclic antidepressants, and benzodiazepines are disposed of largely by liver metabolism, and thus liver disease would increase toxicity of these compounds (Table 8-2).

Many adverse reactions to drugs develop only after their long-term use. Therefore, risk factors should be considered not only in the decision whether or not to initiate drug therapy but also in each subsequent decision to continue treatment. All too often, the decision to continue treatment is made passively. Rational therapeutics dictates that a plan be established, not only as regards expectations and evaluation of efficacy when drug treatment is instituted, but also regarding the criteria for terminating long-term treatment of diseases that undergo partial or complete remission. For example, patients with conditions such as anxiety, depression, schizophrenia, and epilepsy are frequently subjected to drug therapy of indeterminate duration. Little thought is given in many instances to termination of the drug regimen.

Polypharmacy: Pros and Cons

Polypharmacy refers to the simultaneous use of a number of agents belonging either to the same or different classes. The extent to which this occurs among psychiatric patients is very surprising. Ayd [1] reports that the majority of institutionalized psychiatric patients are receiving one or more neuroleptics plus one or more antidepressants, an antiparkinsonian drug, one or more anxiolytics, and a sedative-hypnotic. The out-

Table 8-2. *Central nervous system drugs in relation to liver function*

Prolonged half-life in liver disease
  Barbiturates
  Diazepam and chlordiazepoxide (oxazepam preferred)
  Isoniazid
  Meprobamate
  Narcotics (morphine, meperidine, propoxyphene, pentazocine)
  Phenytoin
  Tricyclic antidepressants (desipramine, nortriptyline)
May cause acute hepatitis
  Acetaminophen
  Ethanol
  Monoamine oxidase inhibitors
  Phenytoin
  Salicylates
May cause cirrhosis
  Ethanol
May cause cholestasis
  Butyrophenones
  Ibuprofen
  Phenothiazines
  Tricyclic antidepressants
May cause liver failure
  Valproic acid

patient, in general, is given fewer prescription drugs but adds to them a variety of self-medications.

It is certain that polypharmacy is practiced far beyond the extent dictated by rational considerations. The result of polypharmacy can be (1) an inability to assess properly the action of any drug independently, (2) a plethora of side effects of equally indeterminate origin, and (3) numerous drug interactions not all clearly understood or elucidated at this time. Moreover, the likelihood of generating an iatrogenic disorder whose cause cannot be determined is greatly increased when many drugs are utilized indiscriminately. Because of these considerations, the rule dictated by prudence is that *a combination of drugs should not be prescribed unless a clear rationale for such a regimen is first established.*

In general, valid rationales for employing more than one agent fall into one of four categories: (1) When a patient exhibits more than one distinct pathologic condition, e.g., epilepsy and schizophrenia; (2) when treatment is essentially symptomatic, i.e., different agents may be required for different symptoms (e.g., levodopa for akinesia and trihexyphenidyl for tremors in parkinsonism); (3) when two therapeutically similar and additive agents have differing, noninteractive side effects (e.g., oxazolidones and succinimides in petit mal); and (4) when the use of one drug increases the bioavailability of another (e.g., carbidopa and levodopa). The use of agents to treat the side effects of other agents, especially prophylactically, is a doubtful practice.

Knowledge of Psychological Factors in Drug Response

Knowledge of all the biologic aspects of drug action will not by itself ensure effectiveness in dealing with patients. Consideration must be given to the psychological factors that contribute to drug response. The psychotherapist, through interactions with the patient, should seek to maximize the effectiveness of the therapeutic process as a whole and the efficacy of the drug aspects of therapy specifically. Increasingly, the science of pharmacology is being forced to acknowledge the importance of personal and social variables in determining drug response.

Placebo Effect

Perhaps the most thoroughly documented example of how psychological elements intrude into the realm of drug therapy is the so-called placebo effect. It is well established that individuals experience a wide range of beneficial or adverse "effects," or both, when given a capsule, tablet, or liquid that they believe to be an active drug but, in fact, is an inert substance, or placebo. The patient's expectations, past experiences, and anxieties—in other words, his or her psychological set—all contribute to the reaction to a placebo. Similarly, the total reaction to an active drug involves not only the specific, physiologic effects of the drug but also its psychological, placebo effects. This has numerous implications for the psychotherapist. To begin with, an accurate evaluation of drug effects must take into account, by means of appropriate experimental design, that not all apparent changes are pharmacologic effects of the drug. Some effort must be made to control for placebo effects.

Second, the therapist must understand that every communication, verbal and nonverbal, has special meaning to the patient, who is often in an emotional state. The therapist's behavior contributes substantially to the patient's psychological set and attitudes toward the drug and nondrug treatment procedures. Every instruction, inquiry, observation, and offhand comment should be moderated by sensitivity to its possible impact on the patient and his or her responsiveness to the therapeutic plan. The therapist should have a keen perception of the feelings of the patient.

A third ramification of the placebo effect is the use of placebo therapy in certain instances. If a patient insists on drug treatment for a condition that either requires none or for which no suitable drug treatment is known, administration of a placebo may be in order. When a placebo is used, the need for a therapeutic rationale for initiation and termination of treatment is no less important than if an active drug were used.

Psychological Toxicity

Another psychological aspect of drug response is "psychological toxicity." When the benefit-risk ratio for a drug is assessed, the risk factor should include the drug's negative effects on the patient's condition and the associated need for hospitalization; namely, separation from loved ones, loss of self-esteem or sense of personal attractiveness, or other changes in life circumstances associated specifically with administration of the drug. The impact of prolonged hospitalization on psychological status is enormous and may, in many patients, exceed that of the combined contributions of the disease state itself and the effects of drugs.

Compliance and Noncompliance

Compliance is another crucially important way in which psychological factors intervene in drug therapy. More often than not, outpatients do not follow prescriptions precisely;

they either omit doses, take incorrect amounts, or improperly space their medications. For conditions such as tuberculosis or depression, where medications have notoriously discomforting side effects, noncompliance can reach astonishing proportions. The likelihood that a given patient is actually complying with his dose regimen cannot be accurately assessed without careful, objective determination. Several studies have shown that neither the physician's judgment as to the patient's degree of compliance nor the patient's verbal report correlates with noncompliance determined objectively [2, 6].

Moreover, noncompliance is not easy to predict. Studies of patient variables such as education, attitudes, sex, age, and disease state have failed to provide consistent insights into all the factors that lead to noncompliance. However, three factors that do seem important are: (1) the number of necessary drugs, (2) the frequency with which the patient must take the drug(s), and (3) the complexity of the drug-taking procedure. Small numbers of drugs, the use of once-a-day regimens, and simplicity of instructions all improve compliance. Even inpatients frequently fail to follow drug regimens reliably, partly because of errors on the part of the staff. Clinical practice must take into account that patients often do not take even aspirin or penicillin as directed. Drugs of marginal value to the overall therapeutic program should be eliminated, and instructions should be simplified.

As patients begin to feel better, they become less motivated to take medication. Sometimes the failure to complete a course of drug therapy is of little significance; at other times, it is of grave importance. In either case, the clinician must be aware that patients frequently do not follow directions and should view the reappearance of symptoms or even absence of side effects as a warning flag that the patient may have ceased taking his or her medication. Noncompliance should be examined routinely as part of the therapeutic plan.

Social Variables

Sociocultural factors in the patient's background, as well as the setting in which the drug is prescribed and administered, affect the outcome in drug therapy. In general, drug-placebo differences prove to be greater among patients of lesser education and in lower socioeconomic levels. The patients who do best on drugs are also found to be older, more likely to have been treated with drugs in the past, and to have more chronic symptoms. Patients with "square" or traditional life-styles, politics, and attitudes are likely to do better on drugs than patients from more "hip" backgrounds. As drug-placebo differences tend to be small for many psychotropics, perhaps a traditional, favorable mind set of "a drug for every discomfort" is needed to enhance the purely pharmacologic action. In all cases it should be remembered that underlying factors in patient response to drugs—intellectual abilities, introspectiveness, and preferred coping behavior, among others—are only roughly correlated with socioeconomic status and other "shorthand" variables employed in most outcome studies.

A laboratory setting or a clinic with a distinctly experimental atmosphere can reduce the success of drug treatment with certain patients. When other influences are ruled out, it seems that the greatest success with drug therapy occurs in charity clinics, the least success in private psychiatric hospitals, with general practice falling somewhere in between.

It has long been known that patients of lower socioeconomic status receive different mental health care than those from a higher status. One difference is that psychotherapy is less available to poorer, less educated patients. Traditional therapy has often been directed to the more verbal and articulate patients, to those with more time and money to invest in a long course of psychotherapy. Psychotherapy resources tend to be concentrated on those who appear to benefit the most from them, which may simply be those whose verbal and interpersonal styles conform sufficiently closely to the models that formed the initial paradigm of a particular school of therapy. Thus poorer, less educated patients have in the past been more likely to be given perfunctory treatment, which often translates into "drugs."

The intriguing conclusion from studies in which sociocultural factors have been a variable is that poor, less educated patients may often be served better by drug therapy (as well as by such practical interventions as those of social workers in their classic role) than by many forms of psychotherapy. The major determinant of this is probably patient expectation regarding drug treatment: whether drugs are desired and whether the patient expects them to help.

Patient Variables

Drugs, particular drugs, and drug-taking mean different things to different people. Effective clinical psychopharmacology must take into account the patient and the personal meanings he or she attributes to things, not just the presenting symptomatology. Thus, patients who expect drug therapy and think that emotional problems should be cured by a physician's actions rather than their own and who have had positive past experiences with psychotropic medication will do better on drug therapy. Such people are more likely to come from a lower socioeconomic level than from a higher one.

It has been suggested that drugs may be contraindicated where they might interact unfavorably with important imagery of the patient [18]. Men with serious doubts about their masculinity and who hold a stereotyped view of passivity as being feminine may see drugs, especially neuroleptics and sedative-hypnotics, as emasculating. This may be most true of men who use intellectual or motor activity or social outgoingness as major elements of personal style or as coping mechanisms. Along similar lines, it seems likely that a highly independent woman who views passivity as stereotypically feminine and unliberated could see some drugs as forcing her back into a mold from which she had escaped.

Very independent persons with very intensive concern for issues of dependence and independence may be poor candidates for "becoming dependent on a drug." In some, drugs would aid and abet a regressive search for dependence, and in others they would induce an extreme reaction against the induced dependence.

People inordinately concerned with body image and the integrity of the body or who might see drugs as either an assault or seduction may present problems when drug therapy is chosen. Patients with a mystical or magical view of the world would also present a problem.

Hollister [8] describes differences in the responses to anxiolytics of "doers" compared with those characterized as "thinkers." Doers, who are extroverted and physically active, may actually become more anxious on an antianxiety drug, apparently because the drug interferes somewhat with a preferred mode of coping with stress, that is, through immersion in activity and relationships. Thinkers, who by contrast are described as tending to be more intellectual, passive, and esthetically oriented, become less anxious when medicated.

A related finding by Rappaport [16] suggests that even when the problem is an acute psychotic episode, certain people may do substantially better without drugs. In his double-blind study of chlorpromazine administered to young schizophrenic males hospitalized for their first or second acute episode, those receiving drugs improved more rapidly at first, while the men given placebos showed greater and more stable long-term gains. Those who benefited most from not receiving medication had been better adjusted prior to the episode and showed more bizarre paranoid symptoms. Apparently medication interfered with their own healthy, though bizarre, struggles to deal with their troubles.

The usefulness of a drug may be dramatically altered by the importance to the patient of the symptom that is ameliorated. The complete removal of a symptom that the patient considers to be of no consequence will be seen by him or her as a failure in treatment, while modest improvement in something given inordinate importance by the patient may be perceived by him or her as an instant cure. Even the latter may be problematical for clinical work, for it may lead to premature termination of therapy by the now "cured" client. An opposite sort of interaction with symptoms of great import to the patient may account for some unusual cases of "adverse reactions," such as paradoxical rage reactions with an agent expected to produce a calming effect.

The meaning to the patient of adverse reactions and side effects may be as important in determining the clinical outcome as the "main" effects of a drug. For some patients, interference with cognitive intellectual functioning could be very anxiety-producing, while for others, autonomic and extrapyramidal motor effects could be more distressing. There may be class differences in this respect. Lower-class patients may complain less about drowsiness from phenobarbital and more about akathisia on fluphenazine than middle- and upper-class patients. Impotence, which can occur as a side effect of neuroleptics, is likely to be of major personal significance to many patients. Elderly patients, perhaps especially those in the early stages of the organic brain syndrome (Chap. 2), may find side effects particularly frightening and become increasingly confused.

Therapist Variables

It is not surprising that the attitude and technique of the physician or psychotherapist can increase or decrease the effectiveness of drug therapy. Regardless of the mode of treatment, with or without drugs, the degree of "therapist comfort" with an assigned treatment method is positively correlated with outcome [19].

In a famous study by Uhlenhuth et al. [20], patients whose physicians took an "experimental" stance, maintaining a skeptical approach to a drug, improved less than patients whose physicians maintained a positive, hopeful, "therapeutic" stance regarding the drug. Placebo responses are also greater with the latter type of physician.

The specific schooling of the therapist or psychiatrist may influence the outcome of drug therapy [7]. Where the physician has been trained in a stance that is traditional, authoritarian, and remote, feedback from the patient may be blocked. The patient may hesitate to communicate his or her reactions or lack of reactions to drugs or to complain of side effects, or to announce discontinuance. In its exaggerated form, this master-slave relationship invites certain resistances that interfere with effective drug therapy.

More "social" and interpersonally oriented therapists have their problems, too, as they are prone to interpret drugs as a sign of the failure of their approach. The newer "humanistic" therapists and the behavior therapists have all but ignored drugs as an adjunct to psychotherapy.

Rickels and Cattell [17] divided therapists into two personality types: the type I therapist, who is authoritarian and extroverted, and the type II therapist, who is low in authoritarianism and more introverted. Testing placebo versus drug with both types, they found that the personality of the psychiatrist was the dominant factor in early progress (at 2 weeks). By 4 weeks, drug-placebo differences were the determining factor, and after 6 weeks the major effects were interactive. Others have reported that patient-therapist interactive effects on drug-placebo differences increase with time. In the long run, the match between therapist and patient determines the outcome. It would appear that when both patient and therapist share a preference for and belief in the appropriateness of drug therapy, psychotherapy has little long-term effect; conversely, when a psychotherapeutic orientation is shared, drugs are irrelevant.

Feedback effects are possible when the patient's complaint and the therapist's concerns escalate a problem. Paranoid behavior on the part of the patient can generate anger, whether conscious or not, in the physician. Control attempts by the physician are met with resistance by the patient. Medication becomes an instrument of control, usually in the perceptions of both patient and physician. In the ensuing power struggle, dosages administered have sometimes been escalated to astronomical proportions [7].

An almost reverse situation is the one in which the physician becomes depressed and discouraged at the lack of progress in the depressed and discouraged patient, consequently terminating or switching drug therapy prematurely, before an adequate trial has taken place. In the extreme, the disappointed physician gives up and lets the patient go.

In yet another type of situation, drugs may be the method by which the physician keeps at a distance a patient whom he or she does not like or is afraid of. The patient, sensing and correctly interpreting the interpersonal meaning of the drug, concludes that he or she is once again unwanted, unworthy, and so on. Or the patient may retaliate, secretly refusing the token of "rejection" by failing to follow the drug regimen.

Adequacy of the Therapeutic Design

After an accurate diagnosis has been made, and all aspects of drug therapy are understood, a third prerequisite for rational therapeutics must be addressed, namely, the necessity for a well-designed therapeutic plan. If each instance of medical intervention is to be considered an experiment in therapeutics, then a systemic program to evaluate the impact of various measures must be undertaken. To be successful, the evaluation procedure requires: (1) anticipation of reactions (both therapeutic and adverse), (2) methodical data collection, and (3) a design that controls for bias, expectations, placebo reactions, and the influence of variables other than the experimental one(s).

Anticipation of Drug Effects

Here, a few observations might be made. The aim of using a given drug should be defined as specifically as possible. Furthermore, when a second or third drug is added to an existing regimen, the expectations for each should also be delineated. In each case, the objective should be realistic and should take into account the established efficacy and limitations of the drug, since exaggerated expectations are frequently the preamble to adverse drug reactions. Consideration should also be given to the possible latency between drug administration and onset of therapeutic effectiveness.

Anticipation of adverse reactions requires sound knowledge of the pharmacology of the drugs utilized and of the established frequency of occurrence of various side effects. It should also take into account the age and sex of the patient, aspects of the disease state that modify drug toxicity, the psychological set of the patient, the route and rate of introduction of the drug, and so forth. When a drug has been given over a prolonged period, the clinician must not forget to anticipate the occurrence of late-developing side effects, such as parkinsonism symptoms in neuroleptic therapy.

Drug Strategy

Criteria for beginning, continuing, and discontinuing drug treatment, as well as for determining the size, frequency, and number of doses, should be established in terms of anticipated therapeutic effects and adverse reactions. Together, these factors determine what is known as the *drug strategy.*

There is considerable variation in the pattern of drug dosage—between classes, sometimes within a drug class, and definitely from physician to physician. For example, the tricyclic antidepressants (such as amitriptyline) are generally started in a standard dosage and gradually increased until the desired degree of symptom amelioration has been achieved. By contrast, therapy with monoamine oxidase (MAO) inhibitors, such as isocarboxazid and phenelzine, is more often initiated with a large dose that is rapidly reduced to a maintenance level.

Determining the Optimal Dosage

Adverse reactions usually limit the maximum therapeutic dose that can be given. The optimum dose strikes a balance between therapeutic effects and adverse effects. Titration refers to the balancing of drug dose against symptoms. Typically, the dose is tested against a certain level of improvement, against the appearance of unacceptable side effects, or against other well-established, though perhaps unrelated, pharmacologic actions, such as signs of sympathetic inhibition (e.g., hypotension, decreased heart rate) with MAO inhibitors. The correct dose is determined in one of two ways. In one method, doses are gradually increased to a level just below that at which adverse side effects occur. This is the most common strategy with neuroleptics. Should unacceptably severe side effects develop before adequate improvement has been achieved, the usual practice is to switch to another drug. In the second method, doses are gradually decreased to a level just above that at which the presenting symptoms reappear. The smallest dose required to maintain the patient in a comparatively symptom-free state is then the correct dose. Since the actions and efficacy of drugs may be different in early and late treatment, both upward and downward gradings may be required in the same course of therapy with one drug. Some drugs are correctly used only for short-term treatments. For example, hypnotics are rarely useful for more than a few weeks of daily administration. Tolerance may develop faster to one effect of a drug than to another. Side effects, which are of major importance in short-term or outpatient use, may decrease or assume less importance with prolonged treatment or in the hospital setting.

Plasma levels of drugs may vary greatly from individual to individual. For example, plasma levels of meprobamate may vary by a factor of 3 among patients given identical doses; with diazepam, by a factor of up to 8. Ideally, the physician would titrate drug dose against plasma concentration as well as against side effects, but for many agents, the necessary laboratory test procedures are too difficult. One exception is lithium, which is frequently titrated against blood concentration. Indications for monitoring plasma levels of a drug are listed in Table 8-3.

Termination of Drug Therapy

Termination of drug therapy is an issue that has been given too little attention in the literature. More often than not, neither clinicians nor pharmacologists have established

Table 8-3. *Indications for monitoring plasma levels of drugs*

1. The relationship between the dose administered and plasma levels is poor
2. The relationship between plasma levels and clinical response is good
3. The drug is being used prophylactically, so that changes in target symptoms are not easy to measure
4. The therapeutic range is narrow; the difference between the therapeutic and toxic blood levels is small
5. Overuse or lack of compliance is suspected
6. Factors modifying normal pharmacokinetics are suspected or known to be present (e.g., tolerance, renal or kidney disease, drug interactions)

clear-cut criteria for termination. Often, there exists a tacit and unquestioned assumption of indefinite continuation. Such an assumption may be reasonable in the case of control of severe epileptic seizures but is of dubious value in the treatment of anxiety. When multiple-drug regimens are used, drug interactions leading to adverse reactions should be reviewed.

Methodical Evaluation of Outcome

Once expectations have been established, a plan for objective measurement of the extent to which those expectations are met must be devised. Too often, therapists rely on clinical impressions as the sole means of assessing drug reactions. Clinical impressions are a poor substitute for systematic evaluation based on objective measures.

Elements of Experimental Design for Drug Testing

On testing a new treatment in a clinical trial, the effect of the treatment is evaluated in a number of patients, called the sample. The selection and size of the sample are important considerations. Thus, the sample of patients should be selected in such a way that the results can be generalized to the larger population of patients having the disease condition in question. Also, where possible, the sample size should be large enough to yield convincing results on statistical evaluation of the data.

When the principles of experimental design are applied to the therapeutic setting, either in a clinical trial or in an individual patient, the *sequential design* is often the most appropriate. In this approach, a given treatment is compared with an alternative one (in a clinical trial) or measured against specific expectations (in an individual patient). The end point of the treatment in question is not a fixed point in time but rather any time at which the difference between the observed effects and the comparison treatment or the criterion expectations exceed(s) a predetermined limit. This approach permits a greater degree of flexibility and discontinuation of treatments that lack efficacy or that involve excessive adverse reactions.

In assessing the efficacy of drug treatment by means of a clinical trial, the influence of both extraneous variables and bias must be controlled for. When therapy is to be administered to a single patient, it is not possible to control for these influences adequately, but every effort must be made to minimize their impact on the outcome of the experimental treatment. In a clinical trial, the contribution of extraneous variables is assessed by use of a control group of patients that does not differ systematically from the therapeutic group except that members of the group are given a placebo or a comparison drug of known efficacy.

One method used to avoid systematic nonequivalency of comparison groups is random assignment. Patients are assigned by random means to one or another group in the study. In this way, the influence of extraneous variables will be approximately equivalent in the therapeutic group and control group. Therefore, any significant difference in response to treatment can be attributed to the difference in drug regimens.

When the efficacy of a treatment in a single patient is being evaluated, the clinician must bear in mind that changes in the patient's condition may be attributable to many factors other than drug treatment. For example, the psychiatric condition may spontaneously improve or worsen, the patient may experience placebo reactions, or uncontrolled changes in the environment may have an effect.

The effect of bias is minimized in a clinical trial by use of the double-blind technique. In this procedure, neither the patient nor the treatment evaluator is aware of the nature of the patient's treatment. As a result, the influence of the patient's expectations, as well as any bias on the part of the evaluator, will not be distributed systematically to one group or the other but rather will fall more or less uniformly upon both groups. The influence of bias and expectation in the assessment of drug treatment in a single patient cannot be reliably eliminated. However, reliance on objective measures and a conscientious evaluative procedure can reduce somewhat the impact of bias on therapeutic decision-making.

To summarize: Drug therapy is an important component of the overall psychotherapeutic plan. Rational drug therapy for psychiatric disorders depends on (1) accurate diagnosis, (2) the application of knowledge in the areas of psychopathology, psychopharmacology, and the psychological aspects of drug therapy, and (3) sound therapeutic design. The psychotherapist who has developed a thorough understanding of pharmacotherapy as it relates to psychiatric disorders will be in a position to interrelate the drug and nondrug components of treatment effectively.

Selected References and Further Readings

1. Ayd, F. J., Jr. Once-a-day neuroleptic and tricyclic antidepressant therapy. *Int. Drug Ther. Newslett.* 7:33–40, 1972.
2. Caron, H., and Roth, H. Patients' cooperation with a medical regimen. Difficulties in identifying the noncooperator. *J.A.M.A.* 203:922–926, 1968.
3. Davis, J. M. Efficacy of tranquilizing and antidepressant drugs. *Arch. Gen. Psychiatry* 13:552–572, 1965.
4. DiMascio, A. Dosage Scheduling. In A. DiMascio and R. I. Shader (Eds.), *Clinical Handbook of Psychopharmacology.* New York: Science House, 1970.
5. Freeman, H. The Utility of Psychotropic Drug Combinations. In A. DiMascio and R. I. Shader (Eds.), *Clinical Handbook of Psychopharmacology.* New York: Science House, 1970.
6. Gordis, L., Markowitz, M., and Lilienfeld, A. The inaccuracy in using interviews to estimate patient reliability in taking medications at home. *Med. Care* 7:49–54, 1969.
7. Havens, L. L. Interaction of Drug Administration with Psychotherapy. In A. DiMascio and R. I. Shader (Eds.), *Clinical Handbook of Psychopharmacology.* New York: Science House, 1970.
8. Hollister, L. E. Uses of psychotherapeutic drugs. *Ann. Intern. Med.* 79:88–98, 1973.
9. Hollister, L. E. Psychiatric Disorders. In K. L. Melmon and H. F. Morrelli (Eds.), *Clinical Pharmacology* (2nd ed.). New York: Macmillan, 1978.
10. Johnson, G., and Gershon, S. Differential Response to Psychotropic Drugs. In D. F. Klein and R. Gittelman-Klein (Eds.), *Progress in Psychiatric Drug Treatment.* New York: Brunner/Mazel, 1975.
11. Klein, D. F. Drug Therapy as a Means of Syndromal Identification and Nosological Revision. In J. O. Cole et al. (Eds.), *Psychopathology and Psychotherapy.* Baltimore: Johns Hopkins University Press, 1973.

12. Klerman, G. L., Paykel, E. S., and Prusoff, B. Antidepressant Drugs and Clinical Psychopathology. In J. O. Cole et al. (Eds.), *Psychopathology and Psychopharmacology.* Baltimore: Johns Hopkins University Press, 1973.
13. Melman, K., and Morrelli, H. (Eds.). *Clinical Pharmacology* (2nd ed.). New York: Macmillan, 1978.
14. Overall, J. E., Henry, B. W., Markett, J. R., and Emken, R. L. Decisions about drug therapy. *Arch. Gen. Psychiatry* 26:140–144, 1972.
15. Paykel, E. S., Klerman, G. L., DiMascio, A., Weissman, M. M., and Prusoff, B. A. Maintenance Antidepressants, Psychotherapy, Symptoms, and Social Function. In J. O. Cole et al. (Eds.), *Psychopathology and Psychopharmacology.* Baltimore: Johns Hopkins University Press, 1973.
16. Rappaport, M. Drugs and schizophrenia. *Behav. Today* 5:252–253, 1974.
17. Rickels, K., and Cattell, R. B. Drugs and Placebo Response as a Function of Doctor and Patient Type. In P. R. May and J. R. Wittenborn (Eds.), *Psychotropic Drug Response.* Springfield, Ill.: Thomas, 1969.
18. Sarwer-Foner, G. J. Psychodynamics of Psychotropic Medication: An Overview. In J. O. Cole et al. (Eds.), *Psychopathology and Psychopharmacology.* Baltimore: Johns Hopkins University Press, 1973.
19. Tuma, A. H., and May, P. R. The Effect of Therapist Attitude on Outcome of Drug Treatment and Other Therapies in Schizophrenia. In P. R. May and J. R. Wittenborn (Eds.), *Psychotropic Drug Response.* Springfield, Ill.: Thomas, 1969.
20. Uhlenhuth, E. H., Duncan, D. B., and Park, L. C. Some Non-pharmacologic Modifiers of the Response to Imipramine in Depressed Psychoneurotic Out-patients: A Confirmatory Study. In P. R. May and J. R. Wittenborn (Eds.), *Psychotropic Drug Response.* Springfield, Ill.: Thomas, 1969.
21. Wing, J. K., Leff, J., and Hirsch, S. Preventive Treatment of Schizophrenia: Some Theoretical and Methodological Issues. In J. O. Cole et al. (Eds.), *Psychopathology and Psychopharmacology.* Baltimore: Johns Hopkins University Press, 1973.

Drug
Abuse
9

Drug Abuse: What Is It?

Drug abuse is a prism of many faces. The light we cast on it emerges at an angle that depends as much on the orientation of the person casting the light as on the prism itself. The definition we prefer is functionalistic: Drug abuse is the self-administration of a chemical substance to an extent that significantly impairs the user's physical or mental health or ability to function in a social context. Thus, cigarette smoking is drug abuse. A smoker is killing himself or herself just as surely, if less rapidly, as a "speed freak" and for essentially the same reason—to get a lift from the drug. Alcohol, although it is legal, remains far and away the number one drug abuse problem in America no matter how you evaluate it—in terms of economic loss, numbers afflicted, physiologic damage, family disruption, or psychological impact. It is clear, therefore, that drug abuse cannot be defined simply in terms of legal versus illegal or even culturally acceptable versus unacceptable.

The definition of *abuse* used in the *Diagnostic and Statistical Manual* (DSM-III) of the American Psychiatric Association is a disappointing one. The three criteria employed in that source are (1) pattern of pathologic use, (2) impairment in social or occupational functioning, and (3) duration of at least 1 month. We would take issue with two points: the emphasis on social costs to the exclusion of considerations of personal well-being (psychological and physical health, financial well-being) and the dubious criterion of at least 1 month's duration. A person who becomes intoxicated on just one night a year and then drives recklessly is, in our view, a drug abuser. The DSM-III definition of *dependence* is likewise marred by acceptance of either tolerance or withdrawal as a basis for establishing the presence of physical dependence. We will show that the potential for withdrawal symptoms, but not tolerance alone, is a sufficient basis for establishing the presence of drug dependence.

A functionalistic definition and approach to drug abuse is especially useful to the psychotherapist who should be able to recognize common psychological, interpersonal, and social elements in cigarette smoking, the use of coffee and tea, and the illicit use of "uppers," along with the difference in the abuse patterns for each drug. He or she should recognize patterns caused by the drug and its action as well as patterns attributable to individual differences. The psychotherapist should also see the mediating social values. In reality, drug abuse is many different things, depending on the individual abuser, the drug abused, and the social milieu in which the abuse occurs. Subsequent sections of this chapter will deal with some of the factors that contribute to the varieties of drug abuse problems, with special emphasis on implications for the psychotherapist.

Pharmacologic Aspects of Drug Abuse

Tolerance

Tolerance is said to occur when the effect of a given dose of a drug diminishes on repeated administration. Another way of saying the same thing is that the dose must be increased in successive applications to maintain a given level of response. The term *tolerance* is reserved for diminished responsiveness occurring on a time scale in the order of hours or days and should not be identified with another pharmacologic phenomenon, tachyphylaxis, which is a diminished responsiveness lasting seconds or minutes after a large dose of a drug.

There are two essentially different types of tolerance. In a particular case, one or both of these may contribute to the development of drug tolerance. *Drug disposition tolerance* occurs when there is an increase in the body's ability to dispose of the drug through increased metabolism or excretion. This type of tolerance generally contributes about 20 percent to overall tolerance. *Pharmacodynamic tolerance* involves some adjustment in the neurochemistry of the brain in response to the continuous or frequent presence of a drug substance that tends to offset the effect of the drug. Because of the brain's adjustment to the presence of the drug, its subsequent absence elicits withdrawal syndrome. It might be said that the presence of the drug becomes the null condition, and absence of the drug becomes a challenge to the system. This may be the pharmacologic analogue of a statement commonly heard from heroin addicts, that they take the drug not to feel high but to feel "normal." This aspect of pharmacodynamic tolerance is closely related to withdrawal.

An unusual variation on the tolerance theme is the rare condition of reverse or negative tolerance. In this situation, the system becomes increasingly sensitive to a drug with repeated administration. This is not to be confused with a "hypersensitivity reaction," which is an immunologic or pathologic response to a drug. Reverse tolerance to the psychic effects of THC, the active principle in cannabis, has been reported.

Withdrawal

Withdrawal or the abstinence syndrome refers to the set of behavioral and physiologic symptoms that occur when drug treatment is withdrawn from a person who has become tolerant to it. The withdrawal syndromes associated with amphetamines, sedative-hypnotics, and narcotics are each distinctive for that class of drugs. Within each class, the syndromes are qualitatively similar but vary in intensity. Not all drugs that produce tolerance have associated withdrawal symptoms. LSD, for example, produces a high degree of tolerance that is of short duration and with no apparent withdrawal symptoms. The characteristics of withdrawal syndromes for various drug classes are described in Table 9-1.

Withdrawal is readily conditionable. Complex or simple stimuli may elicit intensified craving for the drug. The cigarette smoker who regularly lights up after dinner is responding to an urge signaled by internal cues and by the shifting social configuration. A former heroin addict may experience anomalous recurrence of withdrawal-like symptoms months after his or her last drug experience when returning to an old haunt where he or she "shot up" or comes across an old syringe in a drawer. This conditioning phenomenon may well contribute to the cyclical and persistent nature of drug abuse.

Physical Dependence

Physical dependence is a craving for a drug substance as a result of the presence of pharmacodynamic tolerance. It is closely related to the abstinence syndrome, particularly the subjective dysphoria experienced during withdrawal. Its relation to tolerance is the same as the relation of withdrawal to tolerance. There cannot be physical dependence without tolerance but there can be tolerance without physical dependence. Drugs producing the greatest physical dependence do not necessarily produce the highest degree of tolerance (Table 9-2). Physical dependence is not a prerequisite for the occurrence of either addiction or abuse.

Psychological Dependence

It can be said that a person is psychologically dependent if he or she considers the taking of a drug necessary for the maintenance of an acceptable level of well-being. An alternative definition that stresses the behavior of the user is that the psychologically dependent individual is preoccupied with the procurement and taking of a drug to an extent that is detrimental to psychological health and social functioning. Psychological dependence is the sine qua non of addiction. Psychological dependence is the result of the ability of a drug to stimulate the reward system, or suppress the punishment system, or both.

Addiction

Addiction is a term of ambiguous usage and is heavily laden with emotional overtones. We define it as periodic or chronic abuse of a drug, characterized by psychological dependence, generally but not always physical dependence, and a compulsion to continue use of the drug.

The attribute of a drug that most contributes to its *abuse liability* is not its ability to produce tolerance or physical dependence but rather its ability to reinforce the drug-taking behaviors. An important expansion of this concept—and one that has escaped the understanding of many psychotherapists—is that reinforcement of drug-taking behavior need not have any manifestation in conscious experience. Reinforcement of a given behavior *may* be accompanied by subjective feelings of well-being or euphoria (the "rush" or "high," in drug culture jargon), but in other cases drug reinforcement of behavior may occur with little or no subjectively apparent component. Nicotine is an effective reinforcer way out of proportion to its mild subjective effects. (It is interesting in this regard that nicotine has been reported to stimulate the septal area—a limbic system "reward" center.) This is simply an iteration of a theme that will be touched on in several parts of this book. Both conscious and nonconscious brain centers are involved in driving the same vehicle, so to speak.

Of the factors related strictly to the properties of the drug (as opposed to the individual), only the ability of the drug to reinforce drug-taking behaviors contributes initially to drug-taking. A second drug-related factor contributes substantially but still secondarily to maintenance of the drug habit once established, however, and that is the ability of the drug to suspend onset of withdrawal symptoms. Clearly, once the threat of withdrawal hangs over the user's head, the drug's ability to postpone this is a considerable inducement to persist.

Table 9-1. Characteristics of drug withdrawal syndromes

Drug class	Onset	Duration	Symptoms	Clinical management
Sedative-hypnotics				
Barbiturates and similar drugs	8–12 hr	5–10 days	Anxiety, irritability, insomnia, REM elevation, weakness, tremor, nausea, vomiting, hypotension, hallucinations, delirium, convulsions, cardiovascular collapse, possible death	Gradual withdrawal and symptomatic treatment; supportive and psychiatric treatment
Benzodiazepines	2–12 days	9–14 days		For alcohol, in addition to above, substitution of chlordiazepoxide, vitamins (especially thiamine), fluid and electrolytes as needed, diazepam for convulsions
Alcohol	12–72 hr	5–7 days		
Narcotics	2–24 hr	7–10 days	Lacrimation, rhinorrhea, perspiration, mydriasis, yawning, anxiety, irritability, insomnia, REM elevation, anorexia, nausea, vomiting, diarrhea, piloerection, slight hypertension, muscle spasms	Methadone substitution and gradual withdrawal, or clonidine substitution; symptomatic treatment; supportive and psychiatric treatment
Stimulants				
Amphetamine-like drugs	12–24 hr	3–7 days	Fatigue, depression, suicidal ideation, increased appetite, disturbed sleep, REM sleep elevation	Supportive therapy and tricyclic antidepressants for depression if necessary
Nicotine	3–24 hr	1–20 wk	Anxiety, irritability, restlessness, poor concentration, headache, drowsiness, nausea, anorexia	Supportive therapy

			Symptoms	Management
Psychiatric drugs				
Antipsychotics	2–3 days	12–14 days	Withdrawal dyskinesias, nausea, vomiting, diarrhea, sweating, rhinorrhea, increased appetite, insomnia, agitation, delirium, headache, schizoid symptoms	Gradual withdrawal
Tricyclic antidepressants	1–2 days	A few days	Malaise, chills, headache, dizziness, nausea, vomiting, muscle aches, akathisias, anxiety	Resume medication and withdraw gradually
Neurologic drugs				
Antiepileptics	1–2 days	A few days	Seizures, status epilepticus	Resume medication and withdraw gradually
Methysergide	1–2 days	A few days	Headaches	Resume drug and withdraw over 2–3 wk
Endocrine drugs				
Glucocorticoids	A few days	Indefinite	Depression, fatigue, hypotension, anorexia, nausea, vomiting	Resume drug and withdraw gradually over several months
Cardiovascular drugs				
Antihypertensives	2–3 hr	1–2 days	Agitation, insomnia, headache, nausea, hypertension	Resume drug and withdraw gradually; treat hypertension
Antianginal drugs	10 min–2 wk	Variable	Angina attacks, anxiety, trepidation, increased blood pressure	Resume drug and taper slowly

Table 9-2. Drug dependence and tolerance

Drug	Tolerance	Physical dependence	Psychological dependence	Damage to body tissues	Acute psychosis	Death from overdose	Controlled substance
Sedative-hypnotics							
Barbiturates	++	+++	+++	0/+	+	++	Yes
Alcohol	++	+++	+++	+++	+	+	No
Benzodiazepines	+	+	+++	0	+	0	Yes
Stimulants							
Amphetamine-like	+++	0/+	+++	++	++++	0	Yes
Cocaine	+	0	+++ or +*	+	++	+	Yes
Caffeine	+	0	+	+	0	0	No
Nicotine	++	0/+	+++	+++	0	0	No
Narcotics	++++	++++	+++	0/+	0	++++	Yes
Psychedelics							
LSD	++++	0	0/+	0	+++	0	Yes
PCP	+	0	0/+	0/+	+++	++	Yes
Marijuana	+ and −	0	++	0/+	+	0	Yes

0, not occurring or not established; 0/+, little or none; +–++++, from mild or occasional occurrence to intense or frequent occurrence; − (under tolerance), increased CNS sensitivity (negative tolerance) for certain effects.
*Severity of psychological dependence with cocaine is related to route of utilization: +++ if administered IV or by inhalation (smoked); + if administered orally or intranasally (snuffed).

It is difficult to predict the abuse liability of new drugs. The best single test is whether laboratory animals (monkeys are the best subjects for this test) will self-administer and maintain use. The ability of the drug to produce physical dependence or to substitute for known addicting drugs can also be determined, but this is inconclusive, since addiction can occur without physical dependence.

Other Hazards of Drug Abuse

Apart from the risks of psychological and physical dependence, the abuse of any given drug may carry with it one or more additional hazards: damage to bodily tissues, precipitation of acute or chronic toxic psychoses, death from overdose, or legal prosecution. The drugs of abuse differ markedly from one to another as regards the extent to which each of these four hazards is a factor (see Table 9-2). Damage to bodily tissues is most problematic with chronic use of alcohol, nicotine, or amphetamine-like stimulants, but is also relevant to the abuse of cocaine, caffeine, narcotics, and possibly marijuana. Acute toxic psychoses are commonly a consequence of amphetamine, cocaine, LSD, or PCP use and rarely may occur with use of sedative-hypnotics or marijuana. Drugs cause about 6,500 overdose fatalities annually in the United States, in addition to the 5,650 deaths attributed to drug or alcohol dependence (Table 9-3). Non-drug chemicals, including solids, liquids, and gases, add an additional 6,350 substance-induced deaths. CNS drugs account for the lion's share of the drug-related fatal overdoses. Barbiturates are most likely to cause such overdoses, but other drugs with a significant liability in this respect include benzodiazepines, antidepressants, narcotics, alcohol, nonbarbiturate sedative-hypnotics, aspirin, acetaminophen, cocaine, and amphetamines. Alcohol, nicotine, and caffeine are largely unrestricted drugs legally, except that alcohol sale to minors (as defined by each state) is prohibited. The legality of these drugs and the illegality of the others is a societal inconsistency, viewed in terms of medical considerations, but comprehensible (if not defensible) when understood in terms of economic, political, and sociological factors. Misuse of legal prescription drugs is the most common cause of drug-related emergency room admissions, while purchase of street drugs ranks third in cause of admissions, behind over-the-counter purchase.

Psychological Aspects of Drug Use and Abuse

In many ways it can be said that drug abuse has almost nothing to do with drugs and much to do with people! It is clear that psychological and not physical dependence is the sine qua non of addiction. What is it that leads a person from casual or responsible use of drugs to clearly destructive patterns of abuse, to seek the immediate gratification of the "high" or the relaxation of anxieties at the price of dysfunction, disability, or death? The behaviorist talks of drugs as primary reinforcers, the social psychologist reflects upon peer-group pressures and alienation, and the clinician speaks of pleasurable feelings and relief from anxieties. These need not be mutually exclusive viewpoints if they are viewed as components of the metaperspective.

As we have chosen to offer a rather precise functional definition of abuse, it behooves us to differentiate drug use from drug abuse, it being possible that the many contributing factors are of differential importance in these. In fact, we must address three related but distinct issues: the use of drugs, the use of a particular drug, and the abuse of drugs.

Table 9-3. *Approximate incidence of drug or chemical overdoses in the U.S. in 1977*

Drug class	DAWN-network emergency treatments[a]	National Fatalities[b]	National Suicides[a,b]
Sedative-hypnotics			
Barbiturate	13,900	1,200	850
Alcohol	23,800	400[c]	200
Nonbarbiturate	13,700	400	200
Stimulants			
Amphetamine-like drugs	6,500	40	<10
Cocaine	3,600	60	<10
Xanthines	?	10	0
Psychedelics			
Marijuana/hashish	11,100	<10	0
LSD	2,100	0	0
PCP	6,400	50	<5
Other	800	2	0
Psychotherapeutic drugs			
Benzodiazepines	50,200	700	300
Antidepressants	7,000	500	300
Analgesics			
Narcotics	33,600	1,500[d]	300
Aspirin	7,400	150	80
Acetaminophen	4,000	10–75[e]	40
Antiepileptics			
Phenytoin	2,400	2–30	<5
Antihistamines	?	10	0
Other drugs	26,200	400[f]	200
Unspecified drugs	12,400	1,000	600
Total all drug mentions	220,000		
Total all drug episodes	146,000	6,500	3,150
Solid and liquid chemicals excluding drugs		1,850	750
Gases and vapors		4,500	2,600
Total substance overdoses		12,850	6,500
Other specified drug-induced fatalities			
Alcohol dependence		5,100	
Other drug dependences		550	
Delirium tremens		300	
Korsakov's psychosis		15	
Other alcohol psychoses		15	

Table 9-3 (continued)

Drug class	DAWN-network emergency treatments[a]	National	
		Fatalities[b]	Suicides[a,b]
Liver cirrhosis			
Alcoholic		13,000	
Unspecified		14,000	
Homicides by poisoning		46	

[a]Based on data from Project DAWN VI, May 1977–April 1978, United States Department of Justice, Drug Enforcement Administration. Emergency treatment numbers indicate the number of mentions for each drug category for drug overdose episodes reported by participating emergency room and crisis centers in the Drug Abuse Warning Network (DAWN) consisting of 24 metropolitan areas. Data from medical examiner mentions is used to supplement the national figures on use of various classes of drugs for suicides.

[b]Based on data published in the Vital Statistics of the United States, 1977, Vol. II—Mortality, Part A., U.S. Department of Health and Human Services, Public Health Service.

[c]Note other alcohol-related fatalities itemized below.

[d]The figure for narcotic fatalities exhibits substantial discrepancy between the Vital Statistics data and the DAWN Report data, as well as unusual variability from year-to-year in relation to availability of narcotics on the street. The number to unintentional overdoses involving narcotics, reported in the Vital Statistics, reached a high of 1,031 in 1975 and a low of 269 in 1978, for the 1970s.

Acetaminophen appears in many analgesic combinations and thus is often mentioned as a drug involved. It is seldom the sole drug. Ten represents the approximate number of fatalities attributable to acetaminophen alone, 75 the number of fatalities in which acetaminophen was one of the drugs involved.

[f]Noteworthy in this category are cardiac drugs (150–200), autonomic drugs (30–50), and general anesthetics, antimicrobials, cancer drugs, and hormones (20–30 each).

Drug of Choice

The term *drug of choice* is useful in suggesting that the use or abuse of a specific drug by an individual is not merely fortuitous, and that, for the most part, people choose drugs that integrate with their own psychological, constitutional, and social predispositions.

The idea that constitutional factors might influence one's drug of choice is particularly attractive. It has been suggested that a preference for moderate use of drugs that have some anticonvulsant properties—among them the barbiturates and amphetamines—may be a "soft sign" of possible subictal focal EEG activity, cogent only when combined with other signs. People characterized by reticular activating system (intermittent, stimulus)–controlled consciousness dominating the diffuse thalamic system (rhythmic, focused) control are more likely to favor drugs that shift this balance in favor of the latter, e.g., amphetamine at small dosages or cannabis. Genetic predisposition has been suggested by some investigators of alcoholism, and others suggest that alcohol abuse begins as a kind of crude self-medication for chronic anxiety. The full range of constitutional predispositions and their role in drug choice has hardly been scratched but could be a productive area of investigation.

Of course, other influences may and probably do mask constitutional factors. The social influence has often been cited as crucial in juvenile drug abuse. Peer pressure, social drinking, and "toking" at young people's gatherings, and the desire to be "in" and accepted have all been implicated. A young person is most likely to use the current drug of choice of his or her "crowd." The currently endemic shift from teenage cannabis use to alcohol is probably a result, at least in part, of just such social-system amplification of the smaller shifts precipitated by a variety of local influences.

It is naive, however, to talk about such influences only with respect to juvenile drug abuse, for they are certainly powerfully operative in adult social systems as well. The popularity of alcohol is maintained by a complex of integrated social mechanisms that pressure, cajole, tease, and seduce the user into making ethanol the drug of choice. Some of these same semi-institutionalized forces involved in party use of alcohol have probably contributed to the spread of illicit cannabis use among the middle class and the affluent.

We cannot ignore powerful influences of the family system, of influences communicated multigenerationally in what may even take on the character of a "family tradition" in drug use and abuse. The drug-taking behavior itself as well as other stylistic elements are part of the interpersonal learning environment of the family. Alcohol abuse, for example, frequently "runs in families." It is striking how often children of alcoholic parents react adversely to their parents' abuse and vow never to follow suit, yet find themselves having successfully learned the family patterns that favor their own eventual abuse of alcohol.

The effects, both putative and demonstrated, as well as the symbolic meanings of the drugs, differ considerably and are therefore likely to attract people with different personalities, personal styles, and self-images. It is this mechanism that advertisers of legal psychotropics try to manipulate to their own advantage with "Dewar's Profiles," "the Marlboro man," and the "Baby" who has "come a long way." For example, there have been reports of consistent preexisting personality and self-image differences between heroin and cannabis abusers. Although alcohol shares certain pharmacologic properties with the sedative-hypnotics, alcohol use appears to tap into power and control imagery in ways that the barbiturates do not, so that a person with issues in this dimension is a more likely candidate for drinking than pill-popping.

From Use to Abuse

To abuse a drug, a person must first use it. The self-administration of psychotropic drugs seems to be embedded in a complex of intrapersonal, interpersonal, and metapersonal factors.

In the intrapersonal domain, even simple curiosity may lead to experimentation. Much drug use within the "counterculture" seems anchored in a search for the self through altered perceptions of the self. Drugs may generate feelings of self-esteem or self-acceptance that may not otherwise be enjoyed too often. Or drugs may suppress anxieties related to self-doubt. They may lessen inhibitions and free behaviors not usually expressible. Or the taker may feel more capable in social interactions or in performance of solitary tasks.

We regard it as *not* coincidental that these common drug effects are related to the subjective experience of healthy mental functioning as outlined in Chapter 2. One may legitimately infer strong predispositions toward the experience of euphoric self-perception that have an organic basis. It is tempting to juxtapose drug-induced experience of heightened self-esteem and effectiveness with the phenomenon of state-dependent learning. The two phenomena—behavior as response to drug action and state-dependent interference with generalization of responses—strongly mitigate against carry-over into nondrug states and therefore offer a powerful incentive for continued use.

Attention must also be given to drug-taking and subsequent drug-mediated behavior as interpersonal communication. The alcoholic parent expresses to the family an aggressive bid for power while simultaneously demonstrating his or her ineffectiveness. Cannabis use is generally intricately embedded in ritual that serves to declare trust, positive regard, and an interest in meaningful interpersonal contact. Sharing a cup of coffee or a cigarette is a similar, though usually more superficial, method of making contact. On this interpersonal plane may also be included drug-taking as avoidance or escape behavior to deal with upsetting and problematic familial or occupational conflicts.

Finally, in the metapersonal realm, accessibility and peer-group values may intervene. Society reinforces drug-taking patterns in many ways, for example, the smiling and persistent hostess who keeps the glasses filled at a cocktail party. Society may even ensure recidivism by ostracizing the former user to a social milieu where drug-taking is prevalent, such as the local bar, cheap hotels for the unemployed, or the crash pad.

The fact that abuse and addiction have historically been confused, that both have often been described in terms of compulsivity, preoccupation, and driven behavior, suggests that pharmacologic action may play an important role in the transition from use to abuse. While excessive or increased drug use by the individual represents a risk-taking action, it is seldom that the user is truly cognizant or appreciative of the risk involved, denial being found to be a factor in the social abuse of dangerous agents like cigarettes. Three mechanisms already discussed could account for the transition to abuse, given that use can be explained. These are the ability of drugs to function as primary reinforcers of drug-taking behavior, state-dependent learning and behavioral phenomena, and the drug's ability to postpone onset of its own withdrawal syndrome. What these do not explain is why some people remain users and others become abusers. We have no ready, general explanation.

Given its multifaceted nature and persistency as a problem throughout the ages, it is not surprising that drug abuse has given rise to as many treatment approaches as it has, even in the absence of reliable, general theories. Pharmacologic treatment approaches are specific for the drug being abused and are discussed in the chapter on the various drugs. A survey of the myriad psychotherapeutic methods is beyond the scope of this book, but this omission should not be read as a reflection on their import, only that other sources should be consulted.

Drug Abuse Education

How much does ignorance really have to do with the problem of drug abuse? At the least, some deaths from overdoses and emergency room problems can be ascribed in part to naiveté about such matters as dosage, routes of administration, fluctuating tolerance, misrepresentations of drug identity, presence of impurities, and so forth. And certainly, no matter how much the age of drug innocence recedes, there is some age group on the threshold between innocence and sophistication that stands to profit from an effective education program.

Educators in the field of drug abuse have evolved a handful of principles that, it is maintained, contribute to the effectiveness of communication about drugs. For those of you who may someday be called on to participate in drug education programs, or who

Table 9-4. *The eyes have it!*

Ocular symptoms	Possible illicit drugs
Pupil	
Dilated	Amphetamine-like stimulants, cocaine, LSD, anticholinergics
Constricted	Narcotics (unless highly anoxic)
Normal	Barbiturates, marijuana, PCP
Other	
Ptosis	Marijuana
Nystagmus	PCP

are parents wishing to promote the drug education of your children, the rules of thumb that follow may prove useful.

Know your facts about illicit and social drugs! When unsure, admit you do not know! Have a summary table of drug facts handy for reference! Nothing undercuts credibility more quickly than a bald, erroneous statement that your audience knows to be incorrect. Nothing except perhaps your own example, especially as it relates to your own children. When addressing parents, remind them of the importance of role-modeling in determining drug utilization behaviors.

Present a balanced view! This means, among other things, avoiding stereotypes such as the depraved junkie. It also means that when addressing a question such as "Why do people take drugs?", you might want to include answers like "fun," "sociability," and "experimentation" along with the more negatively charged notions of "'in' thing," "escape from reality," "easy solution," and "drug culture."

Avoid scare tactics! Sensational accounts conflict with the firsthand experiences of your audience. Most young people have used one or more psychotropic drugs for social purposes; most of the rest have talked to those who indulge. Therefore, it pays to present the facts as they exist without overstatement.

Avoid trying to defend the laws, especially the state-to-state inconsistencies! You will lose the debate. Besides, it puts you in the position of being "one of them."

Do not neglect discussion of the drugs of abuse accepted by society: alcohol, nicotine, and caffeine! By any accounting, these are the "big three." If your audience is young and you ignore these drugs, your listeners will feel singled out for persecution.

When discussing the research literature relating to adverse effects, acknowledge the vagaries and uncertainties that exist! It is a striking truth that several reviewers of a given body of drug literature can reach starkly disparate and even contradictory conclusions. This is especially true when the drug in question is socially controversial (such as marijuana or LSD) or economically important (such as alcohol or tobacco). Several factors contribute to the apparent and real contradictions in studies of drugs: variations in route, dosage, and dosage form; and matters of experimental design, such as the subject sample and adequacy of controls. One might also add semantics and personal bias. In one study of frequency of "adverse reactions" to marijuana, it was later found that some of the physicians involved in the study construed any effect as an adverse reaction. We can only wonder how reviewers and researchers are influenced by personal biases, such as attitudes toward authority, views on individual rights versus social interdependence, or desires to advance personal or professional interests.

Urge parents to know the telltale signs of drug use! For the parent, teacher, or counselor who wishes to be alert to signs of teenage drug use, the indications are often closer at hand than is commonly appreciated (Table 9-4).

Know how to distinguish casual social use from abuse! For openers, this requires that you internalize a clear definition of abuse that works for you, rationally and intuitively. If you subscribe to a functional definition similar to the one advanced earlier in this chapter, the focus of attention naturally shifts from whether a drug is in use to whether there are signs of impairment of functioning.

Remember and urge others to perceive that drug abuse occurs in an expansive context. It is symptomatic of underlying problems, but is also a problem in its own right. Organic, psychological, and interpersonal systemic factors must all be appreciated and addressed.

Beyond these simple admonitions, you are left to your own wits and accumulated skills as psychotherapists.

Selected References and Further Readings

1. Committee on Nomenclature and Statistics of the American Psychiatric Association. *Diagnostic and Statistical Manual* (3rd ed.). Washington, D.C.: American Psychiatric Association, 1980.
2. Ray, O. S. *Drugs, Society and Human Behavior* (2nd ed.). St. Louis: Mosby, 1978.

Drugs and Arousal State IV

One of the obvious ways in which a pharmacologic agent can affect the behavior of an organism is by an alteration of fundamental arousal state. *An animal can be put to sleep with chloral hydrate, for example. The term* fundamental arousal state *means that under appropriate circumstances an organism can undergo a change in excitability in an across-the-board fashion; that is, the stimulus threshold for all possible responses is altered concurrently rather than each one's being altered independently. An assumption that such a mechanism exists is reflected in our language, and it is interesting that our awareness of the fundamental arousal state predates both the discovery of an anatomic basis for it and its study as a behavioral phenomenon. The terms* uppers *and* downers *and* getting high *are popular expressions that aptly describe the direction of action of stimulants and sedatives respectively, and they present the concept of arousal state as a more or less unitary principle that is subject to chemical modification as a unit. Chapter 10 deals with the physiologic and neuroanatomic bases of regulation of arousal state, while drugs that depress and elevate arousal state are discussed in Chapters 11 through 14.*

The Physiology of Sleep and Arousal

10

℞

It is convenient to model the control of arousal as the function of two distinct interacting subcortical systems acting mutually and reciprocally. The conceptual division in this "dual arousal model" is supported by anatomical, electrophysiological, and functional distinctions. One system, the diffuse thalamic system (DTS), is anatomically associated with various nuclei of the dorsal thalamus, is interconnected with limbic and cerebral cortical areas, and has been functionally equated with cerebral α-wave activity, goal-directed behavior, internalization of attention, and stimulus-processing. The second system, the reticular activating system (RAS), is anatomically associated with the midbrain reticular formation. It interdigitates with the long ascending and descending pathways from and to the periphery and it is functionally equated with cerebral beta-wave activity, arousal of the sympathetic nervous system, externalization of attention, and sensory-mediated behaviors. In the following sections, these two systems will be described, first independently and then as they interact.

The Diffuse Thalamic System

Gross Anatomy of the Dorsal Thalamus

The dorsal thalami, a pair of egg-shaped structures that lie at the very center of the brain, are relay centers that integrate impulses arriving from lower centers and pass on the elaborated information to the cortex or conversely repackage signals received from the cortex for subcortical distribution. Each thalamus comprises eight major nuclear groups, though one of these groups is greatly diminished or absent in humans. Five of these groups contribute directly or indirectly to a profuse system of thalamocortical radiation pathways (Fig. 10-1). Table 10-1 summarizes the functions associated with each of the eight nuclear groups of the thalamus.

Evidence for Thalamic Control of Spindle Activity

The study of the DTS is intimately related to the history of the study of electrical activity in the brain. The existence of cortical electrical potentials as well as the small spontaneous fluctuations thereof, now referred to as the EEG, were first noted by Caton in 1875. (For a full discussion of the EEG, see Electroencephalography.) Early investi-

161

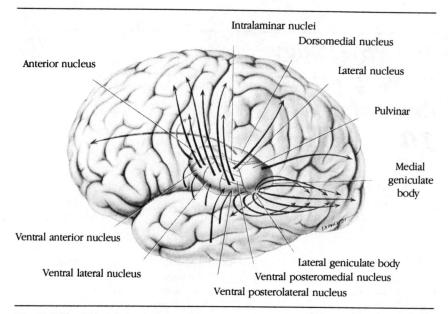

Intralaminar nuclei

Dorsomedial nucleus

Anterior nucleus

Lateral nucleus

Pulvinar

Medial geniculate body

Ventral anterior nucleus

Lateral geniculate body

Ventral lateral nucleus

Ventral posteromedial nucleus

Ventral posterolateral nucleus

Fig. 10-1. *The diffuse thalamic projection system. From S. R. Noback,* The Human Nervous System. © *1974 by McGraw-Hill Book Company, New York. Used with permission.*

gators sought to determine the nature and location of the electrical forces responsible for the rhythmic fluctuations. In the latter part of the nineteenth century, in Krakow, Adolph Beck successfully excluded the possibility that the oscillations were caused by body movements when he made observations in animals treated with curare, a drug that paralyzes skeletal muscles. In 1925, Prawdicz-Neminski of Kiev published the first EEG tracings, and through his experiments he put to rest one of the early speculations— that the oscillations in brain activity were linked to physical pulsations of the brain. He was able to show that asphyxia, which increased brain pulsations, resulted in an elimination of EEG oscillations. Although no clear evidence was available, early assumptions placed the pacemaker for the spontaneous activity within the cortex itself.

In 1929, Hans Berger carried electroencephalography forward two giant steps; the first resulted from his systematic investigation of the human EEG, which gave birth to clinical electroencephalography; the second resulted from his discovery and naming of the human alpha-wave and its differentiation from beta-activity. In subsequent studies, Berger was able to demonstrate that the EEG is generated in the cortices of the cerebrum and that only minute electrical waves could be recorded from underlying white matter. Thus, the question as to the location of the electrical forces responsible for the EEG was settled. Berger was also able to propose that the thalamus might serve as the pacemaker for cortical electrical activity, but it remained for other workers to provide definite supporting evidence for this idea.

In 1935, Bremer showed that sectioning of the brainstem between the colliculi did not impair cortical electrical activity. Three years later, he demonstrated, however, that elimination of all afferents to the cortex did greatly impair rhythmic activity. These two observations showed that pacemaker activity must reside in the diencephalon or at least depend on inputs from the diencephalon for adequate function. The relationship be-

Table 10-1. *Nuclear groups of the thalamus*

Group	Prominent nuclei	Description
Metathalamus	Lateral geniculate nucleus	Relay station for visual system
	Medial geniculate nucleus	Relay station for auditory system
Midline group		Poorly developed or absent in man
Intralaminar group	Nucleus centromedianus	Control center of DTS; some fibers to striatum; highly developed in humans
Nucleus reticularis	Nucleus reticularis	Thin sheet of cells overlying much of thalamus; relay internode in the DTS
Anterior group	Nucleus anterodorsalis	Called limbic thalamus; connect with mammillary bodies of the hypothalamus, the cingulate gyrus, the preoptic area, and the septum
	Nucleus anteromedialis	
	Nucleus anteroventralis	
Ventral group	Nucleus ventralis posterolateralis	Relay of bodily somatesthetic sensations
	Arcuate nucleus	Relay of cranial somatesthetic sensations
	Nucleus ventralis lateralis	Extrapyramidal-pyramidal interconnections
	Nucleus ventralis anterior	Fibers from globus pallidus; function unknown
Medial group	Nucleus dorsomedialis	Related to periventricular system and prefrontal cortex
Lateral group	Pulvinar	DTS projections to associative areas in parietal, temporal, and occipital lobes
	Nucleus lateralis posterior	
	Nucleus lateralis dorsalis	

tween the diencephalon and cortical electrical activity was further elaborated when, in 1941, Adrian recorded rhythmic electrical activity from the thalamus itself and showed that the rhythm persisted even in an animal with cortices completely removed. It therefore became apparent that the property of autorhythmicity resided within the thalami and that cortical rhythmicity required intact thalamocortical radiations.

The idea of the thalamus as pacemaker of cortical electrical activity gained ample support in the subsequent 2-year period (1942–1943) from a series of studies by Morison and Dempsey. They demonstrated that electrical stimulation of certain medially lying nuclei (the intralaminar group) resulted in bursts of synchronous, high-voltage waves in the cortex reminiscent of spindle waves observed during barbiturate anesthesia. They termed this response the *recruiting response*. At the end of the decade and during the 1950s, Jasper and his colleagues further amplified this work by demonstrating that the spread of rhythmic electrical activity in the cortex resulting from midline thalamic stimulation was dependent upon intrathalamic activity involving principally the midline, the intralaminar and reticular nuclear groups of the thalamus, and the nucleus ventralis anterior. Indeed, Jasper regarded this nuclear group, which he termed the *intralaminar system*, as the rostral extension of the RAS that had been discovered in 1949 by Moruzzi and Magoun. In their view, this system is seen as separate from, and independent of, the sensory relay nuclei of the thalamus (the metathalamic and ventral posterior groups). This view gave way in the 1960s to the "facultative pacemaker theory" of Andersen and Andersson [1], whose work showed that the property of autorhythmicity was inherent to many nuclei of the thalamus, including sensory relay nuclei, and that the recruiting response could be elicited in topographically appropriate cortical regions by stimulation of sensory relay nuclei. They postulated that the role of pacemaker (i.e., the "leading focus of activity") may shift from one thalamic nucleus to another as a consequence of changing intrinsic and afferent impulse bombardment.

The Reticular Activating System

Gross Anatomy of the Brainstem Reticular Formation

The reticular formation is a dense, medially lying core of nerve cells that extend from the caudal end of the medulla to the thalamus (Fig. 10-2). It is surrounded along its entire course by the tracts and nuclei of the sensory and motor systems receiving collateral inputs from all the sensory modalities, and in the descending direction it acts as the final common discharge pathway for nearly all extrapyramidal motor influences. Reticular influences on motor function are discussed in Chapter 20.

The ascending influences of the reticular formation seem to be restricted to the rostral pons and midbrain portion of the reticular substance. In particular, a region in the vicinity of the root of the trigeminal nerve, including the ventral portion of the midbrain tegmentum and the nucleus reticularis pontalis oralis, appears to contain the elements necessary for arousal.

Ascending efferents from the reticular formation are, in general, diffuse and multisynaptic. However, two long ascending pathways, the dorsal and ventral tegmental

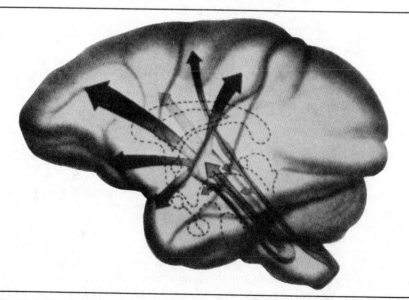

Fig. 10-2. *The reticular activating system. From Lindsley. The Reticular System and Perceptual Integration. In H. H. Jasper et al. (Eds.),* The Reticular Formation of the Brain. *Boston: Little, Brown, 1958.*

tracts, to the subthalamus, thalamus, hypothalamus, basal ganglia, and septum have been identified. There are diffuse direct (nonthalamic) pathways extending to the cortex, including the cholinergic and dopaminergic fiber systems (discussed in Chapter 6), as well as the thalamic projections of the DTS.

Discovery of and Evidence for Reticular Control of Activation

Moruzzi and Magoun opened the era of investigation of the reticular formation in 1949, when they reported that electrical stimulation of this region produced long-lasting activation of cortical electrical activity (β-waves) in an anesthetized animal. Lindsley augmented this finding by his reports that lesions in the reticular formation resulted in a comatose state and elimination of EEG fast-wave activity.

The RAS may be viewed as a general alarm system. It is activated by impulse volleys, along sensory afferents of any modality that reaches it via the collaterals from these tracts. Then, in turn, the RAS initiates diffuse activation of the cortex. To understand the relationship between the RAS and DTS, we need to set the stage by reviewing briefly the nature of EEG recordings, since these provide the most direct means available for assessing the electrical activity of the cerebral cortex in the intact human brain.

Electroencephalography

Definition and Source

The EEG is a recording of spontaneous voltage changes in the cerebrum as measured between two points. Typically, a cup electrode attached to or just under the scalp of a human subject will pick up electrical activity from a circular area of the underlying cortex up to 4 cm in diameter and up to a depth of no more than 3 mm. In experimental animals, depth recordings can be taken at any level by insertion of needle electrodes into the cerebral tissue. The EEG is believed to be an analogue recording of the summed dendritic potentials (excitatory and inhibitory postsynaptic potentials) of cortical neurons.

Aspects of the EEG

Frequency Analysis

The most familiar aspect of the EEG subjected to analysis is the frequency. Wave patterns are commonly identified in terms of four somewhat arbitrary divisions indicated by Greek letters. A frequency of less than 4 Hz is called delta, 4 to 8 Hz is known as theta, approximately 8 to 12 Hz is the alpha range, and frequencies higher than 12 Hz are called beta. There are slight discrepancies in these range definitions, depending on the source. The simplest type of analysis is a qualitative description of an EEG in terms of predominance of one or another of these frequencies. A few generalizations can be made in this regard. Delta activity predominates in infancy, during slow-wave sleep, and in coma. Theta activity is seen in childhood and during emotional states as well as being a characteristic frequency of the hippocampus (Chap. 15). Alpha activity is the "idling" condition of the waking (but nonactivated) cortex. Beta activity is indicative of an alert, activated cortex.

Quantification of the EEG frequency analysis can be accomplished in a number of ways. Some workers report mean frequencies or frequency variability. Another common quantitative method is amplitude integration, which measures the area described by the EEG tracing. Occurrence of waves within a particular frequency band can be examined in terms of the power in the different portions of the EEG spectrum.

Steady Potential

In addition to the rapid, spontaneous fluctuations so often examined experimentally and clinically, several other aspects of the EEG have garnered less attention. One of these, the steady potential (SP, also called DC potential), was actually discovered before the rapid fluctuations but has only recently attracted much interest. The SP denotes the maintained and nonrhythmic difference in potential between the surface of the cortex and the adjacent white matter; *SP shifts* refers to changes in the SP that are not recurrent and that transpire over the course of minutes. They are generally in the microvolt range but may, in extreme cases, reach 2 millivolts in magnitude. A more severe shift in the range of 5 to 10 millivolts occurs in "spreading depression" and is considered pathologic. Shifts in SP involve a local component and a diffuse component of longer latency and duration.

Negative SP shifts occur in response to novel nonreinforced stimuli, but habituate rapidly on multiple presentation. The extent of the SP shift is related directly to the capacity of the stimulus to elicit arousal. Reinforced sensory-evoked SP shifts persist and may be classically conditioned. Positive SP shifts accompany reinforcements such as food and sexual consummation as well as electrical stimulation of self-stimulation centers such as the hypothalamus. Negative SP shifts accompany aversive electrical stimulation. Thus, SP shifts seem to occur in the one direction in response to arousal and in the other direction in response to inhibitory processes.

Steady-potential shifts are mediated through the diffuse thalamic projection system and may be related to hippocampal theta activity. There is a good correlation between the two, and stimuli that block theta activity attenuate SP shifts. It has been hypothesized that SP shifts represent transient integrations of neural relationships critical in the consolidation of cortical events into retained experience. This is certainly plausible in view of the established role of the hippocampus in short-term memory and consolidation of long-term memory.

Cortical Evoked Responses

A third aspect of the EEG subjected to experimental investigation is the cortical evoked response (ER), or evoked potential. An ER is a spike of electrical activation occurring in response to a specific, sensory input such as a tone; ERs occur most obviously in the primary sensory cortex—and, indeed, under pentobarbital anesthesia only in these regions. Interestingly, however, in an unanesthetized animal, ERs that occur in the associative cortex are nonspecific with respect to the modality of the eliciting stimulus, whereas those that occur in the primary sensory cortex are always specific to a particular sense modality. A tone will elicit a response in the auditory cortex, but not in the visual cortex, whereas for a flash of light the result is the reverse.

Evoked responses are often "lost" amidst the spontaneous activity of the EEG. To circumvent this problem, a technique called response averaging may be employed using a computer of average transcients. In this procedure, a series of response tracings are averaged together in order to "average out" activity not linked to the stimulus.

The amplitude of ERs is closely correlated with arousal state in unanesthetized animals. Reticular stimulation or stimulants augment ERs, while CNS depressants diminish them. The amplitude of ERs relates also to stimulus variables, such as stimulus intensity relative to background noise level. Evoked potentials normally habituate when a nonreinforced sensory stimulus of low intensity is repeatedly presented. Depletion of serotonin impairs this habituation process, however.

EEG Correlations with Behavior

Arousal Response (Alpha-Blocking)

When an animal is presented with a startling or threatening stimulus complex, along with the postural and behavior adjustments, there occurs a characteristic EEG response known as the arousal response. If the EEG was predominantly alpha prior to the stimulus presentation, the α-activity immediately gives way to β-activity. The activation may be transient or prolonged, depending on the nature of the stimulus.

Postreinforcement Synchronization

Spindling or bursts of α-activity occur profusely immediately following positive reinforcement. This response is mediated by cholinergic cells in the cortex, since it can be blocked by cholinergic blockers and reinstated by inhibitors of cholinesterase.

EEG Events Accompanying Conditioning and as a Response System

Theta activity occurs in the hippocampus early in conditioning but disappears in later stages. Widespread alpha-blocking accompanies the initial reinforcement of a conditional stimulus, but the activation becomes limited to the applicable primary sensory area once the conditional response is fully established. Positive SP shifts facilitate acquisition of new conditional behaviors, whereas negative shifts inhibit new acquisition.

Aspects of the EEG can be used as responses for conditioning procedures. Steady-potential shifts are readily conditionable, and ERs can be used for conditioning by first habituating the response to the conditional stimulus.

Stimulus Correlates

Complex stimuli (e.g., squares, circles) produce specific and characteristic sensory-evoked responses. The temporal and spatial pattern of neuronal firing elicited by a given stimulus, rather than a particular nerve cell, is the mental unit of representation of that stimulus.

A second type of stimulus correlate that has been identified occurs with rhythmic stimuli such as tones and, particularly, light flashes. The EEG may to some extent mirror the frequency of the stimulus by increasing the amount of wave activity of that frequency. When this occurs, it is known as "driving." If an animal is trained to discriminate between two flicker frequencies and to respond differentially, erroneous responses are accompanied by EEG activity of the "wrong" frequency (the nonpresent stimulus), whereas correct responses are accompanied by EEG activity in the frequency of the stimulus presented.

Clinical Applications of the EEG

Limitations

The EEG is effective diagnostically when used in combination with other established diagnostic techniques, such as neurologic, psychological or mental, and motor tests. Only "positive" results, the presence of EEG abnormalities, can be considered as reliable indications for diagnosis. Negative results frequently accompany known brain pathologic conditions because of the limitations of the EEG. Only a limited area of the brain can be examined by electrodes and only to a very limited depth. Thus, if a focus of abnormal activity lies outside this area, it will go undetected. Furthermore, artifacts from a variety of sources intrude into the EEG and require expert analysis for proper exclusion. The use of leads inserted through the nasal passages increases the effective area under examination. Other procedures that increase the effectiveness of the EEG are the taking of repeated tracings and sleep readings. In spite of its limitations, the EEG remains the single most sensitive measure of cortical function in the intact subject.

The use of the EEG in epilepsy and the 14- and 6-Hz positive-spike pattern will be discussed in Chapter 28. The discussion to follow will be limited to applications in brain damage, psychiatric disorders, and endocrine disturbances.

Application in Brain Damage, Psychiatric Disorders, and Endocrine Disturbances

Cerebral trauma caused by head injury produces EEG alterations proportional to the extent of direct and indirect injury. In severe cases, there is a short period during which there is a generalized suppression of all cortical electrical activity. Alpha activity is slowed into the theta or delta range. As the clinical picture improves, the theta or delta activity increases in rate, and, as it does, a focal abnormality may be revealed. If, on the other hand, further deterioration occurs in the EEG pattern, this is indicative of secondary damage such as cerebral edema.

Localized suppression of electrical activity or slow delta activity is indicative of cerebral damage of a limited nature and may result from the presence of hematomas, tumors, abscesses, severe meningitis, or limited vascular lesions. In general, the EEG abnormalities accompanying tumors and abscesses progress in serial recordings, while those related to vascular lesions usually are less pronounced and may dissipate in a few days.

The EEG can be used effectively in diagnosing cerebrovascular insufficiency. This test is carried out by temporarily compressing one of the carotid arteries while monitoring the EEG. If cerebral blood delivery is impaired because of a diseased carotid or vertebral artery, occlusion of the intact carotid will elicit EEG abnormalities in an appropriate region of the brain.

Hypopituitarism leads to dramatic slowing of the EEG because of the hormonal insufficiency. Conversely, persistent beta activity accompanies acromegaly. In Addison's disease (adrenal insufficiency), the EEG is suppressed; in Cushing's syndrome (adrenal hypertrophy), beta activity is increased. Thyroid dysfunctions produce less dramatic effects; the mean frequency is slightly elevated in hyperthyroidism and slightly decreased in myxedema.

Severe hypoglycemia elicits slow-wave activity of a diffuse, nonfocal nature. If the fall in blood sugar is precipitous, severe neurological and behavioral pathological developments ensue. Symptoms include anxiety, irritability, tremor, agitation or apathy, disorientation, and coma. Because of the rapid onset of symptomatology and the similarity to neurotic disorders, hypoglycemia may frequently be misidentified as a psychoneurotic disorder. Serial laboratory analysis of blood sugar levels should be considered if the abnormal behavioral pattern resembles the hypoglycemic pattern.

A pattern called "mittens," somewhat similar to the spike and dome of petit mal, but with a rounded initial wave resembling the thumb of a mitten, is a frequent correlate of psychiatric conditions. The mitten pattern occurs in only 3 percent of a control population but in about 20 percent of patients with alcoholic dementia, endogenous depression, personality disorder, and/or manic-depressive disorder. It occurs in about 30 percent of patients with organic brain syndrome or paranoid disorder and in about 40 percent of patients with schizophrenia or epilepsy with psychosis.

Functional Interrelationships of the Diffuse Thalamic and Reticular Activating Systems

Alpha-Blocking

The DTS and RAS are intimately related, both anatomically and functionally—so much so that many workers in this field have considered the DTS as simply the rostral extension of the reticular formation. But ablation of portions of the DTS cause synchronization and coma, whereas ablations restricted to the RAS do not necessarily lead to somnolence or coma. Second, although stimulation of the DTS may produce cortical activation, it may produce sleep, as will be shown below. Stimulation of the RAS always produces cortical arousal. Third, the EEG activity generated by DTS stimulation is synchronous, whereas RAS stimulation produces desynchronous (beta) activity.

The best-defined interaction between the two areas is that which is known as *alpha-blocking.* Essentially alpha-blocking, which was first described by Adrian and co-workers, is synonymous with EEG activation. Both terms indicate a sudden shift from predominantly alpha activity to predominantly beta activity. Midbrain reticular stimulation inhibits both the spontaneous and induced firing of intralaminar thalamic neurons—not by direct inhibition of these neurons, as one might expect, but rather by a defacilitation (a "suppression of the depolarizing pressure acting on thalamic neurons").

Sharpless and Jasper proposed in 1956 that arousal mediated by RAS stimulation was tonic (or persistent) activation, whereas that mediated by DTS stimulation was phasic (or transitory) activation related to attention mechanisms. This is consistent with the anatomical specificity inherent to the DTS as compared with the generalized activating effect of RAS stimulation.

Moreover, it is apparent that the two systems can be differentiated on the basis of susceptibility to various pharmacological agents or on the basis of differing responses to a given agent. The response to minor tranquilizers such as chlordiazepoxide is a case in point. Chlordiazepoxide produces an increase in β-activity in the cortex and at the same time decreases the mean frequency of α-activity. This double effect on the EEG has frequently been cited as an argument for postulating two discrete arousal systems.

Dual-Arousal Theory

Routtenberg [13] first formulated his view of two-system control over arousal in 1968, hypothesizing one system associated with the reticular formation maintaining arousal and orientation and a second related to the limbic system controlling incentive-related behaviors. Later he revised this, the reticular formation being viewed as a stimulus-processing system, the second system, associated with response execution, being attributed to limbic and midbrain structures [14]. Deikman's [2] related theory asserts that the human brain performs in two modes: a receptive mode, during which sensory information is gathered and processed, and an active mode, during which the environment is manipulated. These modes correspond to dominance of the stimulus-processing and response-execution systems respectively.

Our own view integrates these views. We postulate that the brain operates in two basic modes: *stimulus-* (or sensory) *processing* and *response-executing.* Each of these modes is itself a dualistic process consisting of two major elements and interconnecting fibers that provide for balance and reciprocal regulation. The dualistic process, which comprises the response-executing mode and is entitled "dual-process theory," is discussed in Chapter 20. The dualistic process involved in stimulus-processing, "dual-arousal theory," grows out of much of what has been said in this chapter.

The two principal systems in stimulus-processing are the DTS and RAS. The DTS is viewed as the system fundamentally responsible for maintaining consciousness. The DTS generates phasic, reentrant activation of groups of neurons within the cortex; it produces only synchronous activity in the EEG. The frequency established by the thalamic pacemaker and imposed on the cortex by the DTS determines whether or not the individual is conscious at a given moment. The possible pacemaker frequencies lie within the delta, theta, and alpha ranges, from zero to approximately 12 Hz. If the pace is in the alpha range (8 to 12 Hz), consciousness occurs. When frequencies fall below about 5 to 7 Hz, consciousness is interrupted. With respect to behavior, the DTS, through its diverse and specific connections, regulates attention and concentration. Attention may be viewed as an internalization of conscious focus. Presumably, intensification of rhythmic, DTS-generated alpha activity increases resistance to the disrupting effects (beta activation) related to novel sensory inputs (arousal stimuli).

Through the agency of the DTS, the capacities of the cerebral cortex for stimulus abstraction, associative learning, and elaboration of behaviors can be brought to bear on the regulatory aims of any of several higher brain centers, in the manner of the time-sharing of a computer. Limbic influences exerted on the DTS (via the anterior thalamus) can direct cerebral cortical activity toward promotion of appetitive or avoidance behaviors. Frontal lobe influences on the DTS can direct cerebral cortical activity toward support of volitional behavioral processes. And the neostriatum and DTS appear to cooperate in circuits that regulate cognitive processes.

Playing against the synchronizing influence of the DTS is the sensory- and drive-related desynchronizing effect of the midbrain RAS. The RAS regulates the extent to which cortical activity is oriented toward environmental stimuli. Activation of the RAS increases externalization of conscious focus, and alpha-blocking of the EEG becomes more likely. Under RAS control, there is also a shift toward elicited (stimulus-controlled) and drive-related behaviors as against the goal-directed behaviors organized by higher brain centers. Reticular activity is a function of the presence of significant stimuli and of escalating primary, homeostatic, and stimulus-related needs, such as hunger, thirst, and sex.

The relationship between the DTS and RAS can perhaps be illustrated better by the following metaphor. Picture a person standing knee-deep in the ocean. Consciousness might be likened to the wave pattern of the sea, the rhythmic pattern of the waves of consciousness being driven by the thalamic pacemaker. The reticular formation is like the person standing in the water. From time to time, this person beats the waves with a plank, with greater or lesser vigor. When the beating of the waves is intensified, the pattern of the waves appears disrupted or desynchronized. If the disruptive activity slows down or stops, the rhythmic pattern reemerges. The ability to disrupt the ocean's intrinsic, rhythmic wave pattern depends on the wave amplitude, for if the waves grow stronger, the disruptive influence will have to be more intense to produce a given degree of desynchronization.

The relationship between DTS and RAS is further illustrated by the four possibilities listed in Table 10-2. Consider for each of the control systems the two ends of the continuum of functional states: for the DTS, pacemaker frequencies in the delta and alpha ranges; for the RAS, an active or an inactive state. Constructing a two by two table, we observe four distinct electroencephalographic-behavioral states. Slow pacemaker activity is associated with sleep (or coma). If this delta activity is paired with RAS inactivity, the observed EEG frequency is delta and the sleep is nondreaming sleep. If, however, the RAS is active, the beta activity superimposed by activity of the RAS on the underlying delta pattern is the observed frequency, and dreaming sleep is the behavioral state. For

Table 10-2. Behavioral states and observed EEG frequencies in
relation to activity of the two arousal systems

DTS (Hz) pace	RAS state	Observed EEG frequency	Behavioral state
≃3	Inactive	Delta	Nondreaming sleep
≃3	Active	Beta	Dreaming sleep
≃ 10	Inactive	Alpha	Awake, relaxed, internalized
≃ 10	Active	Beta	Awake, externalized, stimulus-processing

pacemaker frequencies in the alpha range with an absence of RAS activity, the observed EEG frequency is alpha, and the corresponding behavioral condition is a waking, relaxed state. Superimposition of RAS activity on DTS-induced alpha activity generates a behavioral state in which the individual is alert and actively engaging the environment, and beta activity would appear as the dominant EEG frequency.

The balance between the two arousal systems is regulated by numerous interconnecting pathways. Brainstem regulation of the DTS involves serotonergic, cholinergic, and noradrenergic projections. Reciprocal regulation of the RAS is exercised through descending fibers from the cortex and through limbic discharge pathways.

Imbalance Hypotheses

Several important psychopathologic conditions have been postulated at one time or another to be related to an imbalance between the two arousal systems, the DTS and the RAS.

Hyperkinesis in children has been attributed to late maturation of the DTS and consequent RAS predominance over DTS control of arousal. This would account for the hyperkinetic child's impulsivity, short attention span, hyperreactivity, and explosive irritability. Hyperkinesis will be discussed in detail in Chapter 12.

In early infantile autism, the EEG is persistently desynchronized. This, plus the absence of affectual responding, has led some workers in the field to postulate a sustained suppression of DTS activity [3]. These workers have further postulated that in autism the RAS may function either normally (hyperactive variety) or hypofunctionally (hypoactive variety). This is an attractive hypothesis but one difficult to establish definitely.

Biofeedback

An interesting development of untested potential is the application of biofeedback techniques to conditioning of the human EEG. The public has become intrigued with EEG phenomena, and techniques have become popularized for learning a degree of conscious regulation over alpha activity. Two of these, the Silva mind control technique and transcendental meditation, claim hundreds of thousands of devotees. The laboratory brother of these procedures is the biofeedback technique. With the proper equipment (a filtering system to isolate a selected frequency band), the subject can be presented with a visual or acoustical signal indicating the amount of EEG activity within the selected frequency range. Subjects can rapidly learn to produce the selected frequency at will under such a protocol.

Biofeedback training involving epileptic subjects has been employed and reported by some experimenters with mixed results. Some have noted reductions in seizures with conditioning to nonepileptiform EEGs. A second application of EEG biofeedback procedures has been its use in desensitization of stimulus-provoked anxiety responses or phobias. To our knowledge, EEG biofeedback procedures have yet to be employed in hyperkinesis, schizophrenia, or other imbalance-related psychopathologies, but we anticipate such experiments. In these applications, a subject would be trained to produce slow, DTS-regulated arousal in preference to RAS regulation.

Sleep and Dreaming

Sleep as an Active Phenomenon

We can safely assume that the reader is familiar with the phenomenon of sleep. Despite the universality of this experience, sleep is not easy to define. Sleep is an altered state of consciousness, "a recurrent, easily reversible condition characterized by relative quiescence and by a greatly increased threshold for response to external stimuli" [6]. But defining it gives us no clue as to the functions of sleep; indeed, such clues have been elusive and divergent enough to defy integration.

Sleep was once considered to be a passive phenomenon. In this view, the brain participated only in agreeing not to participate. Reducing the flow of sensory stimuli—by reclining in a quiet, darkened room, for example—was assumed to be sufficient to induce sleep normally. Without an influx of stimuli to maintain wakefulness, the brain would cease to remain active. We now know this view is incomplete and inaccurate. To begin with, sleep can be induced by stimulation of certain brain centers. Moreover, animals or men deprived of sleep may become severely disturbed or even perish. Selective deprivation of one of the sleep stages (desynchronized sleep) produces psychological disturbances. More recently, it has become apparent that lesions in key centers may result in insomnia. Thus, it has become evident that the sleep-wake cycle is a process actively and carefully regulated by the brain.

The Two States of Sleep

Sleep consists of two completely different, though interrelated, substates and five objectively discernible stages (Fig. 10-3). On the basis of EEG patterns, the sleeper is found to progress from the waking state in distinct stages. Stage 1 is characterized by the loss of alpha waves (8 to 12 Hz) in the EEG and the appearance of low-voltage, desynchronized activity, sometimes with low-level (4 to 6 Hz) activity as well. After a few seconds or minutes, the onset of stage 2 sleep occurs, chiefly characterized by so-called "sleep spindles," frequent bursts of 13- to 15-Hz activity. Stage 3 appears in a few more minutes and is recognized by the appearance of delta waves (higher-voltage activity at 1 to 4 Hz). These slow, synchronous waves become the dominant activity in stage 4; hence, this stage is also known as slow-wave (SW) sleep, or synchronized sleep. We will refer to this so-called orthodox or deep-sleep state as SW sleep.

The sleeper typically progresses through four or five cycles of stages 2, 3, and 4 sleep, emerging between times into a markedly distinct state of elevated desynchronized EEG activity, which often contains some slow alpha and occasionally even slower sawtooth-shaped waves. We shall refer to this so-called paradoxical sleep state as D sleep, or desynchronized sleep. Because D sleep is accompanied by rapid eye movements, it is often referred to as REM sleep.

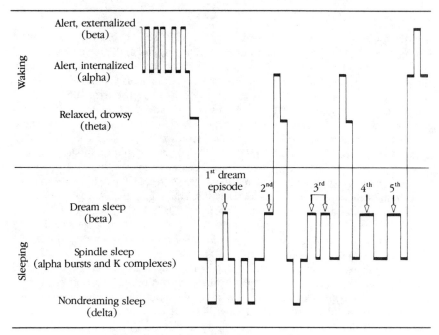

Fig. 10-3. *A typical pattern of stage shifts during the course of a night.*

Slow-Wave Sleep

Traditionally, SW sleep has been termed *deep sleep,* but there are several reasons for regarding D sleep as the deeper state, among them the more relaxed tone of postural muscles and the higher threshold for arousal by external stimuli during D sleep.

Slow-wave sleep is dominated by delta activity in the EEG and is controlled by serotonergic cells in the raphé system. Stimulation of the raphé system, or elevation of serotonin levels, can increase SW sleep; raphé lesions, or depletion of serotonin, on the other hand, produces insomnia. Lysergic acid diethylamide (LSD), believed to be a serotonergic receptor blocker, postpones the onset of sleep that begins with an SW-sleep cycle. There is good reason to believe that SW sleep is generated by the action of the raphé system on the DTS. Stimulation of certain nuclei related to the DTS (intralaminar nuclei of the thalamus) at 3 Hz induces SW sleep, while 8-Hz stimulation induces alpha activity and wakefulness. A hypothesis is that the release of serotonin by the raphé system slows pacemaker activity in the thalamus from alpha to delta frequencies. Some raphé fibers do terminate in the thalamus in an area where serotonin has been identified.

Slow-wave sleep appears to fulfill a physical restorative function, the need for which is manifest as physical tiredness. More SW sleep is needed following increased physical exercise or when catabolism has been increased. Athletes experience more SW sleep than nonathletes. There is evidence of macromolecular synthesis in the anabolic processes of SW sleep; SW sleep probably replenishes supplies of certain macromolecules depleted during waking. Some of the products of synthesis may be used during D sleep, since SW sleep appears to be preparatory to D sleep.

Desynchronized Sleep (D Sleep)

Desynchronized sleep is also known as paradoxical sleep (because of the contrast between elevated EEG activity and muscular relaxation) and as REM sleep (because of concomitant rapid eye movements). Desynchronized sleep is triggered by a nucleus of the RAS (the nucleus reticularis pontis caudalis). It is related to norepinephrine levels but can occur only when serotonin reaches a given level. Because serotonin is required for D sleep but is insufficient to produce it, its function is said to be permissive, and this is related to the postulated preparatory role of SW sleep with respect to D sleep.

The difference between D sleep and SW sleep is not only in EEG activity; in addition to the rapid eye movements that occur during D sleep but not during SW sleep, D sleep is accompanied by deep relaxation of the large muscles of the body and, especially in children, movements of the facial muscles. In SW sleep, either the body may be quiescent, or there may be whole-body spasms. The large muscles, though more relaxed than during waking, are not as deeply relaxed as in D sleep. Penile erections in males accompany most D-sleep periods but do not occur during SW sleep. Pulse and respiration are somewhat faster and more irregular during D sleep than during SW sleep, when they are slow and steady.

Perhaps the most striking aspect of D sleep is dreaming. It now appears that dreaming universally accompanies D sleep, even in subjects who normally report no dreams when allowed to complete their full nightly cycle of sleep. Though it is still possible that there is some form of mental activity during SW sleep, it now seems clear that dreaming occurs largely during D sleep.

Neuroanatomic Centers Regulating Sleep

The neuroanatomic centers involved in regulation of the sleep cycle are illustrated in Figure 10-4. Sleep initiation depends on the combined influence of the midbrain reticular formation and dorsal raphé nucleus. Activation of the brain by the reticular system is minimized when the subject is in a dark, quiet environment. Increased firing of raphé neurons increases serotonin levels late in the evening. In consequence, DTS activity becomes synchronous and slower. When DTS activity falls below about 5 Hz, consciousness cannot be sustained, and sleep has begun. The subject descends through the stages of SW sleep as serotonin levels continue to rise. When serotonin levels reach a critical threshold, autoreceptors on raphé neuron cell bodies in the dorsal raphé shut down the firing activity of raphé cells. The locus ceruleus activates a pontine reticular nucleus (nucleus reticularis pontis caudalis), which controls D sleep. This reticular nucleus stimulates the oculomotor nucleus to trigger rapid eye movements, the midbrain reticular formation to desynchronize the EEG, and the occipital cortex, via the lateral geniculate nucleus, to produce the visual images of dreaming. When serotonin levels drop below a critical threshold, the dorsal raphé resumes firing, inhibiting the locus ceruleus. The dream episode ends abruptly, and SW sleep resumes.

The Function of Dreaming Sleep

The two sleep states appear to serve different purposes. It would be beyond the scope of this book to review all the evidence for the function of dreaming sleep. As that has already been done in a most cogent and systematic manner by Hartmann [6], we will only present what may now be regarded as the most probable hypothesis for the functions of dreaming sleep.

The evidence for the functional role of dreaming comes primarily from observations of situational and constitutional factors that affect the amount of time spent in D sleep

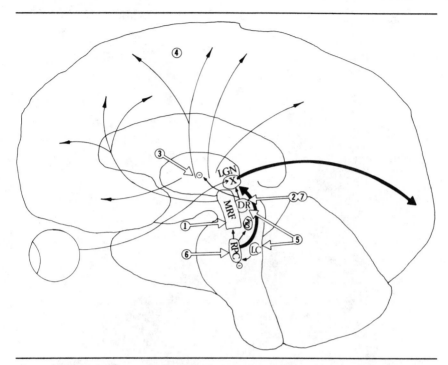

Fig. 10-4. *Neuroanatomic sleep mechanisms. DR, dorsal raphé nucleus; LC, locus ceruleus; LGN, lateral geniculate nucleus; MRF, midbrain reticular formation; OM, oculomotor nucleus; RPC, nucleus reticularis pontis caudalis. (1) A dark, quiet environment minimizes MRF-mediated arousal to facilitate sleep onset. (2) At "bedtime," the firing rate of dorsal raphé cells is elevated, causing serotonin levels to rise (circadian-diurnal rhythm). (3) Serotonin release from raphé nerve terminals in the thalamus and absence of reticular activation combine to suppress relay of sensory afferents and slow the thalamic pacemaker. (4) Cortical wave frequency slows into delta range characteristic of SW sleep. (5) The dream phase is triggered by a feedback action of elevated serotonin levels that shuts down raphé firing and liberates the RPC from locus ceruleus inhibition. (6) RPC discharges are relayed to the occipital cortex via the LGN of the thalamus. These pontine-geniculate-occipital waves are experienced as visual images. RPC discharges to the OM produce rapid eye movements (REMs). RPC discharges to the MRF cause desynchronization of the EEG. (7) When serotonin levels drop below a critical threshold, the raphé resumes firing, and the LC suppresses the RPC (reentry to nondreaming sleep state—step (3) above).*

or, in some studies, REM density and D-sleep latency. There are several ways of evaluating the individual's current "need" for D sleep. REM density is an indication of the intensity of dreaming. Total D-sleep time and the delay before onset of the first D-sleep period (D-sleep latency) are also taken to be indicators. After substantial sleep deprivation or selective deprivation of D sleep, D-sleep latency may drop to zero, for example.

Selective deprivation of D sleep in humans or animals leads to emotional and behavioral disturbances. There is an increase in irritability, defensive behavior, and aggressiveness. The ability to maintain selective attention and goal-oriented activities is impaired. Some studies report hallucinations, delusions, and full-blown psychotic episodes on severe deprivation, but the failure to produce these in some replications leaves such extreme effects in doubt. Indeed, complete, prolonged deprivation may be

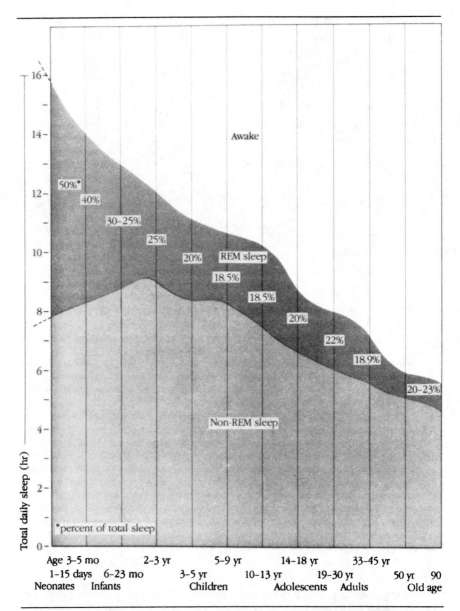

Fig. 10-5. *Changes (with age) in total amounts of daily sleep, daily REM sleep, and in the percentage of REM sleep. Note the sharp diminution of REM sleep in the early years, falling from 8 hours at birth to less than 1 hour in old age. The amount of non-REM sleep throughout life remains more constant, falling from 8 hours at birth to 5 hours in old age. In contrast to the steep decline of REM sleep, the quantity of non-REM sleep is undiminished for many years. Although total daily REM sleep falls steadily during a lifetime, the percentage rises lightly in adolescence and early adulthood. This rise does not reflect an increase in amount; it is because REM sleep does not diminish as quickly as does total sleep. Modified from H. Roffwarg et al. Ontogenetic development of the human sleep-dream cycle. Science 152:604, 1966.* © *1966 by The American Association for the Advancement of Science.*

impossible, since "microsleeps" begin to intrude on waking consciousness, and certain signs of dreaming—penile erections and "phasic pontine-geniculate-occipital spikes" in the EEG—appear during SW sleep after extreme deprivation. There seems to be a strong regulatory mechanism guarding against D-sleep deprivation.

When D-sleep time is temporarily suppressed by any means, a sudden increase in D-sleep time occurs soon after or even before removal of the suppressing influence. This is known as REM rebound or D-sleep rebound. After D-sleep deprivation, D-sleep time may reach as much as 100 percent of total sleeping time, D-sleep latency may drop to nearly zero, and REM density may increase dramatically. Lost SW sleep is not usually "made up for" or recovered in anything approaching a quantitative manner, but the same is not true for D-sleep time.

Many kinds of life stresses may increase the need for D sleep. For example, major life-style changes or periods of stressful personal adaptation are associated with a greater need for D sleep. Greater D-sleep time is associated with emotional stress and stressful learning or intellectual work. Withdrawal from alcohol, barbiturates, or amphetamines is accompanied by markedly increased D-sleep time. Individuals whose personality, or life-style, or both involves continuous change, constant reevaluation, and an emphasis on growth and progress characteristically have patterns of long sleeping with significantly higher D-sleep time than individuals whose lives and personalities are more fixed, stable, and preprogrammed. Infants, whose life stresses and learning requirements are very high indeed, dream during half of their daily sleeping time (Fig. 10-5). The percentage falls to approximately 20 to 25 percent by age 5 or 6, though the absolute value continues to decline somewhat. In the elderly, the need for D sleep as well as total sleep is diminished.

The content of dreams and the effects of sleep deprivation both suggest a restorative function related to the ability to maintain focused attention, the ability to repattern or to consolidate memories and to prepare for new learning, and the integrity of the sense of self, including optimism and positive mood, energy, and self-confidence.

Dreams, Drugs, and Psychotherapy

Many drugs decrease D-sleep time on the first administration, most notably the sedative-hypnotics, barbiturates, and antidepressants. The antidepressants and the MAO inhibitors markedly decrease D-sleep time. Practically the only psychotropic drug that increases D-sleep time is reserpine. The mechanism of these effects is probably related to the role of norepinephrine (NE) in D sleep and/or in the systems affected by D sleep. Artificially elevating CNS NE levels, as with an MAO inhibitor, decreases D-sleep time; diminishing NE levels (e.g., using α-methylparatyrosine) markedly increases D-sleep time. Reserpine reduces NE levels by interfering with storage but also affects other biogenic amines. The levels of NE seem to be part of the chemical feedback loop that controls the duration, frequency, and intensity of D-sleep cycles. That elevating NE levels chemically does not substitute fully for D-sleep time is evident in rebound effects in which D-sleep time is radically increased following withdrawal of these drugs.

Sleep in chronic alcoholic patients is shallow and fragmented, marked by frequent awakenings and stage changes and diminished D sleep and SW sleep. As a result, the chronic use of alcohol is often associated with excessive daytime sleepiness. These sleep disturbances may persist even after 2 years of total abstinence. It is possible that some elements of the sleep disturbance seen in these individuals may have predated the period of alcohol consumption, in which case the alcohol use may be serving as a crude form of self-medication.

Table 10-3. *Sleep and arousal disorders*

Diagnostic category	Type (degree)	Incidence	Sex ratio	Drug treatments
Insomnias				
Psychophysiologic[a]	1	±	F > M	Hypnotics, soporifics, or L-tryptophan
Associated with sleep apneas[b]	1	++	M > F	Imipramine
Associated with nocturnal myoclonus or akathisias	1	?	M = F	Diazepam
Drug-induced[c]	2	+	?	Eliminate drug
Associated with psychiatric disorders[d]	2	+	F > M	Various
Associated with medical conditions[e]	2	+	?	Various
Excessive somnolence				
Excessive daytime sleepiness				
Associated with insomnia[f]	1–2	++	F > M	Determined by type of insomnia (see above)
Associated with insufficient sleep	1	±	?	None
Narcolepsy	1	–	M > F	Stimulants
Sleep drunkenness	1	–	M > F	None
Hypersomnia				
Psychophysiologic hypersomnia[a]	1	±	?	None
Idiopathic hypersomnolence	1	–	?	Methysergide
Intermittent hypersomnias				
Kleine-Levin syndrome	1	–	M > F	None
Menstruation-associated	1	–	F	None
Infectious conditions[g]	2	–	M = F	Antimicrobials
Mixed				
Drug-induced[h]	2	+	?	Dosage adjustment

	1°			
Disorders of sleep-wake cycle				
Transient[i]	1	±	M = F	None
Persistent[j]	1	−	M = F	None
Parasomnias				
Sleepwalking and night terrors (stage 4–related)	1	−	M > F	Diazepam
Nightmares (REM-related)	1	±	M = F	None
Other[k]	1	Varies	Varies	Various

1°, primary; 2°, secondary; +, common; ++, very common; −, rare; ±, rarely of clinical significance but probably common in the overall population.

[a] Stress-related.

[b] Includes central apneas (failure of the medullary respiratory center), upper airway apneas (occlusion), and mixed apneas (combining both).

[c] Withdrawal from sedative-hypnotics (including alcohol) or use of stimulants.

[d] Psychiatric disorders commonly associated with insomnia include mania, depression, acute psychotic states, anxiety disorders, personality disorders, and drug dependence.

[e] Hyperthyroidism, chronic renal insufficiency, and epilepsy, for example.

[f] This is, after all, the usual chief complaint in insomnia.

[g] Trypanosomiasis (sleeping sickness), for example.

[h] Excessive use of depressants or rebound depression after chronic use of stimulants.

[i] Includes jet lag or work-schedule shifts.

[j] Sleep phase syndromes and nondiurnal sleep cycles, for example.

[k] Bruxism, head-banging, painful erections, seizures, and asthma, for example.

The primary functions of D sleep, then, appear to involve learning and restoration in preparation for continued learning: adaption, renewal, or reprogramming of the individual's mechanisms of organization of reality and self, his "maps" of himself in relation to his circumstances. Changes that involve emotion, disruption of usual ways of doing things, and stressful reprogramming during waking hours all require increased D-sleep time for restoration and maintenance of flexible, focused attention, subtle feedback regulation of emotional state, and a continued sense of self and of self-guidance.

At the neurophysiologic level, this appears to involve the repair, reorganization, and formation of new connections in the cortex, stimulated at least in part by the activity of ascending catecholaminergic systems. Though not demonstrated, we may infer the involvement of the dorsal NE bundle of the medial forebrain bundle (a part of the limbic system discussed in Chapter 15) and the DTS.

The function of dreaming sleep under the foregoing hypothesis is intimately related to the goals and processes of psychotherapy. It would seem that D sleep is the neurophysiologic means by which the learning induced by psychotherapeutic intervention may be consolidated and integrated into the client's modes of functioning. That therapy is often stressful and almost invariably emotionally engaging makes it even more likely that D sleep mediates this change process. Hartmann [6] has described the characteristic sleep pattern of long sleepers as having approximately the same SW-sleep time as short sleepers but added D-sleep time, mostly accounted for by an additional D-sleep cycle at the end of sleep. One might even conceive of the therapist suggesting that a client sleep late following particularly meaningful or stressful sessions. Drug interactions with D sleep are therefore potentially of major consequence for psychotherapy. It is a reasonable, though certainly not demonstrated, assumption, then, that drugs that interfere with D sleep might slow the consolidation of changes precipitated by psychotherapy.

Sleep Disorders

Sleep disorders may be primary or secondary. In the latter category, sleep disorders may be related to psychiatric, organic, or behavioral problems. Primary sleep disorders include insomnia, excessive somnolence (excessive daytime sleepiness and hypersomnia), disorders of the sleep-wake cycle, and parasomnias (Table 10-3). Some parasomnias occur during stage 4 of SW sleep (i.e., night terrors, enuresis, and sleepwalking), some during D sleep (e.g., nightmares), and some are not phase-dependent (e.g., bruxism). One form of excessive daytime sleepiness is narcolepsy. The four characteristics of narcolepsy are short, irresistible sleep attacks, cataplexy (sudden loss of muscle tone), sleep paralysis, and hypnagogic hallucinations (onset of vivid dreams before loss of consciousness). The latter two symptoms are less frequent and are not necessary to reach the diagnosis. Narcolepsy occurs in about 0.07 percent of the United States population. Both insomnia and excessive daytime sleepiness may be associated with sleep apneas, that is, disruptions of respiration during sleep. A particularly dreadful variety of sleep apnea is the sudden infant death syndrome (also called Ondine's curse).

Organic problems that often produce sleep disturbances include epilepsy, thyroid dysfunction, and chronic renal insufficiency. The drug-induced sleep disturbances discussed in the preceding section could also be classified as secondary to organic problems.

Sleep disturbances are associated with depression, manic-depressive disorder, schizophrenia, and anxiety states. In depression, sleep disturbance is commonly, but not invariably, present. Most often, sleep is fragmented in major depression, but some depressed patients sleep for excessively long periods during bouts of depression, and still others sleep normally. In manic-depressive disorder, patients tend to sleep more while depressed and less during mania. In schizophrenia, acute psychotic episodes are usually accompanied by insomnia and a lack of D-sleep rebound after deprivation. Chronic schizophrenics exhibit surprisingly normal sleep patterns.

Insomnia is common in patients suffering excessive anxiety, and, indeed, insomnia may be the chief complaint. Insomnias and excessive anxiety disorders are overlapping diagnostic categories; their cause-and-effect interrelationship has not yet been established.

The most widely employed class of drugs for any category of sleep disorders is the hypnotic family. These drugs find widespread use in insomnia, both to induce and to sustain sleep. In the next chapter, this important class of drugs will be addressed.

Selected References and Further Readings

1. Andersen, P., and Andersson, S. A. *Physiological Basis of the Alpha Rhythm.* New York: Meredith, 1968.
2. Deikman, A. J. Bimodal Consciousness. In J. Stoyva et al. (Eds.), *Biofeedback and Self-Control, 1971.* Chicago: Aldine, 1972. Pp. 58–73.
3. Des Lauriers, A. M., and Carlson, C. F. *Your Child is Asleep: Early Infantile Autism.* Homewood, Ill.: Dorsey Press, 1969.
4. French, J. D. The reticular formation. *Sci. Am.* 19615:54–60, 1957.
5. Gillin, J. C., Mendelson, W. B., Sitaram, N., and Wyatt, R. J. The neuropharmacology of sleep and wakefulness. *Annu. Rev. Pharmacol. Toxicol.* 18:563–579, 1978.
6. Hartmann, E. L. *The Functions of Sleep.* New Haven: Yale University Press, 1973.
7. Hauri, P. *The Sleep Disorders.* Kalamazoo, Mich.: The Upjohn Company, 1977.
8. Hughes, R. R. *An Introduction to Clinical Electro-Encephalography.* Bristol, Engl.: Wright, 1961.
9. Jaspar, H. H. et al. (Eds.). *The Reticular Formation of the Brain.* Boston: Little, Brown, 1958.
10. Jouvet, M. Neuropharmacology of the Sleep-Waking Cycle. In L. L. Iversen et al. (Eds.), *Handbook of Psychopharmacology.* New York: Plenum, 1977. Vol. 8.
11. Lindsley, D. B. Attention, Consciousness, Sleep and Wakefulness. In J. Field, H. W. Magoun, and V. E. Hall (Eds.), *Handbook of Physiology.* Baltimore: Williams & Wilkins, 1960. Vol. 3.
12. Noback, S. R. *The Human Nervous System.* New York: McGraw-Hill, 1967.
13. Routtenberg, A. The two-arousal hypothesis: Reticular formation and limbic system. *Psychol. Rev.* 75:51–80, 1968.
14. Routtenberg, A. Stimulus processing and response execution: A neurobehavioral theory. *Physiol. Behav.* 6:589–596, 1970.
15. Weitzman, E. D. Sleep and its disorders. *Annu. Rev. Neurosci.* 4:381–417, 1981.

Sedative-Hypnotics
11

℞

One of the oldest, largest, and best-studied classes of psychoactive drugs are the sedative-hypnotics. Drugs of this class produce a dose-dependent, generalized depression of cellular activity in many organ systems, including the nervous system. The term *sedative-hypnotic* is intended to denote the dose dependency of the effect of these drugs; in general, drugs of this class produce first a sedation at low doses, an hypnosis at intermediate doses, and anesthesia at higher doses. The use of these drugs is now limited, however, with a few exceptions, to the hypnotic action, since more efficacious agents are available both for sedation and for anesthesia.

It should be pointed out that the term *hypnotic,* as employed by the pharmacologist, is unrelated to a "hypnotic state" or trance but simply implies an ability to increase drowsiness, reduce motor activity, and induce and sustain sleep. Two other names that have been used for this group of drugs, *soporific* and *somnifacient,* are perhaps more appropriate and less confusing. *Sedation* implies a reduced excitability and emotionality short of sleep or coma.

The first drug used to induce sleep was opium, but the narcotic stupor induced by opium and opiates is, in fact, distinct from natural sleep. In many species, the effects induced by narcotics and by hypnotics are readily distinguished.

General Pharmacology of Sedative-Hypnotics

Mechanism of Depressant Action

The barbiturates and other sedative-hypnotics are general depressants of cellular function. The activity of nerve cells and all types of muscle cells is depressed. There is a general reduction of oxygen consumption by cells and an inhibition of energy-storing processes. Various peripheral tissues are affected by barbiturates, but the CNS is particularly sensitive. Peripheral effects are substantial only at anesthetic doses but may be a matter of grave concern in cases of barbiturate overdosage.

It is generally conceded that within the CNS the synapse is the site of action of sedatives, since speed of conduction of impulses along nerve axons is not affected. According to a classification by Molitor and Pick, the cerebral cortex is the chief site of action for sedatives that are bromides, alcohols, or aldehydes, while urea derivatives, such as barbiturates and sedatives of related structure (e.g., the piperidinedione derivatives)

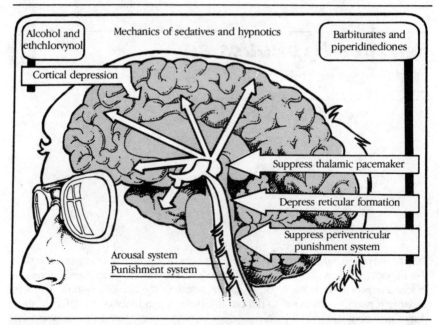

Fig. 11-1. Mechanisms of sedative-hypnotics. Modified from A. K. Swonger, Nursing Pharmacology. Boston: Little, Brown, 1978.

are said to act primarily on subcortical centers (Fig. 11-1). Among subcortical centers, the reticular formation is particularly sensitive to the action of sedative-hypnotics, responding with widespread depression of the firing rates of individual neurons.

One important receptor site for barbiturates is a protein associated with, but not the same as, the gamma-aminobutyric acid (GABA) recognition protein of GABA postsynaptic receptors (Fig. 11-2). The barbiturate receptor is also not the same as the benzodiazepine receptor site, though both receptor proteins appear to be modulatory proteins regulating GABA-binding. The effect of binding of a barbiturate molecule to its receptor is to enhance GABA-binding, a phenomenon called positive cooperativity. Barbiturates also enhance GABA synthesis. Another aspect of the action of barbiturates is a general impairment of excitatory transmission. The barbiturates cause a fluidization of cell membranes that interferes with calcium influx in response to action potentials. The result is reduced transmitter release per action potential and fewer excitatory postsynaptic potentials.

Effects on Sleep

The effect of sedative agents on sleep is complex and multidimensional. Since the induction of sleep and then sustaining it are the most frequent uses of these agents, it is important that their actions on sleep be understood in their entirety.

In addition to altering total sleep time and reducing latency to onset of sleep, sedative-hypnotic drugs may disrupt the relative time spent by the sleeper in each of the two types of sleep: desynchronized (dreaming, or D) and slow-wave (nondreaming) sleep. With their first use or with infrequent use, most sedatives cause a suppression of D-sleep time, so that the usual 20 percent or so of sleeping time spent in D sleep is reduced to 5

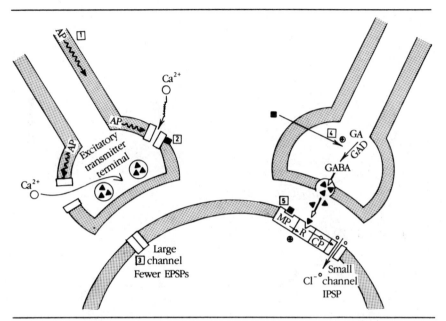

Fig. 11-2. *Neurochemical mechanisms of barbiturates. AP, action potential; EPSP, excitatory postsynaptic potential; GA, glutamic acid; GABA, gamma-aminobutyric acid; GAD, glutamic acid decarboxylase; IPSP, inhibitory postsynaptic potential. (1) Barbiturates do not affect the conduction process. Rather, barbiturates cause "fluidization" of cell membranes, reducing calcium influx (2) in response to action potentials. The result is reduced turnover of excitatory transmitters and fewer EPSPs (3). Barbiturates have more specific interactions with GABA transmission, increasing GABA synthesis (4) and facilitating GABA-binding to postsynaptic receptors (5). The result is increased IPSPs.*

to 15 percent (Fig. 11-3). On the night following a single use of a sedative-hypnotic, the percentage of sleep time spent in D sleep rises above normal. This is called *REM rebound.* Thus, the acute effect of a sedative-hypnotic on dreaming is REM suppression followed by REM rebound.

With chronic use, the initial reduction in D sleep gradually undergoes tolerance over a period of 1 to 2 weeks, and the D-sleep percentage returns to normal (Fig. 11-3). When a person is withdrawn from chronic use of a sedative, there is an elevation in the percentage of REM sleep during the period of rebound hyperexcitability or withdrawal. If the severity of withdrawal symptoms is a frank abstinence syndrome, the REM percentage may rise as high as 100 percent of total sleep time (but total sleep time is sharply diminished during withdrawal from sedative-hypnotics). Thus, the chronic effects of sedative-hypnotics on D sleep consist of REM suppression, followed by tolerance to REM suppression, followed by REM elevation during withdrawal.

The D-sleep effects of sedative-hypnotics as a class are shared fully by alcohol. Two groups of sedatives that are notably exceptional in terms of effects on D sleep are the chloral derivatives and the benzodiazepines, which produce little if any D-sleep suppression. Since there is no REM suppression with these drugs, there is also no REM rebound nor REM elevation during withdrawal.

An oddity with respect to the effect of some sedative-hypnotics is the relatively high frequency of occurrence of so-called idiosyncratic reactions of excitation. This effect,

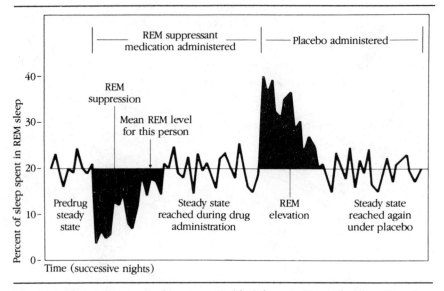

Fig. 11-3. *REM deprivation and recovery. Modified from P. Hauri.* The Sleep Disorders. *Kalamazoo, Mich.: The Upjohn Company, 1977.*

more common in the young than in the old, is reminiscent of excitation produced by alcohol. Although many explanations of this effect have been offered, it is not fully understood. It has been said that these idiosyncratic reactions may contribute to some instances of sedative-hypnotic overdosage. Presumably, users who have taken their nightly dose of sleeping pills might be deluded by such a reaction and the associated confused state into thinking they have forgotten to take them and they may take a second and third dose. This possible happening has been described as "drug automatism," but whether or not it actually occurs is a matter of some controversy.

A user of sedatives may at times awaken with a residual concentration of the sedative in his or her system. Under such circumstances, the user will experience a general intoxication, and feelings of euphoria and great energy. There is some risk that lack of judgment, together with impaired coordination, may result in accidental injury in such cases.

Effect on Respiration

The respiratory center located in the medulla oblongata is another brain region particularly sensitive to the action of sedative-hypnotics. Indeed, depression of respiration is the immediate cause of death in cases of sedative-hypnotic poisoning unless respiration is artificially maintained, in which case cardiovascular complications may precipitate death.

Normally, respiration is maintained by three drives: the neurogenic drive, which refers to the spontaneous rhythmicity of neurons in the respiratory center; the hypoxic drive; and a drive related to pH and levels of carbon dioxide. The neurogenic drive is the one most susceptible to depression by sedative-hypnotics. The hypoxic and carbon dioxide–related drives, however, may also be depressed at hypnotic and higher doses of sedative-hypnotics. The optimal treatment is now considered to be artificial ventilation if such equipment is available. This allows the patient to "sleep off" the drug depression, so to speak. Alternatively, analeptics such as doxapram may be used to stimulate the respiratory center. The antagonism that occurs between sedative-hypnotics and analeptics is considered to be functional (or physiologic) rather than competitive (or pharmacologic) (Chap. 7), so that this is not an ideal approach. Use of analeptics may lead to convulsions if a too large or a too long-acting dose regimen is selected. Administration by inhalation of elevated concentrations of oxygen is considered poor strategy, since this may further suppress any residual hypoxic drive.

Intoxication, Tolerance, and Dependence

Although several nonbarbiturate hypnotics have been initially marketed with claims that they were nonaddicting, such claims have invariably proved false, so that no non-addicting hypnotic is presently known. Indeed, there is very little to choose from among the various sedative-hypnotics as regards severity of abuse liability. All the sedative-hypnotics, barbiturate and nonbarbiturate alike, including alcohol, show cross-tolerance with one another and freely substitute for each other in their ability to suppress symptoms of withdrawal following chronic use. For example, a barbiturate could be used by an alcoholic both to maintain dependence and to postpone the onset of withdrawal.

Barbiturates and nonbarbiturates produce intoxication in the same manner as alcohol. The criteria for establishing sedative-hypnotic intoxication are (1) recent use of a sedative-hypnotic; (2) one or more psychological signs of intoxication (mood lability, disinhibition of sexual or aggressive impulses, irritability, or loquacity); (3) one or more neurologic signs (slurred speech, incoordination, unsteady gait, impairment of attention or memory); (4) maladaptive behaviors (poor judgment or functioning); and (5) lack of an organic or psychiatric etiology.

Dependence does not necessarily follow from therapeutic or limited social use of sedative-hypnotics, but arises as an inevitable consequence of repeated, continuous, immoderate use. Dependence is of both the psychological and physiologic varieties. Psychological dependence is manifested as a strong urge to continue self-administration of the drug in order to reexperience the subjectively perceived effects. Note that this craving is independent of the drug's ability to produce tolerance. Psychological dependence refers *not* to a desire to avoid the subjectively negative experience of withdrawal but rather to the effort to reclaim the subjectively positive "high" that is an immediate consequence of the taking of the drug. The subjective experience with most sedative-hypnotics closely resembles that of alcohol and therefore is "familiar" to most people.

The physical dependence associated with sedative-hypnotics is a particularly serious medical problem. Withdrawal from chronic use of any of these drugs precipitates within 24 hours a "withdrawal syndrome" whose severity is related to the intensity of the addiction. The effects reach a peak between 48 and 72 hours following the last dose of the drug and thereafter subside slowly. The syndrome seen in barbiturate addicts resembles closely that seen in alcohol addicts, the most severe form of which is known as delirium tremens. Depending on the severity of the addiction, any or all of the following may occur: anxiety, involuntary muscle twitches and tremors, muscular weakness, dizziness, nausea, vomiting, insomnia, weight loss, orthostatic hypotension, illusions, delusions, hallucinations, paranoia, delirium, convulsive seizures, and death. The risk of death in withdrawal from alcohol or barbiturates is considerably greater than in narcotic withdrawal. Many nonmedical centers that treat addicts will permit narcotic addicts to undergo withdrawal under their auspices, but wisely refuse to work with barbiturate addicts and alcoholics until they have undergone withdrawal in a medically supervised setting.

All sedative-hypnotics produce tolerance. In the case of barbiturates and several of the other sedative-hypnotics, two independent mechanisms contribute to the development of tolerance. One of these, drug disposition tolerance, will be discussed in the section on drug interactions of sedative-hypnotics. The other mechanism, pharmacodynamic tolerance, is common to *all* the sedative-hypnotic substances. Pharmacodynamic tolerance occurs when the neurochemistry of the brain adjusts to the continuous presence of a drug in such a manner that the drug becomes less capable of modifying brain function. A secondary consequence of this adaptation by the brain is that removal of the drug now "uncovers" the adaptive process and leads to a manifestation of withdrawal symptoms.

Tolerance to sedative-hypnotics develops rapidly but is completely reversible. There is some suggestion that a degree of tolerance may develop to a single dose of a barbiturate, since it has been established that blood levels on awakening from barbiturate-induced sleep are higher than the blood levels at the time of sleep initiation. This phenomenon is known as *acute tolerance.*

Sedative-Hypnotics Abuse

Sedative-hypnotics are widely used and abused. Over 300 tons of barbiturates are manufactured yearly in the United States, and it is estimated that nearly half this amount goes into the black market. Barbiturate addiction is at least as dangerous as opiate addiction, even though it is given less attention. Barbiturates are the most frequently used drugs in suicides and are involved in a fifth of all cases of suicide and in a total of 3,000 deaths per year in the United States. Three of the five most common causes of fatal drug overdosage are sedative-hypnotics: barbiturates, glutethimide, and meprobamate. Alcohol, the nonprescription sedative-hypnotic, poses the preeminent drug abuse problem (Chap. 12).

Drug Interactions of Sedative-Hypnotics

Sedative-hypnotics produce an additive CNS depression when administered along with another CNS depressant such as a tranquilizer or narcotic. Similarly, the depressant effects of alcohol and barbiturates or other hypnotics are additive, and since both are frequently self-administered, this interaction can have tragic consequences.

Many sedative-hypnotics have the capability of "inducing" liver drug-metabolizing enzymes (enzyme induction refers to an elevation of the activity of the drug-metabolizing enzymes of the liver). Thus, administration of a barbiturate, for example, enhances the liver's capacity to metabolize a whole host of drugs and, as a result, decreases the duration and intensity of the action of all drugs metabolized by the liver. Agents thus antagonized by induction of liver enzymes include many analgesics, anticoagulants, antihistamines, anti-inflammatory agents, phenytoin, steroids, meprobamate, and many sedative-hypnotics themselves. Some of these agents are actually inducers of liver enzymes themselves and thus may reduce the action of sedative-hypnotics. A situation in which a drug reduces its own effectiveness by inducing its own metabolism is referred to as "drug-disposition" tolerance.

Early Sedative-Hypnotics

The first sedative-hypnotics employed were bromides and chloral hydrate. The toxic effects associated with bromides have prescribed their use. Because they are slowly excreted, persistent use of bromides produces a buildup of levels in the body, leading to a state of intoxication. Symptoms of bromide intoxication begin with drowsiness, dizziness, impaired memory, and irritability. In some severe cases, intoxication, delirium, hallucinations, delusions, mania, lethargy, and ultimately coma may ensue. Chloral hydrate was introduced into therapy in 1869, and its early use was in the management of psychiatric patients. Actually, chloral hydrate is rapidly converted in the body into trichloroethanol, and it is the metabolite that produces the hypnotic action. Although chloral hydrate is still used to induce sleep, its popularity has suffered since the introduction of the barbiturates. Chloral hydrate has an addiction liability approximately equivalent to that of the barbiturates. Its major disadvantage is that it produces considerable gastric irritation, nausea, and vomiting. It does have one apparent advantage over the barbiturates, however: It produces considerably less suppression of the D-sleep phase of sleep.

Barbiturates

The barbiturates are the most widely used sedative-hypnotics and the best studied. Their actions and side effects may be considered prototypical of the entire class and will therefore be discussed in some detail. Much of what is said concerning the barbiturates can be applied to other sedative-hypnotics except where specific exceptions are noted.

Barbituric acid was synthesized in 1864 by Adolph von Baeyer by the condensation of urea and malonic acid. The first hypnotic derivative, barbital, was first employed therapeutically in 1903 by Emil Fischer. Barbital has for the most part been displaced by derivatives having a shorter duration of action. Phenobarbital was introduced into medicine in 1912 and still enjoys widespread use. In all, more than 2,500 barbiturates have been developed and some 50 marketed.

Classification of Barbiturates

Barbiturates are subclassified on the basis of duration of action because that particular characteristic dictates clinical applications. Duration goes hand in hand with time of onset, the long-acting drugs having the longest latency to onset as well. Four categories are distinguished: long-acting, intermediate-acting, short-acting, and ultrashort-acting. The long-acting group includes phenobarbital and mephobarbital. These drugs find use mainly as antiepileptics and in combinations for asthma and ulcers. Latency to onset is an hour or more; duration of effect is 10 to 14 hours.

The most important intermediate-acting barbiturate is amobarbital (Amytal), known on the street as "blue heaven." It is used as a sleep sustainer, for people who have no difficulty first falling asleep but who are unable to get back to sleep after awakening in the middle of the night. Latency to onset is about 45 to 60 minutes; duration is 6 to 10 hours.

The short-acting category includes pentobarbital (Nembutal) and secobarbital (Seconal), encountered in the black market as "yellow jackets" and "red devils" respectively. Short-acting barbiturates are used as sleep inducers. Latency to onset is about 15 to 30 minutes, and duration is typically 3 to 6 hours. Ultrashort-acting barbiturates, such as thiopental (Pentothal), find use as intravenous anesthetics.

The extent to which a given barbiturate causes residual depression (sometimes called hangover) the morning after being used as an hypnotic is related to its duration of action. Long-acting barbiturates generally cause too much residual depression to be useful as hypnotics. Short-acting barbiturates cause less residual depression than intermediate-acting drugs.

Nonbarbiturate Hypnotics

Piperidinedione Derivatives

The barbiturate domination of the hypnotic market began to erode in the 1950s with the introduction of two drugs from the piperidinedione family. Although nonbarbiturates, the drugs in this group resemble the barbiturates both in chemical structure and in pharmacology. Glutethimide (Doriden), introduced in 1954, and methyprylon (Noludar), introduced in 1955, produce effects barely distinguishable from those of secobarbital.

The piperidinediones have a duration of action and latency to onset equivalent to that of the short-acting barbiturates. In comparison with the barbiturates, the degree of cardiac depression is somewhat greater for these substances in relation to the degree of respiratory depression. Thus, in cases of overdose in which the drug is known to be a piperidinedione, it is important that blood pressure as well as respiration be monitored. For other sedative-hypnotics, it can be assumed that if the patient is breathing without mechanical support, death will not occur from other depressant effects, but with the piperidinediones, circulatory collapse may precede respiratory failure. Another negative characteristic of this family is that acute intoxication is more frequent because absorption of these drugs is irregular. Gastric irritation and rare, but serious, blood dyscrasias are known to occur with the use of glutethimide.

Tertiary Alcohols

A number of tertiary alcohols have been found to be potent CNS depressants. A therapeutically useful agent of this type is ethchlorvynol (Placidyl). Dependence on and withdrawal from this drug resemble closely dependence on and withdrawal from alcohol. Ethchlorvynol is short-acting and has good skeletal muscle–relaxing properties. One advantage of ethchlorvynol is lower incidence of initial excitation or paradoxical reactions. Ethchlorvynol is a distant third to flurazepam and meprobamate in terms of frequency of prescription among sedative-hypnotics.

Methaqualone

Methaqualone (Quaalude) is a substituted quinazalone, several of which have been found to have sedative-hypnotic properties. It closely resembles the barbiturates in its actions, but in addition has antihistaminic activity and potent antitussive properties. It is also structurally related to the benzodiazepines and is a fair, but short-acting, anxiolytic. Latency to onset is about 30 minutes; duration is 5 to 8 hours.

Methaqualone is more effective as a sleep sustainer than as a sleep inducer. Known popularly as the "love drug," it has substantial abuse potential—its illicit use reached nearly epidemic proportions in the United States in 1972–1973 and again in the early 1980s. Its purported aphrodisiac properties reflect only the disinhibition of sexual impulses characteristic of the action of all the sedative-hypnotic drugs.

Minor Tranquilizers

Meprobamate (Miltown, Equanil) and the benzodiazepines can be effective hypnotics, although, with the exception of flurazepam and temazepam, they are more commonly used as daytime sedatives (for a discussion of the latter use, see Chap. 17). The important thing to establish at this point is that minor tranquilizers do not represent a distinct class of drugs at all, but rather are simply those sedative-hypnotics having the greatest preferential antianxiety action as opposed to general sedative action. The benzodiazepines produce little if any suppression of D sleep. Flurazepam (Dalmane) and the new benzodiazepine temazepam (Restoril), are marketed expressly for use as hypnotics. Flurazepam may be considered the current drug of choice as an hypnotic.

Flurazepam

Flurazepam is the most distinctive of the hypnotic drugs, possessing a number of distinct advantages and a smaller number of disadvantages relative to other sedative-hypnotics (Table 11-1). Flurazepam acts as quickly as a short-acting barbiturate, but its effect lasts as long as an intermediate-acting barbiturate. This provides greater flexibility in application, but also means that residual depression is greater than for short-acting barbiturates. Flurazepam is the only hypnotic with demonstrated effectiveness beyond 2 weeks of nightly use. It does not suppress D sleep but decreases stage 4 of slow-wave sleep. Abuse liability is considerably less than with alternative hypnotics. Flurazepam is available in 15- to 30-mg capsules; the hypnotic dose range is 15 to 50 mg. Most patients respond adequately to 15 mg. The common practice of prescribing the 30-mg dose before exploring responsiveness to the lower dose is an unwarranted flirtation with the possibilities of abuse and adverse reactions. Flurazepam has excellent skeletal muscle–relaxing properties similar to other benzodiazepines.

A new benzodiazepine, temazepam, has been marketed as a hypnotic. It is shorter-acting than flurazepam and therefore produces less residual depression.

Antihistamine and Anticholinergic Sleep Aids

Antihistamines are a group of substances commonly used for allergies and in cold remedies. Some newer antihistamines (e.g., chlorpheniramine and phenindamine) produce little if any sedation and may even be mildly stimulatory, but most of the classic antihistamines are sedatives. The degree of sedation varies both with the different drugs and with the biological differences of the users. Tolerance to the sedative effect tends to develop with continued use. A few antihistamines have been expressly employed for their sedative action. Hydroxyzine (Atarax, Vistaril), a prescription drug, is used for anti-anxiety purposes and is discussed in Chapter 17. Throughout the 1970s, most non-prescription sleep aids contained the antihistamine methapyrilene, often in combination with the anticholinergic drug, scopolamine. Methapyrilene was withdrawn from the market when it was found to be potentially carcinogenic. There are currently three antihistamines in use in sleep aid preparations: diphenhydramine in Sominex Formula 2, doxylamine in Unisom, and pyrilamine in most of the remaining formulas (e.g., Sominex Formula 1, Nytol, Sleep-Eze). These sleep aids have the distinct advantages of low abuse potential and no physical dependence, but are only modestly effective.

Scopolamine is an anticholinergic compound that produces EEG synchronization and, at moderate doses, a degree of sedation. At higher doses, scopolamine and other anticholinergics can produce restlessness, agitation, hallucinations, and headaches. The sedative action of scopolamine appears to relate to its direct action on the cerebral cortex, where it inhibits the influence of ACH released by cholinergic neurons that comprise the final link to the cortex for the ascending reticular activating system. Many anticholinergic drugs employed for autonomic nervous system actions have CNS side effects similar to the effects of scopolamine.

Implications for Psychotherapy

Sedative-hypnotics have been known to induce depression that could be mistaken for psychogenic depression. Consequently, the psychotherapist should inquire about the

Table 11-1. *A comparison of attributes of sedative-hypnotics*

Attribute	Flurazepam	Barbiturates		Piperidinediones	Ethchlorvynol	Methaqualone
		Short-acting	Intermediate-acting			
Sleep effects						
Acute effectiveness as sleep inducer	++	++	0	++	++	+
Acute effectiveness as sleep sustainer	++	0	++	0	0	++
Effectiveness after 2 wk	++	0	0	0	0	0
Acute D-sleep suppression	0	++	++	++	++	+
Elevated D sleep during withdrawal	0	++	++	++	++	++
Suppression of stage 4 slow-wave sleep	++	±	±	±	+	±
Abuse potential						
Psychological dependence	±	++	++	++	++	++
Physical dependence	±	++	++	++	++	++
Induction of liver enzymes	0	++	++	++	++	++
Suicide potential	0	++	++	++	++	++
Adverse effects						
Residual depression	++	+	++	+	+	++
Paradoxical excitation	++	++	++	++	+	++
Acute intoxication	0	+	+	++	+	+

0, does not produce indicated effect; ±, equivocal tendency toward effect; +, moderate tendency to product effect; ++, strong likelihood or severity of effect.

use of these drugs in depressed clients. Occasionally, hangover may occur the morning after barbiturate use, as with alcohol use. This is marked by irritability and confusion. At high doses, toxic delirium may occur.

The sedative-hypnotics all possess an exceptionally high abuse potential. This is true also of the so-called minor tranquilizers and of alcohol and the barbiturates. Informal drug sources, the so-called *gray market,* supply many self-administered drugs in these classes. In general, the anxiolytics are thought of as treatment rather than as a problem, but it is entirely likely that the psychotherapist will encounter cases in which their use, even though they are perhaps legitimately prescribed, plays a psychological and interpersonal role analogous to alcohol abuse. Drugs in these classes may be readily prescribed by nonpsychiatric physicians for simple complaints, such as "nerves," "tension," and sleeplessness, making possible marginal and borderline cases between therapeutic use and abusive self-administration. Relevant to their abuse potential is their capacity to function as primary reinforcers, as discussed in Chapter 3.

Chronic abuse of sedative-hypnotics produces a sequence of personality changes related to affectual effects of the drugs. Early effects may be euphoria or depression. If depression occurs, there may be an upsurge of suicidal tendencies. With progressive use, affectual changes may give way to emotional incontinence characterized by lack of motivation, slovenliness, and confusion. Hallucinations may occur in chronic intoxication, and occasionally chronic psychoses develop. In barbiturate intoxication, neurologic concomitants include slurring of speech, double vision, vertigo, and difficulties of visual accommodation and gait. Chronic alcohol abuse may produce a number of neurologic syndromes related at least in part to associated dietary inadequacies.

The severe withdrawal syndromes associated with discontinuance of chronic use of most of the drugs in this class must be taken into account by the therapist who becomes involved in ending use or abuse. Experienced medical supervision is probably called for.

Most drugs of this class suppress dreaming on initial administration, and the large rebound on withdrawal may be interpreted as suggestive of a chronic deficit in D sleep. Drugs that interfere with the D-sleep phase could even interfere with psychotherapy concurrent with their use. If, as noted in Chapter 10, dreaming is essential for mapping of learning in relation to significant life changes, the suppression of dreaming could slow the learning in therapy.

The wide use and easy availability of the barbiturates, minor tranquilizers, and alcohol make them more than usually important from the standpoint of potential state-dependent learning effects (Chap. 3). The effectiveness of barbiturates as internal discriminative stimuli suggests that it is likely that dissociation of learning between the drugged and undrugged states probably occurs with barbiturates. Therefore, the therapist might wish to plan to conduct therapy sessions at times when the patient is not likely to be sedated or intoxicated.

Medically Important Sedative-Hypnotics

amobarbital (Amytal, Tuinal [combined with secobarbital]), a barbiturate sedative-hypnotic: intermediate-acting, used as a sedative and hypnotic. Sedative: 50 to 150 mg. Hypnotic: 65 to 200 mg at bedtime.

chloral hydrate, a sedative-hypnotic: minimal suppression of D sleep. Sedative: 300 to 1,500 mg. Hypnotic: 500 to 1,000 mg at bedtime.

ethchlorvynol (Placidyl), a tertiary alcohol sedative-hypnotic: short-acting. Sedative: 200 to 600 mg. Hypnotic: 500 to 1,000 mg.

flurazepam (Dalmane), a benzodiazepine hypnotic: suppresses stage 4 slow-wave sleep but not D sleep. Hypnotic: 15 to 30 mg.

glutethimide (Doriden), a piperidinedione sedative-hypnotic: principal use is as a hypnotic. Hypnotic: 250 to 1,000 mg at bedtime. Sedative: 250 to 750 mg.

mephobarbital (Mebaral), a barbiturate: long-acting, primarily used as a daytime sedative and antiepileptic, rarely as a hypnotic. Sedative: 50 to 400 mg. Antiepileptic: 100 to 200 mg.

meprobamate (Equanil, Miltown), a propanediol anxiolytic and hypnotic: potent skeletal-muscle relaxant. Anxiolytic: 1,200 to 1,600 mg.

methaqualone (Quaalude, Sopor, Optimil, Parest, Somnafac), a sedative-hypnotic. Sedative: 300 to 450 mg. Hypnotic: 150 to 400 mg at bedtime.

methyprylon (Noludar), a piperidinedione sedative-hypnotic: used primarily as hypnotic. Hypnotic: 200 to 400 mg at bedtime. Sedative: 150 to 400 mg.

pentobarbital (Nembutal), a barbiturate sedative-hypnotic: short-acting, used more as an hypnotic than a sedative. Sedative: 100 to 200 mg. Hypnotic: 100 to 200 mg at bedtime.

phenobarbital (Luminal, Phenaphen [combined with phenacetin and aspirin], Donnatal [combined with belladonna alkaloids], Tedral [combined with ephedrine and theophylline], Pro-banthine [combined with propantheline]), a barbiturate sedative-hypnotic: used primarily as a long-acting daytime sedative, an antiepileptic, and an anticonvulsant, rarely as a hypnotic, and in combinations for asthma and ulcers. Sedative: 30 to 120 mg. Hypnotic: 100 to 300 mg at bedtime.

pyrilamine (Compoz, Dormarex, Nervine, Nytol, Relax-U-Caps, Sedacaps, Sleep-Eze, Sominex, Somnicaps), an antihistamine nonprescription sleep aid. Sedative: 25 to 50 mg.

scopolamine (L-hyoscine), an anticholinergic: used as a sleep aid and in some cold preparation combinations. Typical: 15 mg.

secobarbital (Seconal, Tuinal [combined with amobarbital]), a barbiturate sedative-hypnotic: short-acting, used more as a hypnotic than as a sedative. Hypnotic: 100 mg at bedtime. Sedative: 50 to 200 mg.

temazepam (Restoril), a benzodiazepine hypnotic: shorter-acting than flurazepam. Hypnotic: 15 to 30 mg.

thiopental (Pentothal), a barbiturate: ultrashort-acting, used in anesthesia. Anesthetic: 50 to 75 mg IV.

Selected References and Further Readings

1. Gilman, A. G., Goodman, L. S., and Gilman, A. *The Pharmacological Basis of Therapeutics* (5th ed.). New York: Macmillan, 1980.
2. Nicoll, R. Selective Actions of Barbiturates on Synaptic Transmission. In M. A. Lipton et al. (Eds.), *Psychopharmacology: A Generation of Progress.* New York: Raven, 1978.

Alcohol: The Nonprescription Sedative-Hypnotic

R̴

12

Incidence

Alcohol—or, more precisely, ethyl alcohol—enjoys a unique and extremely important position in the pharmacologic repertoire of our society. Although it is now of limited therapeutic value, its social usefulness and consequences are profound. It is the most frequently self-administered drug, and the associated abuse problems dwarf the abuses occurring with all other drugs combined.

Alcohol is the most widely used psychotropic drug in almost all human societies, although the per capita consumption and the beverage class preference vary from country to country. France has the highest per capita consumption. Other high-consumption countries include Argentina, Chile, Italy, and West Germany. Countries with moderate rates of alcohol consumption include the United States, Canada, England, Sweden, and Peru. Mexico and Finland have low rates of alcohol consumption. In England, 75 percent of alcohol consumption is in the form of beer. West Germany, Canada, and Mexico are other societies in which beer is the main form of alcohol consumed. On the other hand, Italy, France, Chile, and Argentina favor wine—not surprisingly, since these countries are major wine producers. In the United States, beer and spirits compete on equal terms, while wine provides only about 10 percent of the alcohol consumed. In Scandinavian and Central American countries, most alcohol is consumed in the form of spirits.

Alcoholic liver disease (cirrhosis), just one of many kinds of tissue toxicity associated with chronic alcohol ingestion, is now the seventh leading cause of death in the United States. In urban areas it is the third leading cause of death between the ages of 25 and 65 years, a figure that, though staggering, is just the tip of the iceberg of alcohol-related social costs. Willoughby [9] estimates that approximately 60 percent of hospitalizations involve alcohol consumption as a significant factor, though often the role of alcohol is unappreciated by the physician or the patient. The number of victims of alcohol-related homicides, suicides, or assaults is more than twice the number of yearly cirrhosis fatalities. Fatalities from alcohol-related vehicular accidents are more than three times the number of cirrhosis fatalities. And when all the fatalities from alcohol-related cirrhosis, vehicular accidents, homicides, suicides, and assaults are combined, the total is less than the number of fatalities resulting from alcohol-related, nonvehicular accidents.

Approximately 80 percent of cases of liver cirrhosis are alcohol-related. There is a strong correlation between per capita alcohol consumption and the incidence of liver cirrhosis, taken country by country.

The frequency of alcohol-related vehicular accidents has resulted in carefully defined legal limits for the level of blood alcohol permissible while operating a vehicle. Few states have similar laws for other drugs. Most states have adopted a standard of 0.10 percent (100 mg/% or 100 mg/100 ml) as the legal limit (Fig. 12-1). Levels below 0.05 percent are generally safe. A level of 0.5 percent entails outright drunkenness. The approximate fatal level is 0.55 percent.

Acute Pharmacology of Alcohol

Seen exclusively from the point of view of acute pharmacologic actions, alcohol appears an innocuous and somewhat uninteresting drug. The few persisting therapeutic applications of alcohol are related to its acute, local effects on the skin, not to its systemic or CNS effects. At concentrations near 70 percent, alcohol is an effective bactericidal substance. Because of its rapid rate of evaporation, alcohol sponges are used for cooling the skin of patients with fever. Bathing the skin of a bedridden patient with alcohol may help to prevent bedsores, because alcohol hardens and cleans the skin surface.

It is, however, the CNS that is most acutely sensitive to the effects of alcohol. In most respects, the psychotropic effects of alcohol are not unlike those of other sedative-hypnotic substances. There is a general and dose-dependent depression of the CNS, beginning with mild sedation and escalating to anesthesia, coma, and death (Fig. 12-1). The "stimulatory" properties ascribed to alcohol as a result of the popular impression are the consequence of depression of areas of the brain normally responsible for inhibitory control (Fig. 12-2). As a result, some portions of the brain and associated behaviors are released from inhibitory restraint.

The reticular formation is particularly susceptible to the depressant action of alcohol, as it also is to that of the barbiturates. Secondary to this action, there is a slowing of wave frequencies in the EEG and a release of the cortex from the integrating control of subcortical centers. Thought flows freely, but in a disorderly and haphazard flux. The frontal lobe of the cerebral cortex is affected by alcohol blood levels as low as 0.01 to 0.1 percent, resulting in exhilaration, expansiveness, impaired judgment, loquacity, and poor attention. Other cortical regions are depressed at blood levels between 0.1 and 0.3 percent, causing dulled sensibilities, ataxia, apraxia, slurred speech, diplopia, and distorted perception. The cerebellum also responds to levels in the 0.1 to 0.3 percent range, resulting in disequilibrium. The medulla oblongata is least sensitive, fortunately. The fatal effects of alcohol usually stem from depression of the medulla at high concentrations. In the United States the number of such fatalities annually exceeds 300, a rather small number when viewed as a percentage of the total number of alcohol users. Blood levels of about 0.4 percent are necessary before depression of medullary centers becomes noticeable, while levels of 0.55 percent are typically lethal. As with other sedative-hypnotics, there is a euphoriant effect with alcohol. The user becomes self-assured and frequently assertive and loquacious. Despite the increased confidence, motor and mental skills are almost universally depressed.

Although alcohol can be used to produce anesthesia, it is not so used because of its prolonged action and its small margin of safety. The immediate danger in acute intoxication is related to respiratory depression. Analeptics, caffeine, or mechanical respiratory support can be used to counteract this depression. The depressant action of alcohol is additive to that of any other CNS depressant (e.g., narcotics, tranquilizers, antihistamines).

The neurochemical basis for the effect of alcohol is poorly understood. Present evidence suggests that the primary neurochemical interaction is an alteration in

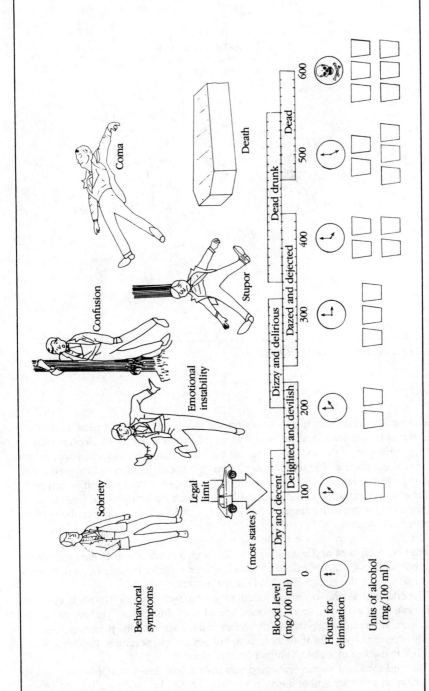

Fig. 12-1. *Stages of alcohol intoxication. A shot of liquor, two glasses of wine, or two bottles of beer constitutes a unit of alcohol.*

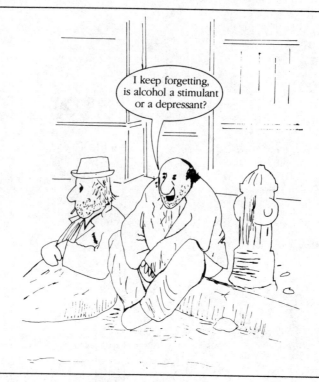

Fig. 12-2. *Alcohol: stimulant or depressant?*

membrane function that sets into motion secondary alterations in neurotransmitter mechanisms and compensatory adaptations. Membrane effects of alcohol include (1) an inhibition of the sodium-potassium exchange pump, leading to an impairment in neural conduction; (2) regional depletion of calcium, leading to increased membrane permeability; and (3) decreases in cyclic adenosine monophosphate and cyclic guanosine monophosphate. Acute or prolonged alcohol administration leads to an increase in norepinephrine turnover. By contrast, acetylcholine turnover in the cerebral cortex is depressed.

Besides its widespread use as a sedative, alcohol is frequently employed by the lay person as an hypnotic and as an analgesic. Although less effective than narcotic or non-narcotic analgesics, alcohol does effectively increase detachment from pain. Alcohol can also elevate the pain threshold about 40 percent.

The effects of alcohol on sexual functioning were well described by Shakespeare in *Macbeth,* in which one character, Porter, speaking of drink, says, "Lechery sir, it provokes and unprovokes; it provokes the desire, but it takes away the performance..." In medical terminology, libido is increased, but sexual functioning is impaired, when alcohol is used in moderate to high concentrations.

The cardiovascular system is affected very little at low doses. Moderate doses cause vasodilation and consequent flushing, warming of the skin, and heat loss.

Chronic Toxicity of Alcohol

The chronic toxic effects of alcohol are widespread, affecting many bodily tissues, and they fall into general categories. To begin with, a distinction can be made between effects that result directly from alcohol consumption and those that are secondary to the nutritional deficiencies that frequently accompany alcoholism. Some examples of tissue toxicity, such as fatty liver, may involve both factors. The primary effects, those related directly to alcohol consumption, can be further clustered into three groups: (1) effects related to alcohol itself; (2) effects related to the acetaldehyde metabolite of alcohol; and (3) effects related to excessive hydrogen formation from the metabolism of alcohol (Fig. 12-3).

Toxic effects related to alcohol itself are prominent in the gastrointestinal tract. Alcohol stimulates secretion of gastric and salivary fluids both through its psychic action and reflexly and thus may exacerbate peptic ulcers. Chronic gastritis, which occurs in a third of all alcoholics, is caused by the irritant action of alcohol on the stomach lining. Alcohol may contribute to acute and chronic pancreatitis.

The other two sets of adverse effects result from the metabolism of alcohol. The first step in the metabolism of alcohol in the liver involves the formation of acetaldehyde from alcohol by the action of the enzyme alcohol dehydrogenase (Fig. 12-4). Hydrogen released in the reaction is used in a reduction reaction in which the oxidized form of the nucleotide nicotinamide adenine dinucleotide (NAD), a cellular energy intermediary, is converted into NADH, the reduced form. Toxic consequences result from both the accumulation of acetaldehyde and excessive conversion of NAD to NADH.

Chronic toxicities related to acetaldehyde include skeletal myopathies (the alcoholic tremor), carditis, and liver inflammation (or hepatitis). Formation of excessive NADH is toxic because the usual hydrogen source for reduction of NAD is the metabolism of fats. When high levels of NADH are formed from alcohol metabolism, the body has no need to metabolize fat. Fat metabolism is inhibited, and lipid molecules accumulate in the blood and liver. Fatty deposits in the liver lead to fatty liver, which often leads to hepatitis and cirrhosis. The level of circulating lipids in the bloodstream also rises, contributing to the development of atherosclerosis and hypertension. Hydrogen formation from alcohol metabolism also has an inhibitory effect on lactate metabolism for the same basic reason that fat metabolism is turned off. Lactate metabolism is another source of hydrogen for conversion of NAD to NADH, but it is an unneeded and unutilized source when large amounts of alcohol are being metabolized. Inhibition of lactate metabolism leads to hypoglycemia and kidney malfunction.

As noted, fatty liver resulting from alcohol metabolism is often a prelude to hepatitis and cirrhosis. Generally, fatty liver, hepatitis, and even the earliest phase of cirrhosis are reversible if alcohol consumption is terminated. However, as cirrhosis continues to develop, it reaches a stage where it becomes irreversible, even if alcohol consumption is terminated. In the most advanced stage, cirrhosis is not only irreversible, but progresses inevitably to death. Cirrhosis involves excessive production of a protein called collagen, an essential constituent of connective tissue and one of the most abundant substances in the body. Overproduction of collagen literally splits apart the liver into nodular islands of cells. Blood flow is impeded and cell death begins to ensue.

Long before the progression of liver injury reaches potentially fatal dimensions, there are significant impairments associated with the liver dysfunction. These impairments include reduced production of serum proteins, clotting defects, jaundice, high ammonia, hypertension, and decreased ability to activate vitamins.

Alcohol supplies a readily usable source of energy for the body. An alcoholic may obtain half or more of his or her caloric intake from alcoholic beverages. Unfortunately,

200

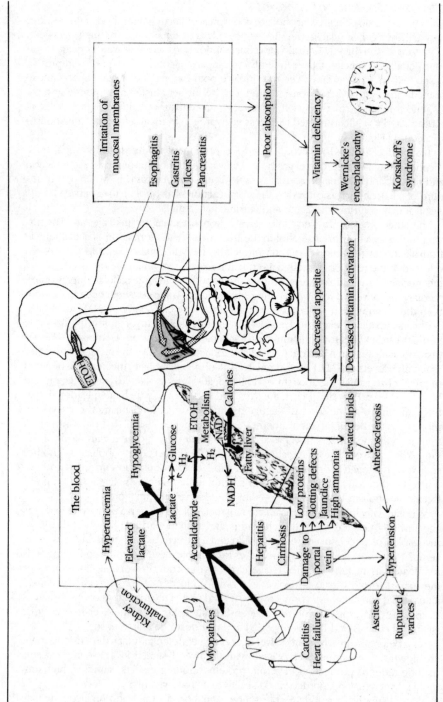

Fig. 12-3. *Tissue toxicities associated with chronic alcohol ingestion.*

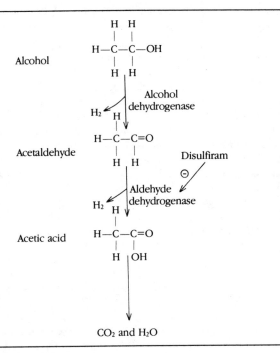

Fig. 12-4. *Metabolism of alcohol.*

such a diet is badly lacking in vitamins. Such vitamins as are ingested may be poorly absorbed because of gastritis or poorly activated because of hepatitis. The result is a functional vitamin deficiency. Various diseases related to vitamin deficiencies are frequently observed in alcoholics. These include liver cirrhosis, nicotinic acid deficiency encephalopathy, and the neurologic disease Wernicke's encephalopathy. The last condition first affects limited brain regions, notably the mamillary bodies of the hypothalamus and the periventricular gray. It may later entail diffuse degeneration of cortical tissue. There is a prominent proliferation and thickening of capillary endothelium in the affected areas. Wernicke's encephalopathy is associated with a behavioral syndrome called Korsakoff's psychosis (or dementia associated with alcoholism). Early symptoms include confabulation and disinhibition. Later, all the classic symptoms of dementia are present.

Alcohol use by pregnant women has been linked to teratogenic effects, called the fetal alcohol syndrome. The birth defects commonly seen in this syndrome fall into five categories: (1) prenatal and postnatal growth deficiencies; (2) craniofacial anomalies (ptosis, intraocular deficits); (3) musculoskeletal anomalies (small nails, diaphragmatic malformations); (4) cutaneous anomalies (hirsutism, pigmentation); and (5) congenital heart disease.

Tolerance and Dependence

The reader should review the discussion of tolerance to and dependence on sedative-hypnotics in Chapter 11, since much of what was said there applies equally to alcohol.

Both the degree of tolerance and the intensity of withdrawal occurring with the use of alcohol are dependent on the quantity of drug consumed and the duration of the pattern of habitual drinking. In its mildest form, the withdrawal syndrome contributes to the well-known hangover experienced the morning after an intoxication. In its most intense manifestation, alcohol withdrawal is called delirium tremens and encompasses the same set of symptoms described for barbiturate withdrawal.

Tolerance to alcohol is mostly of the pharmacodynamic variety. An increase in the metabolism of alcohol contributes only about 20 percent of the overall tolerance to alcohol. Inactivation of alcohol occurs almost entirely by metabolism rather than by excretion of the unchanged drug. Tolerance to alcohol is less than that occurring with many drugs of abuse, for example, the narcotics, amphetamines, nicotine, or psychedelics. Drug-disposition tolerance, related to induction of liver enzymes, may or may not be offset by presence of liver disease.

In the United States, alcohol abuse occurs in about 9 percent of adult males and in approximately 6 million people in all. The exact figures depend in part on one's definition of abuse, and figures as high as 20 million have been suggested. Among the alcoholic population the most frequently encountered personality profile is one of low frustration tolerance and of an inability to persevere in activities. Alcoholics, on the average, have a greater-than-normal impulsiveness and greater-than-normal hostility.

Alcohol abuse involves both psychological and physical dependence. The American Psychiatric Association's *Diagnostic and Statistical Manual* (DSM-III) defines two classifications of alcohol-use disorders: alcohol abuse and alcohol dependence. The latter, but not the former, is characterized by physical dependence. Psychological dependence can vary from mild to strong. The person who becomes highly dependent on alcohol often begins to drink in situations in which drinking is not culturally prescribed, such as drinking alone, and to become obsessed with the obtaining and the taking of the drug.

In Chapter 9, we discussed our reasons for finding the DSM-III criteria for substance-use disorders seriously lacking. Similarly, the stereotyped concept of the "alcoholic" as a skid-row bum is misleading and has the effect of overly restricting our view to those individuals most dramatically impaired by alcohol and least amenable to treatment. A more useful definition is that offered by Willoughby. He suggests substituting for "alcoholic" the phrase "the alcohol-troubled person," whom he defines as "an individual [who] continues to drink when to do so reduces the quality of his or her life in any one (or more) of the following four areas: (1) social, (2) financial, (3) physical, or (4) emotional and cognitive."

Alcohol-Induced Disorders

In addition to the alcohol-use disorders, DSM-III provides six classifications of alcohol-induced disorders: (1) intoxication, (2) idiosyncratic intoxication, (3) withdrawal, (4) withdrawal delirium, (5) hallucinosis, and (6) amnesic disorder. Intoxication is defined by recent ingestion of a typically intoxicating quantity of alcohol and by three additional criteria: maladaptive behavior (fighting, poor functioning, impaired judgment); one or more physical signs (slurred speech, incoordination, unsteady gait, nystagmus, flushing); and one or more psychological signs (mood change, irritability, loquacity, impaired attention). Idiosyncratic intoxication is similar, but involves marked behavioral changes not characteristic of the person, such as assaultiveness.

Alcohol withdrawal is defined by recent reduction or cessation in alcohol ingestion following heavy use, leading to a coarse tremor of the hands, tongue, and eyelids and at least one additional abstinence symptom: nausea, vomiting, malaise, tachycardia, sweating, hypertension, orthostatic hypotension, anxiety, depression, or irritability. As noted, withdrawal delirium (commonly called delirium tremens) is the withdrawal syndrome in its most severe form. Delirium and autonomic hyperactivity are present. Alcoholic hallucinosis is similar, except that hallucinations are present but delirium is lacking. Withdrawal symptoms may first appear in some alcohol users after just a few weeks of alcohol use; on the other hand, some users first experience withdrawal phenomena after 20 years or more of apparently successful social use of alcohol. The transition from use to abuse can occur regardless of how many years of experience the drinker has had.

Alcohol amnesic disorder is what is commonly called alcoholic blackout. It is characterized by periods of amnesia following prolonged ingestion of alcohol. Some theorists believe that alcoholic blackouts may be temporal lobe seizures triggered by alcohol ingestion.

Drug Interactions Involving Alcohol

The widespread use of alcohol ensures a high probability of alcohol interactions occurring with other drugs. Here we will review six important interactions of this kind.

The most common interaction of alcohol is also a rather straightforward one. Alcohol has an *additive depressant effect* with any other CNS depressant. This interaction of alcohol is simply an instance of a very common class of interactions that we defined earlier in a more general form: Any two CNS depressants, of the same or different classes, will have an additive depressant effect. This type of drug interactions is the one most commonly observed of all types of drug interactions. It follows from the preceding definition of this interaction that alcohol will have an additive effect with other sedative-hypnotics, anxiolytics, antipsychotic drugs, antidepressants, lithium, narcotics, anticholinergics, and antihistamines.

Some sedative-hypnotics, notably barbiturates, chloral hydrate, and meprobamate, interact with alcohol by a second mechanism as well. Alcohol and these particular sedative-hypnotics *compete for the same degratory enzymes* in the liver (Fig. 12-5). When alcohol and one of these drugs are simultaneously present in the body, each will slow the other's metabolism. The result is that the two drugs will have a super-additive depressant effect. This phenomenon has been articulated in drug abuse information pamphlets as the "1 + 1 = 3" concept.

When used chronically, alcohol interacts with other sedative-hypnotics and depressants in still another way. Chronic use of alcohol will cause *induction of liver enzymes.* When the liver enzyme system has been induced, the liver metabolizes related drugs more rapidly (Fig. 12-6). The phenomenon of liver-enzyme induction contributes to tolerance to the drug inducer itself (this is the drug-disposition component of tolerance) and also produces a degree of cross-tolerance to certain other drugs metabolized by the same enzymes. When alcohol and another drug metabolized by the liver (e.g., a barbiturate) are present simultaneously in the body, the interaction based on induction is irrelevant because it is quantitatively insignificant compared with the additive and super-additive interactions. But the interaction caused by enzyme induction is important when a chronic drinker uses a barbiturate at a time when little or no alcohol happens to be present in the body. In such a circumstance, the chronic drinker would respond less to a given dose of a barbiturate than would a normal person. On the other hand, if alcoholic liver disease is present, the capacity to metabolize alcohol or barbiturates may be reduced in spite of induction.

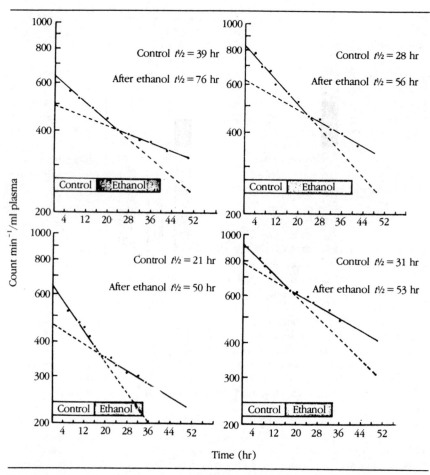

Fig. 12-5. *Effect of acute ethanol intoxication on the disappearance of pentobarbital from the blood of four human volunteers. After ethanol administration (1 gm/kg, followed by 30 gm every 2 hours), the half-life of pentobarbital in the blood was approximately doubled. Solid lines are plotted from data points. Dashed lines are extrapolated. Modified from E. Rubin and C. S. Lieber. Alcoholism, alcohol and drugs. Science 172:1097–1102, 1971.* © *1971 by The American Association for the Advancement of Science.*

The remaining three types of drug interactions of alcohol involve only a small number of specific drugs. Alcohol tends to produce hypoglycemia, which may result in an *additive hypoglycemic action* when insulin or oral antidiabetic drugs are in use. The irritant effect of alcohol on the gastrointestinal system may lead to an *additive ulcerogenic effect* with other ulcerogenic drugs such as aspirin. The final interaction is with the drug *disulfiram* (Antabuse). This interaction warrants special consideration in the next section because of the role of disulfiram in alcohol treatment programs.

A drug interaction of an entirely different nature is the tendency for individuals to become polyabusers. There is a significant correlation between alcohol use and tobacco use. Among alcohol abstainers 30 percent smoke cigarettes, but 51 percent of

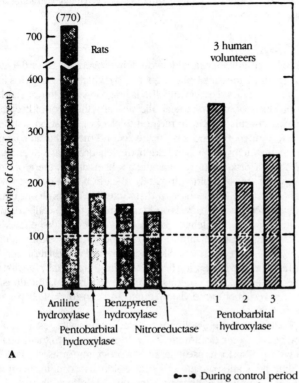

A

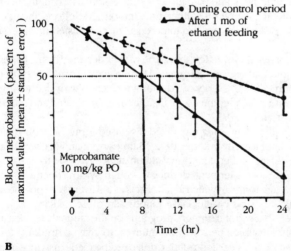

B

Fig. 12-6. A. Effect of chronic administration of ethanol on activities of hepatic drug-metabolizing enzymes in rats and human volunteers. The activity of every enzyme studied was increased by chronic ingestion of ethanol. B. Disappearance of plasma meprobamate in human volunteers before and after chronic administration of ethanol. The half-life of meprobamate in the blood was halved by chronic intoxication. Modified from E. Rubin and C. S. Lieber. Alcoholism, alcohol and drugs. Science 172:1092–1102, 1971. © 1971 by The American Association for the Advancement of Science.

moderate drinkers and 64 percent of heavy drinkers smoke. Heavy drinkers are also more likely to be heavy smokers.

Alcohol and Disulfiram

Disulfiram is an inhibitor of the enzyme aldehyde dehydrogenase. To understand its action, one needs to examine the metabolic sequence by which the body rids itself of alcohol (see Fig. 12-4). As we noted earlier, alcohol is first converted into acetaldehyde and hydrogen. The products of this first metabolic step and the alcohol itself are the three sources of primary chronic toxicity in relation to alcohol ingestion. Subsequent metabolic steps lead to innocuous products. In the second metabolic step, acetaldehyde is converted to acetic acid by the enzyme aldehyde dehydrogenase. Acetic acid is a normal bodily substance, a product of cellular metabolism, and is therefore readily disposed of in subsequent steps, leading ultimately to carbon dioxide and water.

The inhibition of aldehyde dehydrogenase by disulfiram interrupts alcohol metabolism at its most toxic step. Acetaldehyde levels build up, causing the so-called disulfiram reaction, which is, in fact, an acetaldehyde syndrome. Almost all the effects of the alcohol-disulfiram interaction can be mimicked by experimental administration of acetaldehyde. The disulfiram-alcohol reaction includes marked vasodilation, leading to flushing, warm skin, hot face, and a pulsating headache. These are usually the first symptoms. This is followed by nausea and copious vomiting, respiratory difficulties, chest pain, anxiety, confusion, vertigo, blurred vision, thirst, and considerable hypotension. The syndrome may be fatal.

It should be emphasized that the disulfiram reaction occurs as a result of alcohol ingestion in a person who is taking disulfiram. It does not occur when the drug is used by itself, and this fact is the basis for its use in treatment programs. By itself, disulfiram is largely innocuous, although some patients experience skin rash, acneiform eruptions, or urticaria—all allergic symptoms. Other uncommon side effects include fatigue, lassitude, tremor, restlessness, headache, impotence, metallic taste, and gastrointestinal disturbances.

The time course of disulfiram action should be well understood by the patient. About 1 to 2 weeks is required after use is terminated for the activity of aldehyde dehydrogenase to return to normal. The severity of a disulfiram reaction with alcohol ingestion is likely to be still great 3 days after the use of disulfiram is terminated and moderate 7 to 10 days after use is terminated.

Patients using disulfiram must learn to avoid disguised forms of alcohol, since their susceptibility to alcohol toxicity is some 10 to 15 times normal. What would appear to be trivial quantities of alcohol under normal circumstances may be toxic to the person receiving disulfiram. Sauces, fermented vinegar, cough syrups, tinctures, and spirits (the last two are dosage forms in which alcohol acts as a solvent) are potential sources of alcohol. Even alcohol rubs or aftershave lotions can cause toxicity.

Disulfiram is used in alcohol treatment programs on the rationale that it can help to crystallize the alcohol-troubled person's commitment to give up drinking. It is argued that with disulfiram use the decision not to drink need be made just once a day, when the medication is taken, not every time a drink is offered.

Since the disulfiram reaction is potentially fatal, the patients who are to receive the drug must be carefully selected. When disulfiram is used to enforce sobriety in uncommitted subjects—a common arrangement in plea-bargaining situations and in military judicial proceedings—the incidence of disulfiram reactions is high. Some subjects simply continue to believe they can ingest small amounts of alcohol while taking disulfiram. Others discover the possibility of stimulating acetaldehyde activity by mega-doses of vitamin C. Suffice it to say that use of disulfiram is not without significant risks. It should be reserved for patients fundamentally committed to abstinence who feel the need to support that commitment with disulfiram.

Disulfiram may interact with other drugs besides alcohol. It may precipitate phe-nytoin intoxication in patients receiving that drug. In combination with metronidazole or isoniazid, or by itself at high doses, disulfiram has been observed to cause psychotic reactions.

Treatment of Alcohol Withdrawal

Patients presenting themselves to an emergency room with symptoms of alcohol with-drawal are generally dealt with in accordance with a standardized set of procedures established by the facility in question. A typical treatment protocol is discussed in this section. In essence, the protocol involves three steps: (1) obtaining a history, (2) a physical examination, and (3) treatment and disposition.

The history-taking proceeds rapidly, often in conjunction with the physical examina-tion. The clinician seeks to establish the following: (1) the quantity and type of beverage recently ingested; (2) the duration and frequency of drinking during the latest bout; (3) the patient's attitude toward the drinking behavior; (4) the presence of medi-cal complications; (5) any history of treatment for drinking; (6) any history of psychi-atric treatment; and (7) the course and severity of previous withdrawal episodes. Both the patient and anyone who has accompanied the patient to the facility are utilized as sources of information.

Physical examination includes vital signs every 4 hours for 24 hours and blood tests, including purified protein and prothrombin determinations, a complete blood cell count, measurements of blood urea nitrogen, fasting blood sugar, electrolytes, and a liver profile. A chest x-ray and electrocardiogram are obtained.

Treatment begins with the administration of fluids ad lib and diet as tolerated. Forced fluids is common practice but inadvisable. It should be reserved for patients in whom dehydration is significant as determined from the physical examination. Administration of fluids ad lib will correct dehydration in most cases, and some patients enter the emergency room in an overhydrated state. Chlordiazepoxide (Librium), 50 mg, is usually given orally, to suppress withdrawal symptoms. Diazepam (Valium) is used instead or additionally if seizures are present or appear imminent. Thiamine (vitamin B_1) and multivitamins are given to correct the potential vitamin deficiency, but this has little relevance to the acute condition. An antacid might be given for epigastric distress, or acetaminophen for headache. Aspirin is avoided because of its irritant effect on the gastrointestinal system and because it would increase seizure liability. Neuroleptics are avoided because they increase seizure liability, but if delirium is pronounced and not corrected by chlordiazepoxide, thioridazine is preferable to other neuroleptics.

In the best of all possible worlds, one would wish to treat all patients undergoing alcohol withdrawal as inpatients, since the condition is life-threatening. The reality imposed by limited hospital beds requires the application of established criteria to determine which patients are to be admitted. A patient is admitted if any one of the criteria in Table 12-1 is met.

If a patient is to be treated as an outpatient, a typical protocol would call for 1 to 2 hours of observation after treatment with chlordiazepoxide, and release with a 3- to 6-day supply of the drug.

Table 12-1. *Guidelines for determining admission of emergency room patients in alcohol withdrawal*

Admission is indicated if the patient has any one of the following:

Infectious disease

Temperature > 101° or < 95°F

Alcohol-induced disorder (e.g., hepatitis, pancreatitis)

Significant metabolic problem (e.g., acidosis, hypoglycemia)

Congestive heart failure, arrhythmia, significant hypotension

Active gastrointestinal bleeding, significant vomiting, or dehydration

Significant degree of anemia

Alcoholic myopathy

Disulfiram reaction

Hallucinations or delirium

History of recent convulsions

Fluctuating levels of consciousness

Severe depression or suicidal ideation

Lack of satisfactory care as an outpatient

Interpersonal and Systemic Involvement in Alcoholism

Increasing importance is being assigned to the interpersonal functions of alcohol. Alcoholism may be looked at as an anomaly in the individual's participation in social or familial systems. Bateson [1] has suggested that alcohol abuse corresponds to a faulty epistemology in which the alcoholic claims to have personal control over alcohol and, in attempting to affirm this, precipitates his or her own downfall. The highly successful approach of Alcoholics Anonymous amounts to the substitution of an alternate epistemology. Paradoxically, when the alcoholic acknowledges inability to beat "John Barleycorn" and admits defeat, he or she is on the path to victory, because no one component of the system controls the process. Control of systemic process is a function of the totality of relationships between components—in this case the alcoholic and alcohol.

Less esoterically, others have addressed the paradoxical power relationships involved in alcohol use. While the imbiber's perceptions of his or her own power rise, actual power declines. When the drinker becomes intoxicated, it is a strong interpersonal statement, for it requires that others be responsible and take control. Yet this abdication is at the instigation of the alcoholic, who in turn cannot control his or her drinking. The alcoholic protests that he is in control of himself, that he "can hold his liquor," even while demonstrating that he cannot. Families with an alcoholic member are involved in significantly more problematic power transactions than families without an alcohol abuser. Imagery and issues around being in control yet out of control abound in alcoholics.

Implications for Psychotherapy

Alcohol is a drug of paradoxes. It is an unexceptional drug as regards acute effects, but is singularly toxic over time. It is a mild and pleasant euphoriant that frequently kills from within those who indulge too much, through gradual destruction of bodily tissues, and at the same time it threatens even the most absolute teetotaler with the violence of accidents or aggression. It is the drug of parties and sociability that all too often destroys families and fatally impairs social and occupational functioning. The widespread use of alcohol poses a unique dilemma for society.

The therapeutic implications of alcohol are manifold. It has been shown to produce state dependency of learning in humans. It suppresses dreaming sleep and acts as a primary reinforcer. At the organic level of brain functioning, it can produce the neurologic damage of Wernicke's encephalopathy. And its powerful effects on both individuals and families are all too well documented.

Alcohol abuse is unquestionably the most important form of substance abuse. It seems likely that alcohol abuse, high though it is in the population as a whole, is even higher among clients who are undergoing psychotherapy and among the families of these clients. Some psychotherapists have implicated alcohol abuse somewhere in the immediate family or family background of upward of 90 percent of their clients. Both the symptomatic and etiologic nature of alcohol abuse must be considered in addition to the addiction itself. Alcohol use is often found to be intricately imbedded in life experiences that both precipitate its continued use and are the result of the abuse. Simultaneous disentanglement and detoxification may be called for.

Drugs Important in the Treatment of Alcohol Dependence or Withdrawal

ascorbic acid (vitamin C): used in the treatment of severe disulfiram-alcohol reactions. Disulfiram-reaction treatment: 1,000 mg IV.

chlordiazepoxide (e.g., Librium), a benzodiazepine: useful in suppressing severe alcohol withdrawal symptoms. Alcohol withdrawal: 50 mg PO or IM.

diazepam (Valium), a benzodiazepine: useful in treating or preventing "rum fits" (seizures accompanying severe alcohol withdrawal). Anticonvulsant: 10 mg IV.

disulfiram (Antabuse), an aldehyde dehydrogenase inhibitor: useful as an adjunct in alcohol treatment programs to deter use of alcohol. Severe reactions may occur if alcohol is ingested. Management of alcoholic patient: up to 500 mg daily initially; typical maintenance dose, 250 mg daily.

thiamine (vitamin B_1): used in chronic alcoholism to treat associated vitamin deficiency. Thiamine deficiency: 10 to 30 mg.

Selected References and Further Readings

1. Bateson, G. *Steps to an Ecology of Mind.* New York: Ballantine, 1972.
2. Ellingboe, J. Effects of Alcohol on Neurochemical Processes. In M. A. Lipton et al. (Eds.), *Psychopharmacology: A Generation of Progress.* New York: Raven, 1978.
3. Gilman, A. G., Goodman, L. S., and Gilman, A. *The Pharmacological Basis of Therapeutics* (6th ed.). New York: Macmillan, 1980.
4. Greenblatt, D. J., and Shader, R. I. Treatment of the Alcohol Withdrawal Syndrome. In R. I. Shader (Ed.), *Manual of Psychiatric Therapeutics.* Boston: Little, Brown, 1975.
5. Lundwall, L., and Baekeland, F. Disulfiram Treatment in Alcoholism: A Review. In D. F. Klein and R. Gittelman-Klein (Eds.), *Progress in Psychiatric Drug Treatment.* New York: Brunner/Mazel, 1975.
6. Mello, N. K. Alcoholism and the Behavioral Pharmacology of Alcohol: 1967–1977. In M. A. Lipton et al. (Eds.), *Psychopharmacology: A Generation of Progress.* New York: Raven, 1978.
7. Myers, R. D. Psychopharmacology of alcohol. *Annu. Rev. Pharmacol.* 18:125–144, 1978.
8. Rubin, E., and Lieber, C. S. Alcoholism, Alcohol and Drugs. In D. F. Klein and R. Gittelman-Klein (Eds.), *Progress in Psychiatric Drug Treatment.* New York: Brunner/Mazel, 1975.
9. Willoughby, A. *The Alcohol-Troubled Person.* Chicago: Nelson-Hall, 1979.

Stimulants

13

The group of drugs generally labeled CNS stimulants (or psychostimulants) can be subdivided on the basis of any of several characteristics. Various authors have devised taxonomies based on mechanism of action (disinhibition versus activation), therapeutic applications, chemical structure, abuse liability, EEG versus behavioral stimulatory efficacy, or neuropharmacologic interactions. The term *analeptic* may be used for a subset of stimulants that activate the EEG and readily induce seizure activity. All of these are informative, but none of the distinctions emphasized is of obvious preeminence or usefulness in devising a rational classification. We will therefore treat the stimulants in four somewhat arbitrary groups.

It should be noted that stimulants as a class have become of decreasing interest and usefulness from a therapeutic standpoint in recent years. Several early uses for this class have fallen into disrepute—in some cases due to an increasing awareness of the abuse liability and other adverse effects of certain stimulants and in other cases due to lack of efficacy or development of superior treatments. The use of amphetamine as an anorectic (to suppress appetite) is dubious. For one thing, it is ineffective in producing long-term weight loss without accompanying dietary restrictions. For another, it has a severe abuse liability. Tolerance develops to its appetite-suppressing properties as well as to its other CNS effects, and the drug has profound cardiovascular debilitating effects. The use of convulsant doses of pentylenetetrazol as a shock treatment for depressed patients has given way to more subtle and humane approaches. The use of stimulants in parkinsonism has all but vanished with the discovery of levodopa therapy, and their use in depression has been for the most part supplanted by the tricyclic antidepressants. The major persisting applications of stimulants in therapy are in narcolepsy, hyperkinesis, in combination therapies for epilepsy, and rarely for acute treatment of drug-induced respiratory depression. Beyond that there is the enormous and expanding licit and illicit self-administration of stimulants—notably amphetamine, methamphetamine, and cocaine illicitly and caffeine licitly. Caffeine continues to enjoy its unique position as a frequently used and abused mild stimulant. Besides its well-known presence in coffee, tea, and cola, it is found in several over-the-counter (OTC) "cold-pill" combinations and "keep-awake" pills.

Xanthines

Caffeine, theophylline, and theobromine are three closely related derivatives of xanthine and all occur naturally in various plants widely distributed throughout the world.

211

Table 13-1. *Sources and relative potencies of xanthines*

Source and systemic effect	Caffeine	Theophylline	Theobromine
Source	Coffee Tea Cola Chocolate No Doz, etc. Cafergot	Tea Diuretic combinations	Chocolate Athemol (for arteriosclerosis)
CNS stimulation	+++	++	+
Cardiac stimulation	+	+++	++
Diuresis	+	+++	++
Muscle			
Vasodilation	+	+++	++
Visceral smooth muscle relaxation	+	+++	++
Skeletal muscle stimulation	+++	++	+

Least potent (+), most potent (+++).

Caffeine is found in coffee beans or seeds. Tea leaves contain caffeine and theophylline, while cocoa contains caffeine and theobromine. The nuts of the tree *Cola acuminata,* from which cola-flavored drinks are made, also contain caffeine. A cup of coffee or tea contains about 100 to 150 mg of the alkaloid, which approximately equals the therapeutic dose. A 12-oz can of cola contains about one-third that amount. The annual consumption of caffeine in coffee in the United States is about 7 million kg, or about 1 billion kg of coffee.

Of the three common xanthine derivatives, caffeine has the greatest potency as a CNS stimulant, but this same relationship does not necessarily hold for other actions of this class of agents. Caffeine has the least potency of the three in regard to stimulation of the heart and dilation of coronary blood vessels, for example (Table 13-1). Other important peripheral actions of this group of drugs include smooth-muscle relaxation and diuresis. The use of xanthines has been linked to anxiety, increased risk of heart attacks, and pancreatic cancer. The symptoms of caffeine intoxication include restlessness, nervousness, insomnia, diuresis, muscle twitching, rambling flow of thought, cardiac arrhythmias, psychomotor agitation, and periods of inexhaustibility.

Stimulation of the CNS by caffeine occurs particularly in the cortex and the medulla. All regions of the cerebral cortex are stimulated. The cortical action probably accounts for the subjectively experienced effect of the drug, including the feeling of increased alertness, increased speed and efficiency in motor tasks, and enhancement of intellectual processes. The medullary stimulation produced by caffeine is of therapeutic value. Relatively high doses of caffeine can produce a stimulation of the respiratory center in the medulla and can be used to reverse drug-induced depression of respiration.

Caffeine is marketed in the form of OTC tablets (e.g., No Doz) and capsules as an aid in staying awake and restoring mental alertness. A typical oral dose is 100 to 250 mg, taken no more often than every 3 or 4 hours. Caffeine is also found in combination with ergotamine (Cafergot) for use in migraine headaches. Theophylline is used as a diuretic, usually in combination with other diuretics, and as a bronchodilator. Theobromine is marketed for use in arteriosclerosis under the brand name Athemol.

Although the mechanism of action of xanthines is not definitely known, an interesting possibility relates to its inhibition of the enzyme phosphodiesterase (Fig. 13-1). Phosphodiesterase catalyzes the breakdown of an important nucleotide, adenosine 3′:5′-cyclic monophosphate (cAMP). Catecholamines, which are neurotransmitters believed to be involved in regulation of CNS arousal (Chap. 6), are known to stimulate formation of cAMP. Indeed, it has been postulated that cAMP mediates many of the effects produced by catecholamines. It is inviting, therefore, to attribute the actions of xanthines to their ability to increase cAMP levels as a result of inhibition of their breakdown by phosphodiesterase.

Catecholamine-Releasing Stimulants

Amphetamine is the best known and prototypical drug in this subgroup. Amphetamine can also be properly referred to as a sympathomimetic in that its ability to release stored norepinephrine from peripheral nerve terminals of the sympathetic nervous system leads to a stimulation of sympathetically innervated organs and glands. Since the mechanism of action involved in sympathetic and central stimulation by amphetamine is essentially the same, i.e., release of catecholamines from nerve terminals (Fig. 13-1), it is little wonder that there is considerable overlap between the sympathomimetics and CNS-stimulant drug classes. Indeed, one might wonder why the two classes contain different members at all. Nevertheless, some drugs that are effective sympathomimetics possess virtually no CNS-stimulatory properties (e.g., phenylephrine), while certain CNS stimulants of the catecholamine-releasing type are devoid of, for example, cardiovascular effects (e.g., methylphenidate).

Amphetamine exists in two isomers called respectively dextro- (D-) and levo- (L-) amphetamine. The two molecules are identical except that one is the mirror image of the other with respect to three-dimensional configuration. The dextro isomer is about three times more active in the human CNS than the levo isomer. The product Benzedrine consists of an equal (or racemic) mixture of the two isomers (DL-amphetamine). Dexedrine, on the other hand, is the purified dextro isomer and is therefore more potent. Dexedrine is marketed in a time-release (spansule) capsule as well as in tablet form. On the street, Benzedrine sells as "bennies," "hearts," or "peaches"; dexedrine tablets as "oranges" or "footballs"; and dexedrine spansule capsules as "wake-ups," "lid-proppers," or "copilots." Methamphetamine (Desoxyn) is a very potent amphetamine derivative known on the street as "speed."

Amphetamine and its closely related congeners are among the most potent and dangerous of the CNS stimulants. The usual effects of amphetamine include increased motor activity, sleeplessness, agitation, and tremors. There is a pronounced effect on mood, often experienced as an increased confidence, exhilaration, ability to concentrate, and euphoria. There is an enhancement of both mental and physical abilities. Prolonged use of an amphetamine or even a single large dose, however, leads to psychotic-like behavior that is difficult to distinguish from schizophrenia and is followed by a period of depression.

Another major use of catecholamine-releasing stimulants is as anorexics. Amphetamine itself has given way to somewhat less potent stimulants for this purpose, notably diethylpropion (Tenuate, Tepanil), phenmetrazine (Preludin), phendimetrazine (Plegine), benzphetamine (Didrex), and phentermine (Ionamin). All are prescription drugs. Phenylpropanolamine, a sympathomimetic used as a decongestant, is marketed as a nonprescription anorectic.

Amphetamine postpones the need for sleep but not indefinitely. In addition to the overall reduction in sleep time, the pattern of sleep is altered such that the percentage

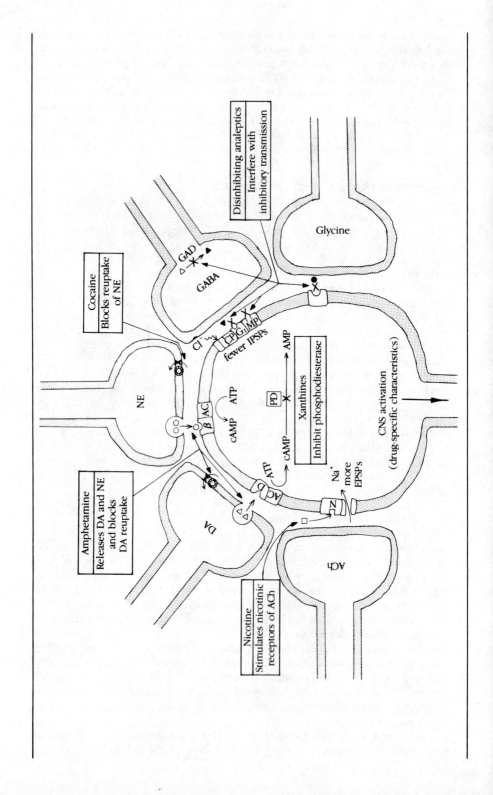

of sleep time spent in desynchronized sleep is reduced to about one-half of normal. The waking EEG pattern is also altered. There is a shifting of EEG frequency distribution toward the higher (beta) frequencies and a lowering of the threshold for EEG activation, that is, alpha-blocking. The action of amphetamine is believed to involve the cortex and the reticular formation. At the reticular level, amphetamine can reverse barbiturate depression of the reticular neurons and by itself increases firing of many individual nerve cells. At least part of the behavioral arousal produced by amphetamine is related to a subcortical site of action, since simultaneous administration with atropine eliminates the EEG activation but not the behavioral arousal produced by amphetamine.

Somewhat paradoxically, amphetamine can be useful in certain cases of epilepsy and in hyperkinesis. Amphetamine eliminates both the seizures and the characteristic EEG abnormalities (3-Hz spike-and-dome discharges) seen in certain cases of petit mal epilepsy in children. Hyperkinesis is discussed in detail in the next section.

Amphetamine can be combined with drugs having both sedative and antiepileptic properties (e.g., phenobarbital) in combination therapies for epilepsy. The stimulant action of amphetamine apparently antagonizes the sedative side effect of the barbiturate at a dose of the stimulant that does not antagonize the desired antiepileptic effect. Amphetamine is used similarly in combination with succinimides and oxazolidones (Chap. 28).

Methylphenidate (Ritalin) is a CNS stimulant of a potency intermediate between that of caffeine and amphetamine. It has a relatively high selectivity for the CNS. Doses that produce substantial central stimulation have little effect on blood pressure. Preliminary indications are that its mechanism of action is similar to that of amphetamine rather than the analeptics. It is currently considered to be the drug of choice in hyperkinesis.

Amphetamines have been widely abused. Acute toxic doses or chronic abuse produces a behavioral syndrome highly similar to that of schizophrenia. Indeed, there have been cases of erroneous diagnosis of people not known to be amphetamine abusers by qualified psychiatric personnel. Amphetamine induces a model psychosis that, though not identical to naturally occurring cases of schizophrenia, indisputably bears a closer resemblance to the disease than do states induced by the so-called psychotomimetics such as LSD. The toxic psychosis related to amphetamine may take the form of delirium or a delusional disorder marked by ideas of reference, aggressiveness and hostility, anxiety, and psychomotor agitation.

The pattern of amphetamine abuse most frequently encountered is dictated by the characteristics of the tolerance induced by the drug. Tolerance to amphetamine develops progressively with chronic use; it is called a "run," and ultimately may reach 100 percent. At this point, withdrawal symptoms can no longer be delayed even if adminis-

---

Fig. 13-1. *Neurochemical mechanisms of stimulants. AC, adenyl cyclase; ACh, acetylcholine; AMP, adenosine monophosphate; ATP, adenosine triphosphate; cAMP, cyclic adenosine monophosphate; β, β- noradrenergic receptor; D, dopamine receptor; DA, dopamine; EPSP, excitatory postsynaptic potential; GABA, gamma-aminobutyric acid; G_1, GABA receptor, type 1; GAD, glutamic acid decarboxylase; IPSP, inhibitory postsynaptic potential; MP, modulatory protein; NE, norepinephrine; PD, phosphodiesterase. Disinhibiting analeptics may block receptors of inhibitory transmitters such as GABA (e.g., muscimol) or glycine (e.g., strychnine), inhibit GABA synthesis (e.g., isonicotinylhydrazide), or inhibit facilitation of GABA-binding by the barbiturate-sensitive modulatory protein (MP) (e.g., picrotoxin).*

tration of amphetamine is continued. Therefore, the abuser may cease taking the drug at the end of a run and may switch to a hypnotic to ease the discomfiture of the withdrawal, or "crash." During withdrawal, the abuser is irritable, unreasonable, and exhausted. He may sleep for several days at a time. At the end of the "crash," tolerance to the stimulant has been lost, and the user may embark on another run. The amphetamine "withdrawal symptoms" are not a true abstinence syndrome, but only a collapse of exhausted neural systems.

The principal dangers of amphetamine abuse are chronic toxicity and violent behavior rather than acute toxicity, although overdosage may occur. In a full-blown toxic syndrome, the user becomes extremely hyperactive and engages in compulsive and stereotypical behaviors, such as sorting and re-sorting, disassembling devices, repetitious short acts, and effusive talking. Memory becomes hazy; the user may become paranoid and brutally and senselessly violent.

In recent years, amphetamine abuse has "progressed" from an oral to an intravenous pattern of administration. Immediately following IV injection of amphetamine, the user experiences a "rush" or "flash" somewhat similar to, but distinguishable from, that accompanying heroin use. The amphetamine "rush" has been described as an abrupt awakening, as opposed to the drowsy drifting effect of heroin. The pleasurable feelings accompanying the "rush" contribute substantially to the risk of abuse. Psychological dependence on an amphetamine is especially strong, and recidivism is high. When amphetamine or cocaine is combined with heroin it is referred to as a "speed ball."

Attention Deficit Disorders

Attention deficit disorders, or hyperkinetic syndrome, is a childhood pattern characterized by impulsivity, elevated motor activity, short attention span and distractability, hyperreactivity, and explosive irritability. Its neurophysiologic reality is demonstrated by a reliable diagnostic test, the photometrazol method. In this technique, the subject is treated with a titrated dose of pentylenetetrazol and stimulated with a stroboscopic light. Hyperkinetic children have a lower-than-normal threshold to seizure discharge activity in the EEG under these circumstances. Both diazepam and trimethadione, which depress thalamic electrical activity, raise the photometrazol threshold to a much greater extent in hyperkinetic children than in normal children. It appears to be easier to overstimulate the thalamic pacemaker in hyperkinetic children than in normal children. This, combined with the fact that focused attention is a function of the diffuse thalamic system (DTS) and stimulus reactivity a function of the reticular activating system (RAS), suggests that hyperkinesis is related to underdevelopment of the DTS relative to the RAS. The fact that hyperkinesis is generally "outgrown" suggests that the DTS is late in maturing rather than permanently defective.

Three categories of attention deficit disorder are differentiated in the *Diagnostic and Statistical Manual* (DSM-III): attention deficit disorder *with hyperactivity* and *without hyperactivity,* and *residual type.* There are six criteria for attention deficit disorder with hyperactivity. Three describe symptom clusters; the remaining three define age of onset, duration, and exclusions (Table 13-2). The criteria for attention deficit disorder without hyperactivity are the same, except that the symptom cluster related to hyperactivity is not present. The characteristics of hyperkinesis have been established empirically by Satterfield et al. (Table 13-3). Their findings suggest some additional means of defining the three symptom clusters.

The recognition that symptoms related to attention deficit disorder may persist into adulthood is an important new development. This has led to the inclusion of the third diagnostic subgroup: the residual type. This person once met the criteria for attention

Table 13-2. *Criteria for attention deficit disorder with hyperactivity*

Inattention (three or more of the following):
    Failure to complete projects begun
    Poor listening ability
    Easy distractability
    Difficulty in concentrating
    Poor stick-to-it-iveness
Impulsivity (three or more of the following):
    Acts before thinking
    Excessive shifting among activities
    Difficulty in organizing work
    Excessive need for supervision
    Frequent calling out in class
    Difficulty in waiting turn
Hyperactivity (two or more of the following):
    Runs or climbs about excessively
    Difficulty in sitting still
    Difficulty in staying seated
    Excessive sleep movements
    Constantly "on the go"
Onset before age 7
Duration at least 6 months
Not secondary to schizophrenia, an affective disorder, or to mental retardation

Table 13-3. *Percentage of differing behaviors* found in hyperkinetic and normal groups matched for age and IQ*

Behaviors	Hyperkinetic boys (N = 14)	Normal boys (N = 14)
Fights with peers	93	7
Unable to take correction	86	0
Rocks, jiggles legs	86	14
Dances, wiggles hands	86	14
Unusually active	86	14
Unable to sit through school period	86	21
Unable to follow directions	79	7
Difficult to get to bed	79	7
Poor relationships with peers	71	0
Temper tantrums	71	7
Does not complete projects	71	7
Hard to get to sleep	71	7
Wakes early	71	7
Defiant	71	14
Unable to sit through meal	64	0
Leaves physician's office	64	14

*p = < .001.
Source: Modified from J. H. Satterfield et al. Physiological studies of the hyperkinetic child. I. *Am. J. Psychiatry* 128:1418–1424, 1972. Copyright 1972, The American Psychiatric Association.

deficit disorder with hyperactivity and currently exhibits social or functional impairment associated with attention deficits and impulsivity, not attributable to schizophrenia, affective or personality disorders, or mental retardation. Hyperactivity is no longer present.

Amphetamine and, more recently, methylphenidate (Ritalin) have been used effectively in alleviating behavioral abnormalities in hyperkinesis. Although this is sometimes referred to as a "tranquilizing" effect, such a characterization is inaccurate. It appears that moderate doses of these drugs exert more stimulatory effects on the DTS than the RAS. The net effect is to enhance concentration, or, in terms of the dual arousal theory (Chap. 10), shift the balance of arousal influences toward internalization, thus protecting the child from being distracted by every novel occurrence in his environment. Hartmann [2] observed that moderate doses of amphetamine in adults also enhance directed attention and increase normal defensive patterns. This drug is widely used illicitly to maintain wakefulness and enhance performance. Stereotypy and psychotic reactions are associated only with extreme dosages.

The effect of the stimulants on NE levels also bears mention in this context. Hartmann noted that the hyperkinetic syndrome is identical to the behavior of normal children when overtired or sleep-deprived. The latter syndrome clears spontaneously when NE levels in catecholaminergic systems are restored by adequate D-sleep time (dreaming sleep is necessary for maintenance of focused attention *and* feedback-regulated emotional control).

Caffeine has also been used successfully with hyperkinetic children. This application grew out of observations that more hyperactive children drank coffee or tea regularly than was expected. Thus, their spontaneous "drug of choice" was a clue to their developmental problem and to a method of treatment.

Cocaine

Cocaine is another stimulant that elevates free catecholamines but by a distinctive mechanism. Cocaine does not release stored catecholamines, but rather prevents the reuptake of catecholamines and prevents their breakdown by monoamine oxidase to some extent as well (see Fig. 13-1). Cocaine also acts as a local anesthetic and is structurally related to procaine and lidocaine, two drugs widely employed as local anesthetics for medical purposes. The stimulant effect of cocaine may relate in part to the local anesthetic mechanism, since procaine produces similar subjective effects but does not block norepinephrine reuptake. Animals self-administer procaine and lidocaine as readily as cocaine.

Cocaine is an ingredient in coca leaves that has been used by native Peruvians for at least 5,000 years, based on archeological evidence. Some 20 million pounds of coca leaves are used yearly by the 2 million Peruvians of the highlands. Coca leaves contain up to 2 percent cocaine. Because coca leaves do not retain their potency very well during long-range transport from South American growing fields, recreational use in Europe and the United States was constrained until the middle of the nineteenth century, when cocaine was isolated from the plant. Freud was an early proponent of the use of cocaine, and the fictional character Sherlock Holmes attributed his magnificent powers of deduction to its use. Cocaine is smuggled into the United States largely by way of distribution points in Colombia. It is sold under such names as "coke," "snow," "gold dust," and "lady" and has the appearance of a white powder. Often, it is diluted with procaine, lidocaine, amphetamine, or other chemicals.

The effects of cocaine are intermediate between the weak stimulatory action of xanthines and the potent action of amphetamine. The effects of intranasal doses of 10

Table 13-4. *Cocaine effects in relation to route of administration*

Form of drug and drug effects		Route of administration		
	Oral	Intranasal	Smoked	Intravenous
Form	Hydrochloride	Hydrochloride	Free base or paste	Hydrochloride
Time to peak plasma concentration	60–80 min	60–80 min	15–20 min	< 5 min
Rebound depression	±	±	++	++
Severity of drug craving	±	±	++	++
Risk of local tissue damage at site of administration	0	+	++	0
Risk of toxic psychosis or death from overdose	+	+	++	++

0, no effect; ±, equivocal effect; +, mild to moderate effect; ++, intense or frequent effect.

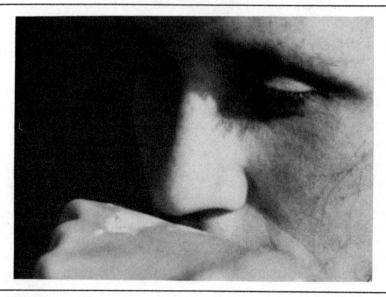

Fig. 13-2. *Snorting cocaine.*

mg are indistinguishable from placebo, but doses of 25 mg and above reliably produce subjective euphoria. The duration of action is much shorter than for amphetamine. Amphetamine effects typically last about 1 to 4 hours; a typical cocaine effect after intranasal administration is only 5 to 15 minutes.

The route by which cocaine is utilized is all-important in defining the risks involved. Four routes are employed (Table 13-4). Most commonly, cocaine is taken intranasally, by snorting (Fig. 13-2). The severity of psychological dependence and rebound depression is minimal when cocaine is used by the intranasal or oral routes. The period of euphoria correlates with the period of rising plasma concentrations of the drug, not the time of peak concentration. A hazard associated with intranasal use is the perforation of the nostrils that can result from repeated snorting. When cocaine is used by the intravenous or inhalation (smoking) routes, the severity of psychological dependence may be marked to the extent of disrupting psychological health and social functioning. For purposes of smoking, cocaine is converted from its usual form as a hydrochloride salt to the free base, or alkaloid, form, which is considerably more heat-stabile. Amateur laboratory kits are available for carrying out the conversion. Cocaine paste, an intermediate product in the manufacture of cocaine hydrochloride in South America, contains about 30 to 90 percent free base and is thus suitable for smoking. A unique hazard associated with smoking cocaine is lung damage resulting from constriction of pulmonary blood vessels.

Physical dependence does not occur, regardless of route. Tolerance develops to the anorectic, convulsant, cardiac, and respiratory effects of cocaine with chronic use. The fact that subjective effects disappear more rapidly than the decline in blood concentrations suggests that "acute tolerance" occurs with respect to the euphoric effects. On the other hand, chronic use is associated with increased CNS sensitivity to cocaine as regards the occurrence of mental alertness and euphoria. At high doses, death can result from convulsions or from cardiac arrest. The latter effect is a consequence of the local anesthetic action of cocaine, which leads to severe myocardial depression.

The cocaine toxic psychosis (cocaine intoxication in DSM-III) resembles that caused by amphetamine. Psychological symptoms include excitement, restlessness, elation, loquacity, grandiosity, anxiety, hypervigilance, and confusion. Physical symptoms include tachycardia, chills or fever, mydriasis, exophthalamos, elevated blood pressure, nausea, and vomiting. Delirium and convulsions occur in severe cases, and coma terminally. The treatment of choice is intravenous diazepam or a barbiturate.

Analeptics

Pentylenetetrazol

The best-studied analeptic is pentylenetetrazol (PTZ) (Metrazol). It produces a diffuse stimulation throughout the CNS by interfering with binding of GABA to its receptors (see Fig. 13-1). Pacemaker neurons of the thalamus are activated by PTZ. When a sufficient level of activation has been elicited by PTZ, convulsions ensue, involving (at low doses) only the head and forelimbs. Convulsions induced by PTZ in mice resemble petit mal attacks in humans, and the two have proved to be susceptible to the same chemotherapeutic treatments. Therefore, PTZ has become a valuable aid in laboratory testing of proposed new antiepileptic agents.

A second application of PTZ is its use as a diagnostic aid in epilepsy. Subconvulsive doses injected intravenously, with or without strobe-light stimulation, can be used to activate latent epileptogenic foci, and these can be monitored by concurrent EEG measurement. This is referred to as the photometrazol test. The photometrazol technique has also been employed in drug evaluation.

Currently, PTZ has no therapeutic usefulness. In its use as a respiratory stimulant, it has given way to new analeptics having better therapeutic ratios, i.e., a greater spread between the dose that stimulates respiration and the dose eliciting convulsions. The current drug of choice for respiratory stimulation following drug-induced depression is doxapram (Dopram).

Nicotine and Tobacco

Another important analeptic of the stimulating type is nicotine. While nicotine has no therapeutic application, its occurrence as a constituent of tobacco makes it one of the most frequently self-administered drugs in our society. Nicotine has widespread effects on the peripheral nervous system. At low doses, it produces a stimulation of both the sympathetic and parasympathetic branches of the autonomic nervous system. At higher doses, the stimulation is short-lasting and is followed by a persistent suppression of autonomic activity. Both the stimulation and the depression are related to an action of nicotine on ganglia. The adrenal medulla and the neuromuscular junctions of the somatic nervous system are subjected to a similar biphasic response to nicotine. Many of the toxic effects of nicotine are related to these peripheral effects.

The CNS is stimulated by nicotine as well, presumably acting on nicotinic, cholinergic receptors (see Fig. 13-1). At increasing dose levels, this stimulant produces tremors and then convulsions. Although the site of action of nicotine in the CNS has not been firmly established, indications from behavioral studies suggest that the DTS arousal system and related limbic structures are involved. In tasks presumably measuring "attention," performance is enhanced by nicotine. Moreover, nicotine has been reported to stimulate the septal area and the hippocampus; a direct action on some cortical neurons has also been reported, however.

The excitation occurring after nicotine administration is followed by a CNS depression. During the excitatory phase, respiration is quickened. During the subsequent depression, respiration is inhibited, which may lead to death after ingestion of toxic quantities of nicotine. In cigarette-smoking, the acute toxic effects (e.g., nausea, especially in novice smokers) are almost exclusively related to nicotine. The chronic effects of cigarette smoking are related only in small part to nicotine, however. Other tobacco constituents, of which some 270 distinct compounds have been identified including 15 known to be carcinogenic, are of more importance with respect to irritation of the respiratory passages and lungs. Nicotine may, however, contribute substantially to the correlation between smoking and various cardiovascular problems. Emphysema has been linked to an action of an oxidant in smoke on a lung enzyme called elastase. Smoke decreases the flexibility of the air sacs, interfering with exchange of carbon dioxide and oxygen. Nitrosamines and other carcinogens in cigarette smoke are implicated in lung cancer. Tobacco constituents suppress the activity of the hairlike cilia of the lungs, thus interfering with the removal of carcinogen-containing smoke particles (tar), microorganisms, and other foreign substances such as dust pollens, and soot, thereby promoting lung cancer and bronchitis. Other forms of cancer that also occur correlatively with tobacco smoking involve cancer of the lips, tongue, mouth, larynx, bladder, and kidney. Nicotine is probably the main component of tobacco that contributes to the cardiac disease, peripheral vascular disorders, cerebrovascular disease (stroke), and ulcers that frequently accompany long-term tobacco use. Tobacco use contributes to a total of about a third of a million deaths per year. There are currently some 65 million smokers in the United States.

Both tolerance and dependence develop with tobacco smoking. Nicotine dependence is both physiologic and psychological, and abstinence is marked by indications of withdrawal, including restlessness, inability to concentrate, and irritability. Other withdrawal symptoms include a craving for tobacco, anxiety, headache, drowsiness, and gastrointestinal disturbances.

Strychnine

Were it not for the occasional occurrence of strychnine poisoning and the adoption of this drug as a lacing agent by black marketeers, the disinhibiting-type stimulants would be of no more than heuristic interest. Strychnine is a naturally occurring alkaloid found in nux vomica, the seeds of a tree found in India (*Strychnos nux-vomica*). It is employed as a poison for rats and has been frequently encountered as an additive in marijuana in the United States. These two sources account for most occurrences of strychnine poisoning.

It is unlikely that anyone would be administered strychnine for any therapeutic purpose, for there is no rational therapeutic application. While it is sometimes employed in "tonics," the actions ascribed to it either simply do not occur or occur only at doses that are potentially toxic.

Research interest in strychnine centers around its rather unusual mechanism of action. Strychnine interferes with the inhibitory influences exerted on nerve cells throughout the brain and particularly in the spinal cord. It is generally believed that strychnine is an antagonist of glycine (see Fig. 13-1), a central transmitter substance found in high concentration in the brainstem and spinal cord. Normally, electrical activity in the CNS is confined to appropriate pathways, in part by tonic inhibition exerted on other nerve cells. When this tonic inhibition is lifted, as by strychnine, impulses course without restriction throughout the brain. At toxic doses, strychnine elicits a characteristic convulsion that can be distinguished from that produced by PTZ or other excitatory analeptics. Reflex responses to sensory stimulation become greatly exaggerated, and convulsions may be precipitated by a loud noise or a tactile stimulus. Rapid intravenous administration of a short-acting barbiturate or a centrally acting skeletal muscle relaxant such as mephenesin (Tolserol) is effective antidotal therapy. Stomach lavage soon after ingestion of strychnine can be accomplished with potassium permanganate solution.

One of the active toxins in tetanus infection, tetanospasmin, produces a strychnine-like toxicity pattern, although the latency of onset of its action is much longer than for strychnine.

Implications for Psychotherapy

Apparent schizoid behaviors may in fact represent manifestations of amphetamine toxic psychoses. The associated paranoid ideation and hallucinations may be indistinguishable from schizophrenia, particularly the paranoid variety, although it is said that visual hallucinations are more prominent in the drug-induced psychosis. Amphetamines also may precipitate psychotic episodes in latent schizophrenia. A less severe reaction is a transient delirium marked by confusion and partial amnesia. A still milder response may involve slight agitation, talkativeness, insomnia, and restlessness. Neurologic manifestations of amphetamine abuse may include headache, vertigo, and tremors.

Abstinence symptoms may accompany withdrawal from stimulants and appear as psychopathologic states. A pronounced depression, or "crash," may accompany withdrawal after prolonged amphetamine use. Abstinence from caffeine or nicotine in heavy users of these drugs may appear as agitation or restlessness. Heavy doses of caffeine (1,000 mg or 7 to 10 cups of coffee) may produce restlessness and excitement progressing to mild delirium, sensory disturbances such as ringing in the ears, and muscular shaking. Misdiagnosis of acute caffeine toxicosis (from "keep awake" pills) as psychoneurotic anxiety and hysteria has been reported. Some patients seeking treatment for chronic anxiety prove to be heavy caffeine users who have failed to relate the toxic symptoms to their coffee- or tea-drinking.

Stimulants are powerful primary reinforcers. Continued abuse of stimulants may mitigate against therapeutic efforts. State dependency has been definitely established with respect to many of the stimulants, so that transfer of learning may be limited between the drugged and undrugged states. Whether this applies to mild stimulants such as nicotine or caffeine is not scientifically established. On the other hand, stimulants have been shown to enhance learning while the subject is on the drug, especially when motivated or focused attention is called for.

The use of coffee and tea by children may be a possible "soft sign" suggestive of hyperkinesis. Therapy with hyperkinetic children and their families is probably the context in which the therapist is most likely to encounter ongoing use of major stimulants. There is little doubt that the hyperkinetic behavior pattern can be as difficult in the therapy setting as it can be in the conventional school. Some nondrug interventions have proved useful in both contexts. Taking account of the child's easy distractability by simplifying the environment is one such approach. Another effective strategy is to adapt the environment to the activity and shifting interests of the child.

One researcher, noting a preference among hyperkinetic children for rhythmic rocking to and fro when attempting to concentrate, hypothesized a deficit in such stimuli. In fact, hyperkinetic children may respond exceptionally favorably to, and spontaneously engage in, rhythmic rocking, swinging, swiveling, or even just stroking of the limbs, which can sometimes bring about a dramatic, almost immediate, change in behavior and ability to attend. We would reinterpret these observations in light of the imbalance theory given earlier in this chapter, however. Rhythmic inputs at or near a subharmonic of the thalamic pacemaker in the diffuse thalamic system can "drive" its oscillations and thus reinforce DTS predominance over the RAS. The therapist may wish to try simple mechanical and environmental techniques and, when they prove effective, consider them as possible alternatives to continued medication with amphetamine, methylphenidate, or other stimulants.

Reports of widespread, possibly indiscriminate, administration of stimulants to school children at least support the possibility that some children receiving them are not actually hyperkinetic. The therapist probably should look into the basis of the diagnosis, and when a photometrazol test has not been performed, suggest that it be conducted.

Medically Important Stimulants and Analeptics

amphetamine (Benzedrine), a stimulant: primarily used for narcolepsy and hyperkinesis, largely superseded as anorectic and antidepressant. Narcolepsy: 20 to 100 mg. Hyperkinesis (children over 5): 10 to 30 mg.

caffeine (theine), a xanthine stimulant: bronchial asthma, migraine (cranial vasoconstriction), and mild stimulation. Stimulant: 500 to 1,000 mg.

dextroamphetamine (Dexedrine), a D-Isomer of amphetamine (see amphetamine above).

diethylpropion (Tenuate, Tepanil), an amphetamine-like stimulant: used as anorectic. Anorectic: 75 mg.

doxapram (Dopram), an analeptic: used in respiratory depression. Analeptic: 0.5 to 1.5 mg IV.

ephedrine, a sympathomimetic stimulant: nasal decongestant; CNS side effects resemble those of amphetamine but are less pronounced; common in cold and asthmatic combinations.

methamphetamine (Desoxyn, Syndrox, Methedrine, and others), an amphetamine-derivative stimulant: see amphetamine; also used in acute hypotension. Narcolepsy: 5 to 60 mg. Hyperkinesis (children over 5): 5 to 20 mg.

methylphenidate (Ritalin), an amphetamine-like stimulant: used in mild depression (but see text), hyperkinesis, narcolepsy. Hyperkinesis and narcolepsy: 10 to 60 mg.

pentylenetetrazol (PTZ) (Metrazol), an analeptic: diagnostic use to activate EEG, hyperkinesis, and epilepsy.

theophylline, a xanthine stimulant: various peripheral uses, including bronchial asthma, angina pectoris, and as diuretic; milder CNS effects than caffeine: 500 to 1,000 mg.

Selected References and Further Readings

1. Gilman, A. G., Goodman, L. S., and Gilman, A. *The Pharmacological Basis of Therapeutics* (6th ed.). New York: Macmillan, 1980.
2. Hartmann, D. L. *The Functions of Sleep.* New Haven: Yale University Press, 1973.
3. Iversen, L. L., Iversen, S. D., and Snyder, S. H. (Eds.). *Handbook of Psychopharmacology.* Vol. 11: Stimulants. New York: Plenum, 1978.
4. Jaffe, J. H., and Jarvik, M. E. Tobacco Use Disorder. In M. A. Lipton et al. (Eds.), *Psychopharmacology: A Generation of Progress.* New York: Raven, 1978.

5. Satterfield, J. H., Cantwell, D. P., Lesser, L. I., and Podosin, R. L. Physiological Studies of the Hyperkinetic Child: I. In D. F. Klein and R. Gittelman-Klein (Eds.), *Progress in Psychiatric Drug Treatment.* New York: Brunner/Mazel, 1975.
6. Weiss, G., Minde, K., Douglas, V., Werry, J., and Sykes, D. Comparison of the Effects of Chlorpromazine, Dextroamphetamine and Methylphenidate on the Behavior and Intellectual Functioning of Hyperactive Children. In D. F. Klein and R. Gittelman-Klein (Eds.), *Progress in Psychiatric Drug Treatment.* New York: Brunner/Mazel, 1975.
7. Zarcone, V. P., Jr. Diagnosis and treatment of excessive daytime sleepiness. *Clin. Neuropharmacol.* 2:87–97, 1977.

who
Ripped
This
Out?
Rude!

The DSM-III definition of PCP intoxication centers on five criteria: (1) recent use of the drug; (2) two or more physical symptoms (nystagmus, increased heart rate or blood pressure, numbness or hypoalgesia, ataxia, or joint aches); (3) two or more psychological symptoms (euphoria, psychomotor agitation, anxiety, emotional lability, grandiosity, slowed time, or synesthesias); (4) maladaptive behaviors (belligerence, impulsivity, assaultiveness, impaired judgment); and (5) lack of alternative organic or psychiatric causes. An acute toxic psychosis may occur in the form of delirium, which may progress to organic delusional disorder.

Other True Psychedelics

Except for LSD, dimethyltryptamine (DMT) is the best-known drug among the substituted indoles. The subjective effects are similar to those of LSD but of shorter duration, usually only 1 to 2 hours. Psilocybin and psilocin are found in mushrooms, such as the *Psilocybe mexicana* and *Stropharia cubensis*. Mushrooms containing these hallucinogens grow in the northwestern United States and in Central America as well as in other parts of the world. Bufotenin is found in *Amanita muscaria*, in secretions of the skin and parotid glands of toads, and in the seeds of a Haitian and Venezuelan tree, *Piptadenia peregrina*. A chemical related to LSD, lysergic acid amide, is found in the seeds of the morning glory (ololiluqui). Still another indole psychedelic is harmine, a commonly used laboratory drug and a constituent of a Middle Eastern plant, *Peganum harmala*.

Mescaline is found in the peyote cactus (*Lophophora williamsii*), a plant common in the southwestern United States and Mexico. Peyote has been used for centuries by certain Indian tribes for religious purposes, and that use is sanctioned by U.S. federal law.

Psychedelics that are phenylethylamine derivatives (group B) produce a marked pupillary dilation and are more likely to induce nausea and vomiting than the tryptamine derivatives, reflecting their relatively greater autonomic activity. Paranoid and aggressive responses are more likely with this group. Psychedelic reactions may be long-lasting—up to 72 hours. Blood pressure may soar because of activation of the sympathetic nervous system.

The benzilic acid ester derivatives (group C) are extremely potent central anticholinergic compounds. It has long been known that large doses of the more familiar anticholinergic drugs could produce psychic manifestations characterized by confusion, dizziness, delirium, hallucinations, and memory distortions. The benzilic acid ester derivatives, of which the most familiar is Ditran (really a combination of two such derivatives), produce marked CNS as well as autonomic nervous system effects, including elevated blood pressure, increased heart rate, pupillary dilation, ataxia, confusion, inability to focus attention, delirium, and distortions of time and space. Hallucinations are frequent and dramatic, and reality contact may disintegrate.

Cannabis

Characteristic Effects

Many pharmacologists prefer to classify cannabis and its active constituent tetrahydrocannabinol (THC) as a sedative rather than as a psychedelic. Like sedatives and unlike LSD, cannabis prolongs barbiturate sleeping time; however, cannabis also prolongs amphetamine-induced stimulation, as does LSD and unlike sedatives. Suffice it to say that cannabis does not fit perfectly into either group, but rather shares some properties with each.

Cannabis produces sedation and ataxia in human subjects, monkeys, dogs, and in most laboratory animals, although only at somewhat higher per kilogram doses. In human subjects, this is accompanied by a mild euphoria and altered perceptions of space, time, and sensory information. The physiologic effects in monkeys and dogs most closely parallel those in humans. There is a general decrease in spontaneous activity, hypothermia, and suppression of the corneal reflex. Heart rate is quickened in all species except rats, and this is experienced by human subjects as palpitations. Human subjects also experience dryness of the mouth and an increased appetite. A drooping of the eyelids (ptosis) is a characteristic sign of cannabis intoxication. Street names of marijuana include "pot," "grass," "weed," and "Mary Jane." Marijuana cigarettes are called "joints" or "reefers."

Factors Influencing Cannabis Potency

Cannabis potency varies markedly based on a number of factors. Assessment of the extent of drug influence that an individual experiences must therefore take into account not only frequency of use but also the nature of the product in use.

Marijuana refers to the dried, chopped-up parts of the *Cannabis sativa* plant. The cannabis contains several pharmacologically active substances. The main component contributing to subjective effects in humans is called Δ^9-THC (or by another system of nomenclature, Δ^1-THC). Two other contributors are Δ^8-THC (Δ^6-THC) and cannabinol. Another ingredient, cannabidiol, has an antagonist action, diminishing the action of the other constituents. Cannabis exists in a male and in a female variety (Figure 14-2). The male plant is generally inactive or poorly active because of either too little THC or too much cannabidiol. The male plant is relegated to the making of a kind of rope, called hemp. It is the female plant that is generally used in marijuana preparations.

Within the female plant, there is considerable difference in concentration of the active ingredient from one plant part to another. Roots, seeds, and large stems have little or no active ingredient; leaves have substantial levels. The flowering tops, or bracts, of the female plant and the plant resin are the most potent. The resin may be gathered in a gooey, brick-like mass and, as such, is called hashish. Marijuana from which seeds and stems have been removed is more potent, while marijuana low in bracts is weak.

Other factors influencing marijuana potency include genetics, climate where grown, and the time it is picked in relation to the growing season. Marijuana potency may vary from year to year, even if genetic and location factors are controlled, much as grapes grown for wine vary in relation to annual growing conditions. Generally, marijuana grown where the season is long (near the equator), and picked late in the season is strongest.

The various active components apparently contribute in differing proportions to marijuana's various pharmacologic actions. Thus, two samples of marijuana, when tested in mice, will have different ratios of potency for inhibiting the corneal reflex and for suppressing aggression.

Adverse Effects with Chronic Use

There are inconclusive indications that cannabis use may be associated with a behavioral pattern referred to as an "amotivational syndrome." Even if such a syndrome does occur correlatively with cannabis use, the direction of causality has not been

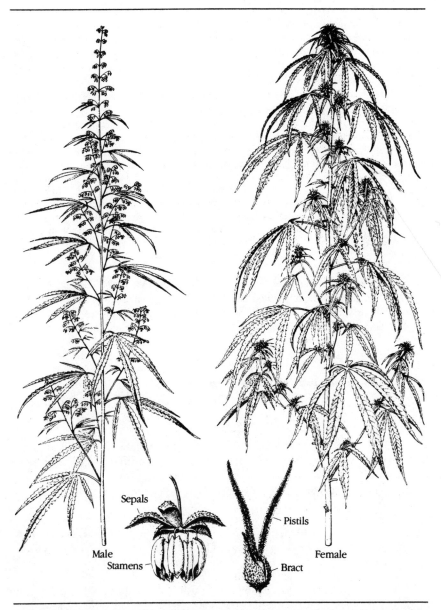

Sepals

Pistils

Male
Stamens

Bract

Female

Fig. 14-2. *Hemp plant* (Cannabis sativa) *is a common weed growing freely in many parts of the world, where it is used as a medicine, an intoxicant, and a source of fiber. It is classified as a dioecious plant, that is, the male reproductive parts are on one individual (left) and the female parts are on another (right). Details of the two types of flower are shown at bottom. The active substances in the drug are contained in a sticky yellow resin that covers the flower clusters and top leaves of the female plant when it is ripe. (Modified from L. Grinspoon. Marihuana. Sci. Am. 221:17–25, 1969. © 1969 by Scientific American, Inc. All rights reserved.)*

established. Other reputed adverse effects include lowered testosterone levels in males, brain damage, carcinogenicity, and leukopenia. It is clear that each of these effects occurs at the high concentrations used in toxicity studies, but it has not been demonstrated that such effects occur at relevant doses. The problem associated with such studies can be illustrated by a study reporting brain-wave changes in rhesus monkeys exposed to marijuana smoke. The following comments on that study were made by Dr. Julius Axelrod, a 1970 Nobel prize–winning pharmacologist, speaking before a Congressional subcommittee investigating marijuana:

One of the fundamental principles in pharmacology is the amount of a compound or drug that enters the body. You could take the most poisonous compound, and if you take too little, there is no effect. One may take a very supposedly safe compound, and if you give enough of it, it will cause toxic effects. This, I think, all pharmacologists recognize. I respect Dr. Heath; he is a fine neurologist; but the doses he has given for the acute effect, for example, would be equivalent to smoking 30 [marijuana] cigarettes, a very heavy dose of [marijuana]. And the amount he has given for the chronic effect represents smoking 30 [marijuana] cigarettes three times a day for a period of [6] months. The results indicate that [marijuana] causes an irreversible damage to the brain. But the amounts used are so large that one wonders whether it is due to the large toxic amounts Dr. Heath has given.

Unfortunately, this kind of study is characteristic of research in the field. The lack of conclusive evidence of adverse effects with chronic marijuana use does not in any sense establish that it is a safe drug. As with any instance of nonmedical drug use, frequent use combined with behavioral indications of psychopathology should be cause for concern.

Intoxication, Tolerance, and Dependence

Marijuana intoxication is defined in the DSM-III on the basis of six criteria: (1) recent use of cannabis; (2) tachycardia; (3) one or more psychological symptoms (euphoria, intensification of perceptions, slowing of time, and apathy); (4) one or more physical symptoms (conjunctival swelling, increased appetite, dry mouth); (5) maladaptive behaviors (anxiety, suspiciousness, paranoid ideation, impaired judgment or functioning); and (6) lack of an organic or psychiatric cause. Acute toxic psychoses are rare when marijuana is smoked, but may occur when hashish is used. The toxic psychosis is a delusional syndrome.

The issue of tolerance to cannabis is complex. The peripheral effects (e.g., on heart rate) undergo tolerance development with habitual use similar to that occurring with many other psychopharmacologic agents. On the other hand, the psychic effects undergo a reverse or negative tolerance, so that experienced or chronic users require a smaller dose to "get high" than does the naive user.

There is no withdrawal syndrome following chronic use of cannabis, and there is no physical dependence. Psychological dependence occurs in some users, however.

A recent survey found that approximately 16 million Americans had used marijuana in the preceding 30-day period.

Mechanism of Action

Cannabis has anticholinergic properties, and some of the effects of cannabis are related in part to that action. Memory impairment, for example, is probably an anticholinergic action on the hippocampus (see Fig. 14-1). Another component of the effect of marijuana is a low-level anesthetic action, somewhat like that produced by nitrous oxide. Marijuana is said to cause a fluidization of cell membranes, which produces a general impairment of neural function.

Legal Status of Marijuana

The penalties for possession or casual transfer of small amounts of marijuana vary widely from state to state, and the statutes involved are badly in need of standardization. Federal regulations (the Comprehensive Drug Abuse Prevention Control Act of 1970) provide that mere possession or casual transfer is a misdemeanor, and maximum penalties are set at $1,000 or 1 year in jail for first offenses. Cultivation, importation or exportation, sale, distribution, or possession with intent to distribute are all felonies punishable by imprisonment up to 5 years for the first offense. The imposition of laws restricting personal freedoms and the attachment of severe penalties would seem to require a justification that is lacking from objective studies of the societal and personal hazards attendant on marijuana use. Marijuana is singularly lacking in acute toxicity, and, thus far, concerns about chronic toxicity have not been borne out by either laboratory studies in this country or epidemologic studies in Jamaica, Costa Rica, and Greece. Recommendations for relaxing the legal strictures for possession of marijuana were published in 1894 (*The Indian Hemp Drugs Commission Report*), in 1944 (*The La-Guardia Committee Report*), and in 1972 (*National Commission on Marihuana and Drug Abuse*) by government-appointed study groups. Thus far, less than a dozen states have decriminalized the possession of marijuana.

Possible Medical Uses of THC

A number of medical uses have been established or suggested for marijuana. The most valuable application to date is for alleviation of nausea in conjunction with cancer chemotherapy. Marijuana is as good or better than the conventional drug, compazine, for this application. It is useful in glaucoma in cases refractory to the conventional drug, pilocarpine. Marijuana has antianxiety properties, but has not been tested against conventional anxiolytics in controlled studies. It is only moderately effective in asthma and not even as effective as conventional treatments. Other proposed applications seem largely unfounded.

Implications for Psychotherapy

Acute or chronic psychotic episodes have been reportedly precipitated by LSD. The therapist should become aware of the patient's drug history in much the same manner as he or she determines other relevant history that might contribute to a neurolopathologic state. On the other hand, the patient's limited experience with psychedelics should not be assumed to have contributed to psychopathology in the absence of causative indications. In fact, LSD has been successfully employed as an adjunct in psychotherapy where insight generation seemed indicated.

The possibility that chronic use of cannabis leads to an "amotivational syndrome" remains largely unsubstantiated but nevertheless a possibility. Cannabis is presumably an effective primary reinforcer, and its continued use, *if* linked to dysfunctional behavior, may compromise therapeutic effectiveness. On the other hand, it is apparent that cannabis has been used by many individuals in the absence of, and without leading to, pronounced psychopathology.

Dissociation of learning has been reported with cannabis and may be presumed to occur with other psychedelics. Mescaline has been used in laboratory studies as a discriminative stimulus.

Selected References and Further Readings

1. Bateson, G. *Steps to an Ecology of Mind.* New York: Ballantine, 1972.
2. Bloomquist, E. R. *Marijuana, the Second Trip* (2nd ed.). Toronto: Glencoe, 1972.
3. Braude, M. C., and Szara, S. (Eds.). *Pharmacology of Marihuana.* New York: Raven, 1976. Vols. 1 and 2.
4. Gilman, A. G., Goodman, L. S., and Gilman, A. *The Pharmacological Basis of Therapeutics* (5th ed.). New York: Macmillan, 1980.
5. Grinspoon, L. *Marihuana Reconsidered.* Cambridge, Mass.: Harvard University Press, 1971.
6. Harris, L. S. Cannabis: A Review of Progress. In M. A. Lipton et al. (Eds.), *Psychopharmacology: A Generation of Progress.* New York: Raven, 1978.
7. Hollister, L. E. Psychotomimetic Drugs. In L. L. Iversen et al. (Eds.), *Handbook of Psychopharmacology.* New York: Plenum, 1978. Vol. 11.
8. Jones, R. T. Marihuana: Human Effects. In L. L. Iversen et al. (Eds.), *Handbook of Psychopharmacology.* New York: Plenum, 1978. Vol. 12.
9. Kaplan, J. *Marijuana: The New Prohibition.* Cleveland: World Publishing, 1970.
10. Sankar, D. V. S. (Ed.). *LSD—A Total Study.* Westbury, N.Y.: PJD Publishers Ltd., 1975.

Psychiatric Disorders and Drugs V

℞

In Part IV, control and drug-induced modification of the basic arousal state were discussed. In Part V, a second fundamental aspect of psychic function susceptible to drug alteration—affect—is considered. As suggested in Chapter 2, of the elements of psychic functioning often involved in a problem situation, affect (or mood, emotional state) is the usual one modified by drug therapy. It is therefore not surprising that in this part of the book most of the drugs that are employed in the treatment of psychopathologic conditions will be discussed. We will look at the antipsychotics (Chap. 16) and anxiolytics (Chap. 17), which attenuate disturbed affect. Next, the antidepressants, which elevate mood, will be considered (Chap. 18), and finally, drugs used in cyclic disturbances of affect (Chap. 19) will be discussed. As has been the procedure in previous parts of the book, we will begin with a review of the neuroanatomic basis of affect, focusing on the systems that govern emotional behavior.

Neuroanatomic Bases of Emotion

15

Emotional behavior is largely associated with the functioning of a brain system called the limbic system. The concept of a limbic system had its origins in the ideas of J. W. Papez, first published in 1937. Although much of the detail of Papez's formulation was erroneous, it nevertheless was an incredible piece of speculation, and its basic premise had the effect of sparking research and theorizing that continues today. Noting the rich interconnections between the hypothalamus, anterior thalamus, and phylogenetically older regions of the cortex called the juxtallocortex and allocortex, Papez proposed that these structures constituted a circuit that was involved in emotional behavior and acted as a staging area for passage of emotional signals to the cortex. Although ideas about the nature of limbic function have grown ever more complex since Papez's day, the fundamental observation of the high degree of interrelationship of the various limbic regions has progressively been strengthened by subsequent experimental data.

The exact boundaries of the limbic system vary somewhat according to the usage of a particular author. We use the term to include the cingulate and hippocampal gyri, the hippocampus, amygdala, septal area, olfactory bulb and tubercle, habenula, interpeduncular nucleus, limbic midbrain, and the many interconnecting fiber bundles of each hemisphere (Fig. 15-1). We exclude the hypothalamus, anterior thalamus, mamillary bodies, and granular frontal cortex, although each of these regions interacts substantially with the limbic system proper.

To the student first encountering the notion of the limbic system, it might well seem strange that the many diverse and anatomically distinct structures that constitute the limbic system should have come to be thought of as a system at all. And it is true that no other system we consider in this book includes structures quite so separated in the spatial arrangement of the brain. The overriding reasons for treating these structures as a unit are the abundance of anatomic interconnections and the considerable similarity of function that exists between various pairs of limbic structures. Both these ideas will become self-evident in the discussion of the individual limbic system structures.

General Functions of the Limbic System
Olfaction

Another term often applied to the limbic system is *rhinencephalon*, which means literally "nose-brain." This term derived from early recognition of the connection between limbic structures and the olfactory sense. The olfactory bulbs comprise clus-

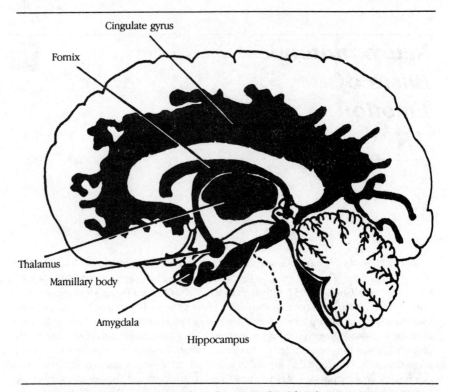

Fig. 15-1. Brain regions constituting the limbic system. (Modified from J. R. Smythies. Brain Mechanisms and Behaviour. *New York: Academic, 1970.)*

ters of nerve cells, called mitral cells, which are the secondary neurons of the olfactory system. The neurons located in the olfactory bulbs are innervated by axons extending from primary sensory neurons located in the nasal mucosa and whose dendrites comprise the hair-like endings that are activated by chemicals. The mitral cells project centrally, mainly via the lateral olfactory stria to the amygdalae and via the medial olfactory stria to a portion of the septal area (Fig. 15-2) called the parolfactory region. Olfactory connections proceed from the parolfactory septum via the stria medullaris thalami to the habenulae and thence to the interpeduncular nucleus.

It is not without significance that olfaction is so closely tied to limbic function. Of the sensory modalities, it is hardest in the case of olfaction and taste (which is in part related to olfaction) to separate affective tone (attraction-revulsion) from the purely sensate component. Usually, the odor or taste of an object determines in us a direction of movement with respect to the object, either away from or toward. We cast away that which gives a bitter or too sour taste or foul odor. If the sensation is accompanied by a positive affective tone, we may approach the object and take it up. Much of our spontaneous orientation toward things around us derives from the feeling tone associated with these two senses. Visual and auditory sensations by contrast possess such direct affective tone only when the level of receptor stimulation is of a magnitude as to threaten the integrity of the sensory system. The relationship between olfaction and the limbic system is further discussed under Conditional Behavior and Prepared Learning.

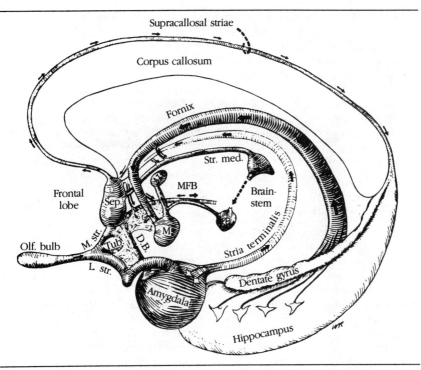

Fig. 15-2. *Principal limbic interconnections. MFB, medialoforebrain bundle. (Modified from P. D. MacLean. Psychosomatic disease and the visceral brain. Psychosom. Med. 11:338–353, 1949.)*

Emotional Behavior

Ever since Papez first proposed that the limbic system played a role in emotion and emotional behavior, it has become increasingly apparent that this system is of preeminent importance both with respect to innate patterns of emotional behavior and conditional behavior. In this section, we will consider the role of the limbic system in innate patterns of emotional behavior and mood, while its role in conditional behavior will be taken up later.

In 1937, Klüver and Bucy described a syndrome occurring in monkeys after bilateral removal of the temporal lobes. Later, it was found that the syndrome was related specifically to removal of the amygdalae, which lie at the basal tip of the temporal lobe. What they described has become known as the Klüver-Bucy syndrome and is characterized by compulsive oral responses, a tendency to shift attention from object to object in a stereotyped pattern, loss of fear and aggressiveness, and hypersexuality. After removal of the amygdalae, an animal appears to lose appreciation for the meaningfulness of objects. A monkey, after such a lesion, will no longer demonstrate a fear response to a snake and will pick up and bite objects that he would not normally attempt to eat. It has been found that wild animals, such as wild cats, can be tamed by removing their amygdalae.

On the other hand, rage responses can be elicited by lesions of the septal region or the hypothalamus or by electrical stimulation of appropriate hypothalamic or amygdaloid regions. Later in the chapter, the control of aggressive behavior will be considered in some detail with respect to each of the individual structures. Suffice it to say that this is an important aspect of limbic function.

Different from both these innate behavioral patterns and from the conditional behaviors that will be discussed is mood. *Mood* is a psychic state that for an indefinite period of time influences responses to various situations. It is analogous to the tonic innervation of groups of muscles that determine a certain bodily stance and may be considered the psychological posture of the individual. The subjective reports of patients who have undergone brain stimulation experiments as well as reports by temporal lobe epileptic patients implicate the limbic system in regulation of mood. Beyond that general statement, however, little can be said with any degree of certainty as regards the role of other brain regions or specific limbic structures with respect to mood.

Response Modulation

The limbic system plays a crucial role in many behaviors involving preferential suppression and facilitation of response tendencies. This is true not only for conditional behaviors but also for certain spontaneous behaviors. An example of spontaneous behavior controlled by the limbic system is spontaneous alternation, which refers to a tendency of animals to alternate choices of alleyways in exploration of a T- or Y-maze. It has been found that this alternation occurs because the subject suppresses the choice of returning to the alley most recently visited using whatever cues—such as odor trail, position, and appearance of the alleys—are available to determine which alley that is. An equivalent phenomenon has been demonstrated in humans. Bilateral hippocampal lesion blocks spontaneous alternation, so the hippocampus is apparently involved in this inhibition of the "repeat" choice.

A broader statement of this aspect of limbic function is that the limbic system controls habituation of behaviors elicited by stimuli. If a given elicited behavior is not reinforced, it rapidly ceases to recur or recurs at a reduced intensity. This widespread and divergent phenomenon is referred to as *habituation*. Bilateral limbic lesions of the septal region or the hippocampus prevent, in many cases, habituation of behaviors.

From a functional point of view, the limbic system and associated thalamic nuclei constitute a second-level "paleomammalian" processing system that modulates the more primitive "protoreptilian" brainstem system. The activities generated by the paleomammalian system are what behavioral psychologists call appetitive and avoidance behaviors, behaviors resulting from selective facilitation and suppression of innate, learned, and haphazard response patterns to achieve either drive reduction or avoidance of punishment.

Conditional Behavior and Prepared Learning

Many types of conditional behavior are impaired following limbic lesions or drugs thought to alter limbic system activity. This is true both of conditional behaviors requiring suppression of an innate response tendency and those requiring execution of an active response. Conditioned avoidance-responding, such as in a shuttle box, is impaired by lesions of the cingulum especially. Passive avoidance, such as a step-down paradigm, is sensitive to hippocampal and septal lesions. Conditioned emotional responses may be prevented by drugs known to inhibit hippocampal activity. Many types of learning are impaired by hippocampal lesions. Deficits occur in successive discrimination tasks and alternated bar-pressing.

An interesting paradigm, which may reveal something about the extent and limits of limbic control of behavior, is the "go-no-go" paradigm. A go-no-go paradigm is one in which the subject is required on alternate trials to execute or withhold a given response for reward. It is known that hippocampectomy *enhances* performance in certain go-no-go tasks. Now assume for the moment that the animal's decision to respond or not is determined at each trial by two competing factors: (1) the animal's expectation of reward or lack of reward as suggested by his learning of the sequence; go, then no-go; and (2) the expectation based on the recent memory of the outcome of the immediately preceding trial. Obviously, the first of these competing influences is leading the animal to respond correctly, while the second is encouraging it to respond incorrectly. The enhanced performance following hippocampectomy could be explained by postulating that the second of these two influences is intimately connected to limbic (specifically hippocampal) function, while the first is considerably less so. If this is so, hippocampal lesion would block the influence leading to the incorrect choice and increase the domination of the correct-leading influence, thereby improving performance.

This type of extracted evidence, together with observations that some degree of learning does still occur after hippocampal lesion, has led to recognition that the limbic system, while important in regulation of behavior, is not the exclusive anatomic substrate for learning. *The limbic system appears to regulate behavior on the basis of recent memory traces and ongoing affectual state or mood.* Learning that is well established (either overlearned or not recently learned) and perhaps learning requiring abstractions such as spatial or temporal alternations may be less related to limbic function.

A peculiar special case of conditioning is the phenomenon referred to as *prepared learning.* This is what has popularly been called "the sauce-béarnaise syndrome." Having experienced an upset stomach several hours after eating, along with more familiar foods, some sauce béarnaise, a person may find himself or herself unable to eat it again. This type of circumstance illustrates the unusual aspects of prepared learning compared with other types of learning: association to very specific stimuli, a long delay to negative reinforcement, and learning after only a single "trial."

Under certain circumstances, a particular unconditional response will become associated not with just any contiguous conditional stimulus, as is usually the case, but with only a select subset of all possible stimuli. One associates gastrointestinal disturbances (an unconditional response) only with taste or olfactory cues. Visual, auditory, or somesthetic cues do not become conditioned to gastrointestinal upset. Thus, in prepared learning, not all possible associations are equally likely, and the principle of equipotency of stimuli is inoperative.

In addition to this deviation from the laws of conditioning, prepared learning exhibits other unique attributes. The maximal interstimulus interval that can occur in prepared learning is orders of magnitude greater than that which occurs in unprepared learning. In unprepared conditioning procedures, the maximal delay between conditional stimulus and unconditional stimulus can be no more than several seconds, and the optimal delay is generally less than 1 second. In prepared learning, interstimulus intervals as great as 8 hours have been reported.

Prepared conditional learning occurs with extreme rapidity and is very resistant to extinction. A single trial is frequently enough to establish a learned aversion to an unusual taste stimulus. When such an aversion has been established, it may persist without further reinforcement years later or in the face of many opportunities for extinction.

Taste is intimately associated with olfaction. Taste per se involves only the sensations of salty, sour, sweet, and bitter. Much of what we call taste is really olfaction. Conditioned taste aversion occurs most readily to unfamiliar-tasting substances, so that the phenomenon most certainly involves the olfactory component of "taste." Olfaction is, of course, intimately interwoven with the limbic system. It is entirely appropriate that the sense associated with the limbic system should be capable of extended interstimulus intervals, because the limbic system is also involved in memory function.

In lower species, the olfactory function of the limbic system is more developed, and the behavioral and memory functions are less developed. With progress up the phylogenetic scale, there is a progressive shift in emphasis from olfactory to behavioral and memory involvement. It is entirely possible that memory was a phylogenetic outgrowth of olfaction, with the selective impetus being the capacity for prepared learning.

In general, the impact of significant, threatening visual or auditory cues is felt within a matter of seconds or not at all. In contrast, olfactory cues display their consequences only after many minutes or a few hours as a rule. Therefore, the selective pressure to develop memory most probably centered around the olfactory system. The hippocampus in particular is involved in short-term memory and consolidation of learning into long-term memory. This function was discussed in detail in Chapter 3.

Functions of Specific Limbic Structures

Hypothalamus

Interconnections

The hypothalamus is a collection of densely packed nuclei (Fig. 15-3) lying ventral to the thalamus. Rich interconnections pass between it and many other brain regions. Inputs come principally from the limbic structures, prefrontal cortex, general and special sensory systems, thalamus, globus pallidus, and reticular system. Outputs go principally to the anterior nuclei of the thalamus, pituitary gland, cranial nerve nuclei of the brainstem, subthalamus, and reticular formation.

Functions

We will discuss only the function of the hypothalamus as a whole. The breakdown of functions by individual nuclei is summarized in Table 15-1.

The hypothalamus may be considered the principal output center for the limbic system. As such, it is capable of organizing complex response patterns that utilize sympathetic, parasympathetic, and somatic effector mechanisms. The impetus for emotional behavior arises in the limbic system, and the behaviors then are expressed through the response-organizing mechanisms of the hypothalamus. Cortical suppression of emotional behavior is exerted by way of fibers running from the prefrontal or granular cortex to the hypothalamus.

Four key homeostatic processes of the body are regulated chiefly by the hypothalamus: energy balance, water balance, temperature regulation, and sexual activity. The lateral nucleus of the hypothalamus is postulated to be a center regulating food intake. Lesions of the lateral nucleus produce avoidance of eating and consequent emaciation.* The ventromedial nucleus is believed to be a satiety center that inhibits the lateral nucleus when intake of food is adequate. Cells in the hypothalamus monitor blood sugar levels and possibly other chemical parameters as well. The hypothalamus also controls utilization of energy stores by its influence over the autonomic nervous system and through regulation of growth-hormone release and thyroxine levels.

---

*This postulate has been called into question because lesions in this area also sever the nigrostriatal dopaminergic fibers, and there is some indication that this pathway may be involved in feeding behavior.

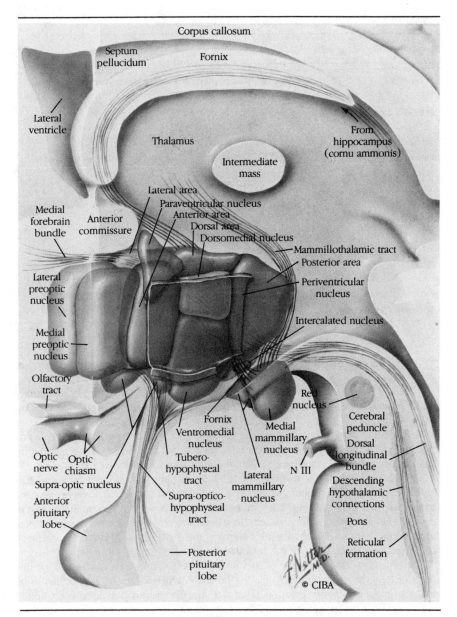

Fig. 15-3. *Reconstruction of the hypothalamus and major interconnecting fiber bundles. (Copyright © 1965 CIBA Pharmaceutical Company, Division of CIBA-GEIGY Corporation. Reproduced with permission from the CIBA Collection of Medical Illustrations by Frank H. Netter, M.D. All rights reserved.)*

Table 15-1. Principal nuclei and regions of the hypothalamus

Region	Functions
Anterior area	Heat dissipation; thermostat; sex drive and mating behavior
Dorsomedial nucleus	Rage behavior
Infundibulum	Releasing factors for control of anterior pituitary: includes arcuate nucleus (A_{12})
Lateral area	Appetite; preconsummatory reward
Limbic midbrain	Area of interconnection between hypothalamus and midbrain
Mamillary bodies	Olfactory circuit; arousal (via diffuse thalamic system); biologic periodicity
Paraventricular nucleus	Regulates oxytocin synthesis and release
Periventricular nucleus	Part of punishment system
Posterior area	Heat conservation
Preoptic area	Connected with prefrontal cortex, septum, and periventricular system
Supraoptic nucleus	Regulates antidiuretic hormone synthesis and release
Tuber cinereum	Development of reproductive organs via releasing factors
Ventromedial nucleus	Appetite and rage suppression

Water balance is monitored by the hypothalamus by means of volume and osmolality sensors. In response to signals from these units, the hypothalamus controls water intake and water retention. Hypothalamic lesions produce adipsia (cessation of drinking). Water retention is regulated through the control of release of antidiuretic hormone by the pituitary.

Temperature regulation involves the anterior and posterior regions of the hypothalamus. The anterior region controls heat dissipation (sweating, panting, cutaneous vasodilatation, and piloerection), while the posterior region controls heat conservation (shivering and cutaneous vasoconstriction). Temperature-sensitive neurons in the anterior thalamus act as a central thermostat, and cutaneous hot and cold receptors contribute information regarding skin temperature. During fever, the central thermostat is displaced in an upward direction; aspirin and related antipyretics reset the thermostat to its normal setting. Anesthetics, neuroleptics, and sedatives may impair the temperature-regulating mechanism of the hypothalamus.

Sexual and mating behavior is also under hypothalamic control. Lesions of the anterior hypothalamus obliterate mating behavior, whereas electrical stimulation of this region leads to penile erection, mounting, and ejaculation in male animals. Copulation and orgasm are associated with high-amplitude slow waves in the hypothalamus and hippocampus.

The hypothalamus exerts direct neural control over the posterior pituitary gland. Neurons lying in the supraoptic nucleus of the hypothalamus synthesize antidiuretic hormone. The hormone flows down the axons of these cells along their course into the posterior pituitary gland. Neurons in the paraventricular nucleus of the hypothalamus similarly synthesize and deliver oxytocin. Stimulation of one of these nuclei produces pituitary release of the corresponding hormone. Antidiuretic hormone increases resorption of water in the tubules of the kidney and is instrumental in the regulation of water balance. Oxytocin controls lactation and uterine contractions.

The hypothalamus exerts endocrine control over the anterior pituitary gland. Releasing factors are secreted by the infundibulum and tuber cinereum regions of the hypothalamus and are transported by the blood to the anterior pituitary. There, the releasing factors stimulate release of corresponding anterior pituitary hormones: growth hormone, thyroid-stimulating hormone, adrenocorticotropic hormone, and sex hormones.

The hypothalamus is closely involved in mechanisms of reward and punishment. The lateral nucleus is a potent self-stimulation site, while the posterior area is an aversive stimulation site. It appears that the hypothalamus regulates *pre*consummatory reward mechanisms, a distinction that was amplified in Chapter 3.

Amygdala

The amygdaloid complexes are closely situated bilateral nuclear groups lying at the base of the temporal lobe. Interest in the amygdala stems from the 1937 observation by Klüver and Bucy that temporal lobe lesions produce a loss of fear and aggressiveness, hypersexuality and increased activity, compulsive oral responses, a stereotypical shifting of attention, and so-called psychic blindness. This last symptom refers to a seemingly lost appreciation of the meaning of objects. Subsequent observations associated these changes in behavior with removal of the amygdala.

The amygdala is functionally divisible into two major regions: the corticomedial and the basolateral regions. The corticomedial region receives the lateral olfactory stria. It lies proximal to the caudate and putamen nuclei of the corpus striatum and is functionally related to them. Presumably, the corticomedial portion of the amygdala modulates appetitive behavior in relation to olfactory cues, including pheromones.

The basolateral portion of the amygdala has no olfactory connections but is continuous with the hippocampus. Stimulation of the basolateral complex produces a characteristic "searching response." The animal arrests all ongoing activity, raises its head, its eyes open wide and dilate, and its ears become more erect. More intense stimulation initiates defensive aggressive reactions. The basolateral portion can be further broken down into an area that facilitates attack behavior and another that inhibits it, presumably by inhibiting the attack facilitory region. Aggression elicited by stimulation of the amygdala utilizes a pathway that runs directly to the hypothalamus. The basolateral portion of the amygdala is involved in generating all kinds of defensive behaviors, including the orienting response, aggression, flight, active and passive avoidance behaviors, and adrenocortical and sympathetic activation.

Lesions of the amygdala produce, in addition to the Klüver-Bucy syndrome, deficits in avoidance learning and stimulus discrimination. There is also an increase in stimulus generalization and changes in social dominance hierarchies in monkeys. The amygdala has a characteristic fast rhythm, in the range of 40 to 45 Hz, which is evoked by meaningful or noxious stimuli.

Hippocampus

The hippocampus is a nuclear mass located in the depths of the temporal lobe. A large fiber bundle called the fornix projects from the hippocampus to the mamillary bodies of the hypothalamus and ultimately to the brainstem and diffuse thalamic projection system. The hippocampus has a characteristic electrical activity called the theta rhythm, which occurs in response to arousal stimuli and, according to Grastyán, signals possible or received reinforcement. Theta activity can be observed in the neocortex waxing and waning with the hippocampal theta. This neocortical theta is called the isohippocampal rhythm, and it appears just before lever-pressing for a food reward or just after successful avoidance. The pacemaker for hippocampal theta activity resides in the septal region.

Functional Hypotheses

In 1963, Carlton [3] formulated a view that the hippocampus acts as a "second system," exerting response selectivity by means of inhibitory influences on the reticular formation. He further postulated that this hippocampal system was essentially cholinergic. In support of his view, one can point to the many types of studies indicating that hippocampal lesions and anticholinergic drugs impair behaviors requiring response inhibition. For example, either treatment produces hyperactivity and deficits in successive discrimination, extinction, alternated bar-pressing, spontaneous alternation, and passive avoidance. In Carlton's early formulation (and in Douglas's [7] 1967 review), the hippocampal inhibitory system is described as mediating the effects of nonreinforcement; i.e., conditioned drive reduction. Later revisions by Carlton [4] and Bignami and Rosic [2], however, so generalized the view, so that the second system is now described as regulating response inhibition in general.

Not all capacity to inhibit particular responses selectively resides in the hippocampus, however. Single-alternation tasks can be learned (albeit slowly) after hippocampal lesion and, once learned, are not disrupted by cholinergic blockers. Thus, it is apparent that other brain regions in addition to the hippocampus contribute to shaping of responses. Our view is that the hippocampus shapes responses related exclusively to goal-directed (or emotional) behavior by means of selective response inhibition.

A second function closely linked to the hippocampus, at least in humans, is memory. Milner [10] postulated that the hippocampus is involved in short-term memory and the consolidation process by which short-term memory is translated into long-term memory stores. In support of this view are the pronounced memory deficits that occur in humans when the hippocampus is damaged. Already established memories are not lost, but new events are not retained. Neurosurgeons have reported that electrical stimulation of the hippocampus and related temporal cortical regions can elicit complex and specific memory traces. The memory process may be ancillary to the response-shaping aspect of hippocampal function, i.e., a recording of response executions that was reinforced. The role of the hippocampus in learning and retention was discussed in Chapter 3.

Septal Region

The septal area is a portion of the telencephalon lying medially and just anterior to the lateral cerebral ventricles. It is connected with the hypothalamus, hippocampus, midbrain reticular formation, amygdala, olfactory system, and thalamus.

The septal area (or septum) has been called the "pleasure center," because stimulation of this area in humans produces a feeling described as "peaceful euphoria" or "well-being." Animals will press a lever for stimulation of the septal region but not as incessantly as for lateral hypothalamic stimulation. The septum appears to be related to consummatory reward mechanisms.

The septal area is closely related in some of its functions to the hippocampus. The septum acts as pacemaker for the hippocampal theta activity. Lesions of the septal region block the theta rhythm of the hippocampus and produce behavioral changes

Table 15-2. *Nuclei of the septal region*

Nucleus	Likely function
Septal nuclei	
Dorsal septal nucleus	Pleasure center
Lateral septal nucleus	Consummatory reward
Medial septal nucleus	Pacemaker for hippocampus; cholinergic, noradrenoceptive
Nucleus of diagonal band	Same as above
Bed nucleus of stria terminalis	Suppression of aggression
Nucleus septalis fimbrialis	Olfactory influences on behavior; cholinergic
Nucleus septalis triangularis	Same as above
Adjacent nuclei and regions	
Nucleus accumbens septi	Possibly implicated in schizophrenia; dopamiceptive
Substantia innominata (basal olfactory region)	Relay station for ascending RAS; cholinergic, cholinoceptive
Anterior perforated substance and olfactory tubercle	Related to olfactory system

similar to hippocampectomy. For example, there is an inability to suppress emotionality and startle responses. There are deficits in conditional emotional responses (freezing responses to shock or shock-paired conditional stimuli) and passive avoidance. And the general activity level is increased. In humans, the "septal syndrome" may occur when tumors impinge on the septal area. Such patients become irritable and are likely to display outbursts of aggression or uncontrolled emotionality, as well as a heightened sensitivity to sudden noises.

The septal region is a complex of seven nuclei (Table 15-2). The dorsal septal nucleus receives afferents from the hippocampus by way of the fornix and projects in turn to adjacent septal nuclei. The lateral septal nucleus receives additional hippocampal afferents and discharges to the adjacent medial septal nucleus, the hypothalamus, and brainstem centers. The dorsal and lateral nuclei are the ones that produce self-stimulation behavior and thus are involved in consummatory reward mechanisms.

The medial septal nucleus and the nucleus of the diagonal band of Broca form the medial nuclear group of the septal complex. The medial group contains many cholinergic cells and projects to the hippocampus. It is this portion of the septal region that serves as pacemaker for the hippocampal theta activity. The medial group receives afferents from the medial olfactory stria, the basolateral amygdaloid complex and surrounding cortex, the lateral septal nucleus, and the hippocampus. The medial group also receives noradrenergic fibers from the locus ceruleus. The projections from the medial group reach other limbic and brainstem centers in addition to the hippocampus.

The bed nucleus of the stria terminalis serves as an aggression-suppressing center. It is connected with the central nucleus of the amygdala, as well as many limbic, hypothalamic, and midbrain nuclei.

The last two nuclei, the nucleus septalis fimbrialis and nucleus septalis triangularis, are cholinergic nuclei that relay signals received from the fornix to the habenular nuclei via the stria medullaris thalami.

Adjacent to the septal complex is the nucleus accumbens septi. It receives dopaminergic inputs from the midbrain and other inputs from the bed nucleus of the stria terminalis and amygdala. It is currently the subject of intensive interest because of its having a possible role in schizophrenia. Autopsy studies have revealed an increased number of dopamine receptors in the nucleus accumbens septi of schizophrenic patients.

The caudal extension of the septal region is a large, gray mass of cells called the substantia innominata. It stretches beneath the putamen and globus pallidus to separate these nuclei of the corpus striatum from the preoptic area of the hypothalamus. The substantia innominata is a relay post in ascending cholinergic projections of the reticular activating system (see Fig. 6-4). The rostral end of the substantia innominata underlies the anterior perforated substance. In species with highly developed olfactory senses, but not in humans, the anterior perforated substance forms a prominent eminence called the olfactory tubercle.

Cingulate Gyrus and Related Cortical Areas

The cingulate gyrus and related orbital, temporal, and insular regions of cortex constitute the innermost layer of the cerebral cortex. Much less is known about the function of these regions than is known regarding the limbic structures thus far discussed. Many of the responses that occur on cingulate gyrus stimulation resemble those occurring with vagal stimulation. In general, there is an arrest of spontaneous muscular activity, including respiration. Cingulate lesions tend to produce excess freezing behavior or an inability to suppress such responses. As a result, conditional avoidance-responding is impaired. On the other hand, passive avoidance performance may be enhanced. Too little is known about the function of these regions of the cortex to begin development of a functional theory.

Limbic Midbrain

The limbic midbrain refers to the region just posterior to the hypothalamus where massive two-way interconnections occur between the reticular formation, on the one hand, and the hippocampus, septum, hypothalamus, and amygdala, on the other hand. Stimulation of this area elicits cortical desynchronization and disrupts recent memory. Lesions on the other hand produce an unresponsive animal. This region is a potent negative reinforcement area with respect to self-stimulation.

Descending Discharge Pathways

In addition to the multitudinous interconnections of the limbic midbrain, four major discharge pathways extend from the hypothalamus and descend into the midbrain and hindbrain. The anterior, posterior, and dorsal hypothalamic-tegmental tracts descend to tegmental nuclei of the midbrain. The dorsal longitudinal fasciculus is part of the periventricular system, which is described on page 34 as a punishment system.

Ascending Regulatory Pathways

The midbrain exerts widespread regulatory influences over the limbic system by means of ascending amine pathways. Adrenergic pathways of the medial forebrain bundle (MFB) are involved in some way with reward. Dopaminergic pathways extend to the septal region and amygdala, but their function is unknown.

Serotonin-containing fibers from the raphé nuclei run adjacent to the MFB and innervate most limbic regions as well as the thalamus, corpus striatum, hypothalamus, and portions of the cortex. There is considerable evidence suggesting that these serotonergic pathways help to regulate, on the one hand, the balance between the inhibitory activity of the limbic system and the response facilitory activity of the descending reticular formation and, on the other hand, the balance between the diffuse thalamic system and the ascending reticular arousal system.

Selected References and Further Readings

1. Angevine, J. B., Jr., and Cotman, C. W. *Principles of Neuroanatomy.* New York: Oxford University Press, 1981.
2. Bignami, G., and Rosic, N. The Nature of Disinhibitory Phenomena Caused by Central Cholinergic (Muscarinic) Blockade. In O. Vinar et al. (Eds.), *Advances in Neuropsychopharmacology.* Amsterdam: North-Holland, 1971.
3. Carlton, P. L. Cholinergic mechanisms in the control of behavior by the brain. *Psychol. Rev.* 70:19–39, 1963.
4. Carlton, P. L. Brain-Acetylcholine and Inhibition. In O. Vinar et al. (Eds.), *Reinforcement: Current Research and Theories.* Amsterdam: North-Holland, 1969.
5. Carpenter, M. B. *Human Neuroanatomy* (7th ed.). Baltimore: Williams & Wilkins, 1976.
6. DeFrance, J. F. (Ed.). *The Septal Nuclei: Advances in Behavioral Biology.* New York: Plenum, 1976. Vol. 20.
7. Douglas, R. J. The hippocampus and behavior. *Psychol. Bull.* 67:416–442, 1967.
8. Eleftheriou, B. E. (Ed.). *The Neurobiology of the Amygdala: Advances in Behavioral Biology.* New York: Plenum, 1972. Vol. 2.
9. Isaacson, R. L. *The Limbic System.* New York: Plenum, 1974.
10. Milner, B. Disorders of memory after brain lesions in man. *Neuropsychologia* 6:175–179, 1968.
11. Reichlin, S. et al. (Eds.). *The Hypothalamus.* New York: Raven, 1978.
12. Seligman, M. E., and Hager, J. L. The sauce-Béarnaise syndrome. *Psychology Today* 613: 59–61, 84–87, 1972.
13. Shepherd, G. M. *The Synaptic Organization of the Brain.* New York: Oxford University Press, 1974.
14. Smythies, J. R. *Brain Mechanisms and Behavior.* New York: Academic, 1970.

Psychosis and Antipsychotic Drugs

16

℞

The terms *antipsychotic, neuroleptic,* and *major tranquilizer* have been used somewhat interchangeably to distinguish agents that produce a calming of agitated subjects and lessened reactivity to emotional stimuli with little overall effect on consciousness. This class is distinct both from the sedative-hypnotics, which produce a change in emotional reactivity only at doses that depress consciousness, and from the so-called anxiolytics, or minor tranquilizers. The main use of neuroleptics is in treatment of psychoses, especially schizophrenia. Before examining the antipsychotic drugs, let us review the diagnostic classifications for which these drugs are employed.

Classification of Psychoses

Excluding drug-induced psychoses and organic brain syndrome, there are three diagnostic categories that designate the psychoses in the latest edition of the *Diagnostic and Statistical Manual* (DSM-III) [3]: schizophrenic disorders, paranoid disorders, and other psychotic disorders. The label *schizophrenia* is the single most widely employed diagnostic label for first admissions to mental hospitals. Schizophrenic disorders are further divided into five subcategories: disorganized, catatonic, paranoid, undifferentiated, and residual. In addition to identifying a subcategory, the clinician may further specify the time course, using the terms *subchronic, chronic, subchronic with acute exacerbation, chronic with acute exacerbation,* or *in remission.*

Schizophrenia

Schizophrenia is diagnosed when the patient profile meets five conditions (Table 16-1). The first and foremost condition is the presence of one or more of the overt symptoms that characterize the disorder. These include delusions, hallucinations, incoherence, affective disturbances, catatonia, and disorganized behavior. It is not necessary—and indeed is unlikely—that a given individual exhibit all these symptoms. The delusions of the schizophrenic generally involve beliefs that are absurd, such as being controlled by forces or being capable of supernatural powers (e.g., thought broadcasting). Often, the delusions are grandiose, religious, or nihilistic in nature. Persecutory or jealous delusions are not sufficient in and of themselves to dictate a diagnosis of schizophrenia, since such delusions are characteristic of paranoid disorders. Halluci-

Table 16-1. Diagnostic criteria for schizophrenia

At least one of the following symptoms during a phase of the illness:
  Delusions (bizarre or grandiose ideas)
  Auditory hallucinations
  Incoherence
  Blunted, flat, or inappropriate affect
  Catatonia or grossly disorganized behavior
Deterioration of previous level of functioning
Duration at least 6 months
Onset before age 45 years
Exclusions
  No preceding depressive or manic episode of extended duration
  Not secondary to organic brain syndrome or mental retardation

nations in schizophrenia are characteristically auditory, usually experienced as hearing one or more voices. Incoherence is a marked loosening of associations in which thinking becomes highly illogical. Affective disturbances common in schizophrenia include blunted or flat affect, extreme ambivalence, or affective incongruity. Catatonia is a state of elevated muscle tone and rigid posture.

The other criteria that must be met are deterioration of previous level of functioning (work, social relations, self-care), duration of at least 6 months (including the prodromal phase), onset before age 45, and exclusion of preceding depression, mania, organic brain syndrome, or mental retardation.

The psychotherapist would do well to become especially familiar with the prodromal symptoms of schizophrenia, so that patients exhibiting the potential for schizophrenia can be recognized. Prodromal symptoms are listed in Table 16-2.

Schizophrenia is an episodal condition. Some patients experience recurrent acute episodes (nervous breakdowns, in common parlance), separated by periods of more or less normal functioning. Even in chronic schizophrenia, periods of acute worsening may alternate with periods of relative remission. The episodal nature of schizophrenia dictates three rather distinct modes of application of antipsychotic drugs to treatment of the condition. First, a neuroleptic may be employed for the duration of an *acute* episode, withdrawal of medication following somewhat after remission of symptoms. Second, patients prone to repeated acute episodes may receive *maintenance* doses, usually one-third to one-fifth the doses used acutely or in chronic schizophrenia. This tactic has proved enormously successful in reducing the frequency and severity of subsequent episodes with minimal risk of adverse effects. Third, neuroleptics may be given for years on end for treatment of *chronic* schizophrenia as a means of providing symptomatic relief.

Schizophrenia is widely believed to be related to an elevation in dopamine activity in the brain. It is probably not true that schizophrenia is caused by an elevation in dopamine activity as was implied in the early formulations of the dopamine hypothesis of schizophrenia. But it is probably accurate to state that some of the symptoms of schizophrenia (e.g., catatonia, aggression, paranoia) are attributable to the elevated dopamine activity that accompanies schizophrenia. The dopamine hypothesis and other neurobiologic theories of schizophrenia are discussed subsequently in more detail.

Table 16-2. *Prodromal (or residual) symptoms of schizophrenia*

Social isolation or withdrawal
Impaired functioning
Peculiar behavior
Impaired personal hygiene
Flat or inappropriate affect
Digressive, overelaborate speech
Bizarre ideation
Recurrent illusions, delusions, or hallucinations

Table 16-3. *Diagnostic criteria for paranoid disorders*

Persistent delusions with persecutory or jealous content
No affective, associative, or behavioral disturbance except in relation to the delusional system
No prominent hallucinations
Duration at least 1 week
Exclusions
   No preceding full depressive or manic syndrome of extended duration
   No organic brain syndrome

Paranoid Disorders

The psychoses belonging to the second group of diagnostic categories are the paranoid disorders. Here, there are four categories available: paranoia, shared paranoid disorder, acute paranoid disorder, and atypical paranoid disorder. The diagnostic criteria for this group are six in number (Table 16-3). The *sine qua non* is the presence of persistent delusions having persecutory or jealous content. The paranoid disorders are considerably less common and much more limited in symptomatology than schizophrenia: there is an absence of affective or behavioral disturbance, except as related to the delusional system. Hallucinations are also absent or rare. The duration must have reached at least a week, and depression, manic-depressive syndrome, and organic brain syndrome must be excluded. The subcategory "shared paranoid disorder" involves a delusional system that has developed as a result of a close relationship with a person suffering persecutory delusions, the well-known *folie à deux.*

Other Psychotic Disorders

The third group of psychotic disorders not classified elsewhere includes schizophreniform disorder, brief reactive psychosis, schizoaffective disorder, and atypical psychosis. The first two are distinguished in part by duration. *Schizophreniform disorder* is used for conditions meeting all the criteria of schizophrenia except that duration is more than 2 weeks, but less than 6 months. *Brief reactive psychosis* is restricted to psychotic conditions of more than a few hours, but less than 2 weeks; the crucial distinction, however, is that the term is applied only to psychotic states following an identifiable calamity that would evoke signs of distress in almost anyone. *Schizoaffective disorder* is used when a patient exhibits symptoms of schizophrenia together with pronounced symptoms of mania or depression, provided it is unclear whether or not the schizoid or the affective symptomatology is secondary. The use of this category should be avoided whenever possible, because it encourages overindulgence in multiple-drug regimens. *Atypical psychosis* is a catchall for psychotic conditions not meeting the criteria for any of the specific categories.

Neurobiologic Theories of Schizophrenia

Two issues arise in considering the causes of schizophrenia. One is the nature versus nurture debate; that is, the question of the relative importance of organic and psychological-interpersonal factors in the etiology of the disorder. Most workers in the field now concede that organic factors have a preeminent significance in schizophrenia, at least to the extent of creating a predisposition or vulnerability to schizophrenia. Nonorganic factors are nevertheless important, most obviously in acute reactive psychosis. The once-popular view that schizophrenia might be related to contradictory messages conveyed from parent to child is now largely in disrepute.

The second issue concerns the nature of the organic alterations culminating in schizophrenia. The three theories currently under active consideration are the dopamine hypothesis, the transmethylation hypothesis, and the autoimmune hypothesis.

Dopamine Hypothesis

At present, the dopamine hypothesis has the strongest support. The evidence is largely pharmacologic. Virtually all drugs that are effective in controlling the symptoms of schizophrenia interfere with dopamine activity, whether by blocking dopamine receptors or by depleting the storage vesicles of the transmitter. Drugs that elevate dopamine activity, on the other hand, often generate schizoid symptoms. For example, amphetamine, which releases dopamine, causes an acute toxic psychosis that closely resembles schizophrenia. Levodopa, the precursor of dopamine, may likewise cause schizoid reactions.

Autopsy studies have been of limited value in providing evidence for or against the dopamine hypothesis, since most schizophrenics have received long courses of neuroleptic treatment prior to death, rendering it inconclusive whether the observed differences are due to the disease or to the drug treatment. There is evidence that the number of binding sites for dopamine is increased in the brains of schizophrenics, notably in the nucleus accumbens, a target site of the mesolimbic dopamine pathway.

There seems to be little doubt that dopamine is implicated in the *pathogenesis* of schizophrenia. It seems equally clear, however, that altered dopamine function is not the fundamental *cause* of schizophrenia. Dopamine-blocking drugs suppress some of the symptoms of schizophrenia, but do not eliminate the condition. Some symptoms are remarkably improved, while others remain essentially unchanged. Thus, the dopamine hypothesis is simply a valuable piece of a largely unsolved puzzle.

Transmethylation Hypothesis

The transmethylation hypothesis proposed some 30 years ago by Osmond and Smythies makes note of the structural similarity between catecholamine transmitters and certain psychedelics (e.g., mescaline). An error in brain metabolism, it is supposed, might lead to production of endogenous psychotomimetic substances, i.e., trans-methylated catecholamines. Thus far, the theory remains an appealing speculation, since no evidence of synthesis or accumulation of such substances has been forthcoming.

Autoimmune Hypothesis

The autoimmune hypothesis, first proposed by Heath in 1954, suggests that antibodies react to antigens found in neurons of the nucleus accumbens septi. Fluorescent antibodies were found to accumulate in this region in brain specimens from schizophrenics but not from normals. Efforts to confirm these findings have been unsuccessful. Thus, the hypothesis, like the transmethylation theory, remains only plausible.

Antipsychotic Drugs

History

Since the introduction of the first phenothiazine derivative in 1954, antipsychotic drugs—particularly chlorpromazine (Thorazine)—have been among the most-studied and most-prescribed drugs. The year following the introduction of chlorpromazine marked the first year in which the historical trend of an increasing population in psychiatric hospitals was reversed (Fig. 16-1), and there is probably a direct relationship between the two events. Antipsychotic drugs provide the possibility of deinstitutionalization for some patients who would otherwise remain institutionalized indefinitely. The symptomatic relief afforded by neuroleptics may mean the difference between the patient's being manageable or unmanageable in a home environment. Since institutionalization has been found to be the single strongest negative variable in determining the prognosis in schizophrenic patients, the ability of neuroleptics to facilitate return of the patient to a community environment is perhaps the greatest benefit conferred by the medication.

There is great similarity among the drugs currently in use as antipsychotic medications, especially as regards efficacy. Chlorpromazine remains among the most frequently prescribed, though not the most specific, of the neuroleptics.

Mechanism of Action

The gross behavioral effects of chlorpromazine and similar drugs, referred to as the neuroleptic syndrome, include a slowing of motor activity, a decrease in emotionality, and an indifference to external stimuli. At high doses, spontaneous motor activity ceases, and the body becomes rigidly fixed, an effect known as *catalepsy*. In human subjects, there is a diminished ability to perform tasks involving motor coordination, such as pursuit-rotor tests but less effect on purely intellectual tests.

The neuroleptic activity of antipsychotic drugs is related to a central reduction in dopaminergic activity (Fig. 16-2). The ascending reticular activating system is depressed, and there is a related decrease in cortical release of acetylcholine. In contrast to barbiturates, phenothiazines depress arousal brought about by sensory stimulation but not by direct electrical stimulation of the reticular formation. Barbiturates depress arousal induced by either technique. This suggests that chlorpromazine blocks the ability of sensory inputs to activate the reticular system via the sensory collaterals to the reticular formation, but that, unlike the barbiturates, it does not depress the reticular formation itself.

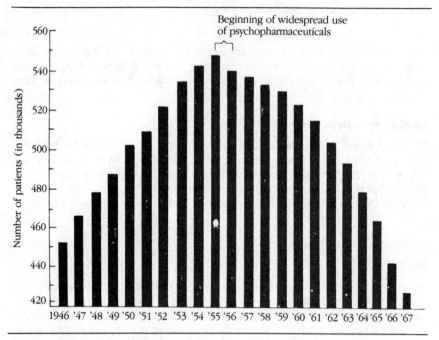

Fig. 16-1. *Number of resident patients in state and local government mental hospitals in the United States (based on U.S. Public Health Service figures), 1946–1967. (Modified from N. Kline. Presidential Address. In D. Efron (Ed.),* Psychopharmacology: A Review of Progress, 1957–1967. *Washington, D.C.: U.S. Government Printing Office, 1968.)*

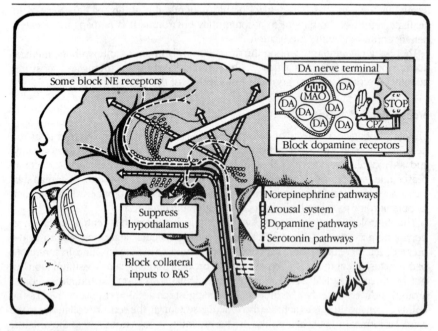

Fig. 16-2. *Mechanisms of neuroleptics. NE, norepinephrine; DA, dopamine; MAO, monoamine oxidase; CPZ, chlorpromazine; RAS, reticular activating system. (Modified from A. K. Swonger.* Nursing Pharmacology. *Boston: Little, Brown, 1978.)*

Antipsychotic potency is related to the ability of neuroleptics to block dopamine receptors. The ratio of dopamine–receptor blocking to norepinephrine receptor–blocking activity for a given drug can be ascertained by means of specific behavioral tests or receptor-binding studies. Butyrophenones and piperazine neuroleptics have substantially greater specificity for dopamine receptors than do other phenothiazines. Some neuroleptics, such as the diphenylbutylamines, have virtually complete specificity for dopamine receptors. The latter agents are devoid of norepinephrine sedative and autonomic side effects.

There are five identified dopamine pathways in the brain, and each accounts for an effect of antipsychotic drugs. The mesolimbic dopamine pathway is most probably involved in the antipsychotic efficacy of neuroleptics. The nigrostriatal dopamine pathway is implicated in the extrapyramidal side effects. The mesocortical pathway is probably involved in the sedative action of neuroleptics, and the hypothalamic-hypophyseal and incertohypothalamic pathways are responsible for the neuroendocrine side effects caused by neuroleptics. Of the two clearly distinguishable classes of dopamine receptors, the D_2 type would appear to be of greater relevance with respect to antipsychotic efficacy and extrapyramidal symptoms, since the relative binding affinity for haloperidol versus chlorpromazine at the D_2-receptor parallels the order of clinical potency (haloperidol > chlorpromazine). At D_1-receptors, the relative affinity of these two neuroleptics is the reverse.

The conventional view that defines the mechanism of action of neuroleptics as related to their ability to acutely block dopamine receptors fails to account for the delay in clinical efficacy that is observed. It requires 3 weeks or more of neuroleptic treatment to produce amelioration of psychotic symptoms, but blockade of dopamine receptors is an immediate biochemical effect. To explain the delay in clinical efficacy, it is necessary to look beyond the acute action of neuroleptics and examine the compensatory adjustments that occur with chronic use (Fig. 16-3). Psychosis is seen as associated with (not necessarily caused by) an elevation in dopamine activity, in keeping with the modern version of the dopamine hypothesis. The immediate effect of neuroleptics is the blockade of dopamine receptors, as described in the classic view of the neuroleptic mechanism. Both postsynaptic and presynaptic receptors are subject to the antagonistic action of neuroleptics. Blockade of presynaptic receptors initiates a short-term compensatory adjustment in which synthesis and release of dopamine are elevated. The increased turnover rate of dopamine is also related in part to multineuronal feedback mechanisms stimulated by the lack of activity in the postsynaptic cell. These short-term compensatory measures largely offset the blocking action of the neuroleptics.

After 2 to 3 weeks of treatment, long-term adaptations begin to supplant the short-term compensations. Postsynaptic receptors develop a supersensitivity that helps to offset the blocking action of the neuroleptic. On the other hand, presynaptic receptors also begin to become supersensitive, overcoming the presynaptic antagonistic action of the neuroleptic. Renewed activity of the presynaptic receptors begins to bring synthesis and turnover rates back to normal levels. The composite result of the direct and adaptive activities after 2 to 3 weeks is a reduction in transmitter-binding to the postsynaptic receptor, only partially offset by postsynaptic receptor supersensitivity. Short-term compensations, which more completely offset the postsynaptic blocking action of the neuroleptic, have undergone tolerance.

Clinical Indications for Antipsychotic Drugs

The clearest indication for neuroleptics is for psychotic conditions. The evidence of efficacy for these compounds in schizophrenia is stronger than is the case for antidepressants in depression or, for that matter, any other psychotherapeutic agent in its

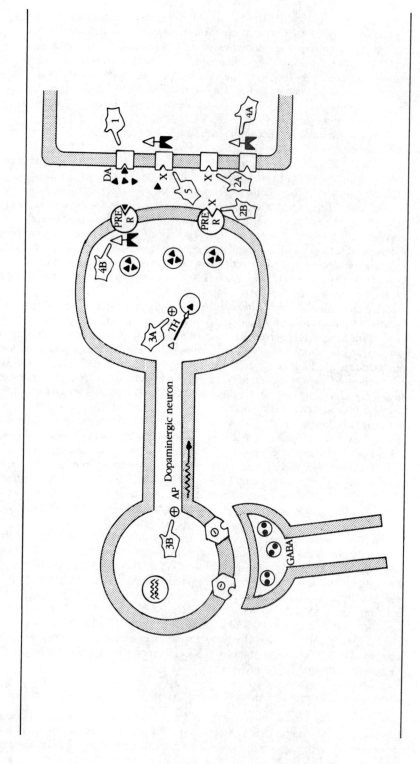

designated application. Numerous studies have indicated superiority of neuroleptics relative to placebo, and studies that have failed to demonstrate the therapeutic effectiveness of neuroleptics have either utilized too-few subjects, too short a duration, or too-low doses [4]. The rate of spontaneous remission from schizophrenia is less than 25 percent. Effective pharmacotherapy can yield remission rates greater than 75 percent.

Neuroleptics are useful in acute mania. Lithium is clearly preferable to a neuroleptic for manic-depressive disorder, but acute mania responds more rapidly to neuroleptics. Phenothiazines have been used for management of belligerence and explosive hyperexcitability in children exhibiting conduct disorder of the aggressive, undersocialized type.

Psychotic symptoms often accompany chronic organic brain syndrome, whether due to senility or arteriosclerosis. Neuroleptics may be used successfully in such patients, but at smaller doses, since the depressant effects of the drugs will aggravate the cognitive and functional impairment associated with organic brain syndrome. A rare illness called Gilles de la Tourette syndrome is treated with haloperidol and will be discussed later.

Neuroleptics are frequently employed in depression in which agitation, anxiety, or tension is a marked component. This form of depression, formerly called depressive neurosis, is now called dysthymic disorder. Neuroleptics are effective in short-term treatment of this condition. Alternative treatments include anxiolytics or antidepressants. Small doses of neuroleptics are also sometimes employed as a kind of placebo therapy in generalized anxiety disorder, as an alternative to the use of potentially addictive anxiolytics. If the patient is liable to abuse, or is insistent about wanting drug treatment beyond the time limit of anxiolytic effectiveness, low-dose neuroleptic treatment is a reasonable approach. The use of an actual placebo may not serve as well, because patients often check out drugs they have been prescribed in drug information sources. All but the most sophisticated patients will be reassured to learn that they are receiving a "tranquilizer." Few will examine the dose prescribed in relation to the effective dosage range.

Several of the neuroleptics, most notably prochlorperazine (Compazine), have uses that are entirely unrelated to psychiatric disorders. These applications include sup-

---

Fig. 16-3. *Mechanism of action of neuroleptics. DA, dopamine; GABA, gamma-aminobutyric acid; TH, tyrosine hydroxylase. Psychosis is associated with elevated functional activity in the dopamine system [1]. Stress events may play a role in precipitating an attack in some instances. The primary and immediate biochemical effect of neuroleptics is to block DA receptors, postsynaptically [2A] and presynaptically [2B]. This potentially beneficial acute effect is largely offset in the short run by compensatory adjustments in the DA transmission process. The blockade of presynaptic receptors leads to an increase in activity of the synthetic enzyme TH [3A], the rate-limiting enzyme in DA synthesis. Multineuronal feedback loops, generally involving GABA in the last step, are suppressed [3B], freeing the DA neuron from feedback inhibition, resulting in an increased firing rate and turnover of DA neurons. These compensatory mechanisms negate the primary blocking effect of neuroleptics on postsynaptic DA receptors and delay clinical efficacy. With chronic administration of neuroleptics, adaptive changes begin to emerge after 2–3 weeks. Postsynaptic [4A] and presynaptic [4B] receptors undergo up-regulation, the latter resulting in a return to normal synthesis and turnover rates. Up-regulation of postsynaptic receptors only partially compensates for receptor blockade. The net effect is a reduction in transmitter access to postsynaptic receptors [5]. The time course of clinical efficacy correlates with the occurrence of the long-term adaptive changes.*

pression of nausea and vomiting (e.g., associated with cancer chemotherapy, motion sickness) and suppression of severe itching (the so-called antipruritic action). Dosages for these purposes are at the low end of the dosage range.

Adverse Effects of Neuroleptics

The adverse effects of neuroleptics are of particular importance because (1) they are severe enough to weigh heavily on risk-benefit considerations in reviewing therapeutic options, and (2) differing patterns of side effects constitute the main basis for selecting a particular drug for a particular patient. Before comparing the various neuroleptics with one another, we will examine the general character of the side effects observed with neuroleptics as a class. By and large, individual drugs within the class vary only in the relative frequency and severity of particular side effects, not in the kinds of side effects encountered.

Adverse reactions to neuroleptics can be grouped into three clusters: (1) "early" side effects, which generally occur soon after initiation of therapy; (2) continuing side effects, to which tolerance does not develop; and (3) multifaceted extrapyramidal side effects, three forms occurring early in treatment and one late in treatment (Table 16-4).

Early Side Effects

Early side effects of neuroleptics fall into four categories: anticholinergic side effects, sedation, orthostatic hypotension, and blood cell disorders. The anticholinergic side effects are a cluster of autonomic and CNS symptoms related to a weak blockade of cholinergic receptors of the muscarinic type. Anticholinergic effects include dryness of the mouth, blurred vision, glaucoma, mydriasis, constipation, urinary retention, and tachycardia. Generally, neuroleptic drugs having the most intensive anticholinergic properties produce fewer early extrapyramidal side effects, a fact that is consistent with the efficacy of anticholinergic drugs such as benztropine in both organic and drug-induced parkinsonism. At the same time, there is some evidence that anticholinergic properties have a negative effect on antipsychotic potency, which is also consistent with the observed interaction of benztropine with neuroleptic therapy.

The sedation produced by neuroleptics is due to the combination of anticholinergic, antidopaminergic, and antinoradrenergic actions. All three of these transmitters are involved in CNS arousal networks. Orthostatic hypotension is partly a central (antinoradrenergic) action, partly a peripheral action on blood vessels, and partly a direct depressant effect on the heart. Tachycardia occurs in part because of the anticholinergic action but also partly as a reflex reaction to falling blood pressure. Tolerance develops to the orthostatic hypotension after several weeks of chronic treatment.

Blood dyscrasias and allergies are two types of blood cell disorders occasionally observed with neuroleptic medication. Leukopenia, a drop in the number of white blood cells, particularly granulocytes, may occur suddenly, usually between the fourth and twelfth weeks of treatment. At the first sign of upper respiratory infection, a complete blood cell count should be ordered. Fortunately, severe agranulocytosis occurs in only 1 in 10,000 patients.

Allergies (hypersensitivity reactions), largely related to lymphocytes in the blood, occur in a wide variety of manifestations. The mildest form of allergy to neuroleptics is skin rash, which is also the most common, occurring in about 5 percent of patients receiving chlorpromazine. Dermatologic reactions may occur from contacting the drug on the skin surface as well as from ingestion. Allergic jaundice is a more severe allergic

Table 16-4. Time of maximal risk of various neuroleptic side effects

Type of side effect	Period of maximal risk
Early	
Anticholinergic	First few weeks; tolerance develops
Sedation	First few weeks; tolerance develops
Orthostatic hypotension	First few weeks; tolerance develops
Blood cell disorders	
Dyscrasias	4–12 weeks
Allergies	1–8 weeks
Persistent	
Lowered seizure threshold	Anytime
Hypothalamic	Anytime
Extrapyramidal	
Pseudoparkinsonism	5–30 days
Tardive dyskinesias	After months or years
Akathisias	5–60 days
Acute dystonic reactions	1–5 days

reaction. Photosensitivity is also seen. The two manifestations of photosensitivity are susceptibility to sunburn and pigmentary retinopathy. Protective clothing and sunglasses can be useful. Pigmentary retinopathy may be particularly pronounced when high doses of thioridazine are used. Allergies generally occur within the first 8 weeks of treatment and abate if the drug is discontinued. Allergic manifestations may or may not recur when drug therapy is reinstituted.

Continuing Side Effects

Some of the CNS side effects of neuroleptics do not exhibit tolerance. Many of the neuroleptics lower the seizure threshold. When a neuroleptic is to be used in a seizure-prone patient (e.g., in epilepsy or delirium tremens), care should be taken to select a drug with minimal effect on the seizure threshold (e.g., molindone or thioridazine).

Another cluster of side effects of neuroleptics relates to the hypothalamic-pituitary axis. Neuroleptics suppress the temperature-regulating mechanism, so that a patient taking a neuroleptic is more than usually susceptible to cold exposure or heat exhaustion. This loss of temperature-regulating ability is called poikilothermy. Appetite is often altered by neuroleptics, most drugs increasing appetite, some (e.g., haloperidol) suppressing appetite. Secretion of pituitary hormones regulated by dopamine, as might be predicted, is altered by neuroleptic therapy.

Growth hormone–releasing factor, secreted in the infundibular region of the hypothalamus under the influence of dopaminergic neurons, is suppressed by neuroleptics. Consequently, release of growth hormone from the pituitary is diminished. When neuroleptics are used in children, drug "holidays" must be provided to minimize stunting of growth. Prolactin secretion is inversely related to dopamine activity, in that release of prolactin inhibitory factor is regulated by dopaminergic neurons. The stimulatory effect of dopamine-blocking drugs on prolactin release causes pseudolactation.

Tolerance does not develop to the prolactin-stimulating action of neuroleptics. Other effects on reproductive functioning include anovulation in women and impotence and retrograde ejaculation in men. Antiadrenergic neuroleptics, such as chlorpromazine, also suppress secretion of adrenocorticotropic hormone and antidiuretic hormone.

Extrapyramidal Side Effects

The extrapyramidal side effects of antipsychotic drugs are of four types: pseudoparkinsonism, tardive dyskinesias, akathisias, and acute dystonic reactions. The period of greatest risk of pseudoparkinsonian symptoms is between 5 to 30 days after initiation of therapy. These appear as akinesia, muscle rigidity, tremors, and other motor symptoms. (The appearance and treatment of drug-induced parkinsonism are discussed in detail in Chapter 21.)

Tardive dyskinesias are late-occurring and persistent side effects. The risk that tardive dyskinesia will develop increases with the duration of treatment as well as with the dosage. Tardive dyskinesias appear as gnawing or curling, twisting movements of the tongue. This form of extrapyramidal disorder is a particularly undesirable side effect because therapeutic response options are severely limited (Chap. 21). Akathisias are symptoms of motor restlessness, easily mistaken for agitation. They develop most commonly after 5 to 60 days of treatment. Acute dystonic reactions appear as facial grimacing or muscle spasms involving the tongue, face, neck, and back. These generally appear during the first 5 days.

Anticholinergic drugs are useful in treatment of the tremor and rigidity of pseudoparkinsonism and acute dystonic reactions but aggravate tardive dyskinesias and do not affect akathisias or akinesias. Anticholinergic drugs should not be used prophylactically in anticipation of extrapyramidal reactions.

Variations Among Neuroleptics

Distinguishing features among the various groups of neuroleptics as regards selective therapeutic spectra have been exaggerated as a result of pharmaceutical manufacturers' advertisements. A principal aim of advertising is to establish product differentiation, and in this respect the drug houses have succeeded far beyond the degree warranted by objective, large-scale tests of relative efficacy. Among the antipsychotic drugs, no one is clearly superior in efficacy at therapeutically equivalent doses. Some researchers consider the dopamine-blocking action of neuroleptic drugs to be the crucial characteristic conferring neuroleptic potency, and they believe that the norepinephrine-blocking action contributes only to the autonomic and sedative side effects. If one accepts this viewpoint, the neuroleptic of choice might be expected to be one having the highest ratio of antidopamine to antinorepinephrine properties. Extrapyramidal symptoms were once regarded as inseparable from therapeutic effectiveness. However, newer antipsychotics, the so-called atypical neuroleptics, provide substantial efficacy with little risk, or even no risk, of extrapyramidal reactions. The butyrophenones and the piperazines have greater specificity for dopamine receptors than do the older aliphatic phenothiazines.

Clinical studies and experience have generally failed to substantiate the superiority of neuroleptics with higher dopamine specificity. Representative members of various subgroups, including chlorpromazine, perphenazine, prochlorperazine, trifluopromazine, thioridazine, haloperidol, and thiothixine, have, in general, produced comparable results in clinical trials. There has been some indication that thioridazine may be more effective in less severe cases and less effective in more severe cases [6].

On the other hand, there are definite differences in the occurrence of side effects among the various neuroleptics (Table 16-5). Insofar as side effects may interact with a given pathologic condition under treatment, particular neuroleptics are preferentially used in certain conditions. Thus, while the alternative neuroleptics are pharmacologically equivalent with respect to their primary therapeutic action, they may at times be clinically distinguishable on the basis of their side effects.

Phenothiazines

The phenothiazine class comprises three subgroups: the aminoalkyls (or aliphatics), the piperazines, and the piperidines. Chlorpromazine is an aminoalkyl phenothiazine. The aminoalkyls produce considerable sedation and hypotension and some intellectual impairment. They predispose epileptics to seizures and produce, correspondingly, an increase in spike-and-burst activity in the EEG. On the other hand, extrapyramidal side effects are moderate in intensity and frequency. The concomitant sedation with this group has led to their effective use in agitated rather than withdrawn schizophrenic patients. Chlorpromazine is frequently used in drug-induced psychoses (LSD, mescaline, amphetamine).

The piperazine subgroup causes less sedation and less impairment of performance in motor and cognitive tasks. There is considerably less hypotension and fewer skin reactions to the piperazines, but extrapyramidal effects, particularly the acute dystonic reactions, are a greater problem than for the aminoalkyls. Prominent members of this subgroup include prochlorperazine (Compazine), trifluoperazine (Stelazine), fluphenazine (Prolixin, Permitil), perphenazine (Trilafon), and acetophenazine (Tindal). The piperazines have less effect on the seizure threshold than the aminoalkyls. The lack of sedative side effects has led to the use of this group of drugs in dull, withdrawn, or apathetic schizophrenic subjects. In neurotic patients, perphenazine has also been found useful and preferable to chlorpromazine. Piperazines are particularly effective in suppressing vomiting brought on by drugs or pathologic conditions.

The third subgroup, the piperidines, comprises only three prominent members: thioridazine (Mellaril), piperacetazine (Quide), and mesoridazine (Serentil). Thioridazine produces little jaundice or rash and few extrapyramidal symptoms, but is especially prone to produce pseudolactation, inhibition of ejaculation, and pigmentary retinopathy. Thioridazine is employed in withdrawn and hypoactive schizophrenic subjects, autistic children, dysthymic disorder, delirium tremens when a neuroleptic is required, and the positive-spike pattern syndrome (Chap. 28).

Rauwolfia *Alkaloids*

Reserpine was introduced almost simultaneously with chlorpromazine and is one of several *Rauwolfia* alkaloids tried therapeutically as antipsychotics. Unlike chlorpromazine, reserpine is no longer used as a neuroleptic. Reserpine acts by depleting the CNS of its stores of catecholamines and serotonin. Unfortunately, the depletion of catecholamines is not confined to the CNS, and depletion of peripheral stores of norepinephrine leads to extensive autonomic side effects because of diminished sympathetic activity. In addition, reserpine may produce an initial agitation prior to the tranquilizing effect. It is still widely used as an antihypertensive agent, but as a neuroleptic is now only of historical and experimental interest.

Table 16-5. *Side effects of various neuroleptics*

Subgroup	Relative dose[a]	Anti-cholinergic[b]	Sedation	Orthostatic hypotension	Blood cell disorders[c]	Lowered seizure threshold	Hypo-thalamic[d]	Extra-pyramidal
Phenothiazines								
Aminoalkyl								
Chlorpromazine	100	+++	+++	+++	++	+++	++	++
Piperazine		+	+(+)	+	++	+	++	+++
Acetophenazine	20							
Fluphenazine	2							
Perphenazine	10							
Prochlorperazine	15							
Trifluoperazine	5							
Piperadine		+++	+++	++	+[e]	+[e]	+	±
Mesoridazine	50							
Piperacetazine	10							
Thioridazine	100							

	Dose[a]					(↓ Appetite)	
Butyrophenones							
Haloperidol	2	0	+	+	+	+++	+++
Thioxanthenes							
Thiothixene	5	+	+	++	+	++	+++
Dibenzoxazepines							
Loxapine	10	+	+	++	+	+	++
Indolics							
Molindone	10	+	+	+	0/+	+	+
Diphenylbutylpiperidines							
Pimozide (experimental)	2	+++	+++	++	+	±	+
Dibenzodiazepines							
Clozapine (experimental)		+	++	++	+	±	0
Benzamides							
Sulpiride (experimental)		+	±	±	+	++	+

0, does not produce effect; ±, little or no tendency toward effect; +, mild tendency toward effect; ++, moderate tendency toward effect; +++, severe tendency toward effect; no symbol, propensity for effect not established.

[a] Dose equivalent to 100 mg of chlorpromazine.

[b] Anticholinergic side effects include dryness of the mouth, blurred vision, mydriasis, acute glaucoma, constipation, urinary retention, sweating, mental confusion, and tachycardia.

[c] Blood cell disorders include blood dyscrasias and allergies.

[d] Hypothalamic side effects include poikilothermy, appetite changes, sexual dysfunctions, growth hormone suppression, etc. (see text).

[e] Retinopathy and sexual dysfunctions occur frequently with piperidine phenothiazines.

Butyrophenones

The butyrophenones are closely related to the phenothiazines. Haloperidol, the prototypical butyrophenone, is known to be a rather specific blocker of dopamine receptors. Not surprisingly, therefore, the extrapyramidal effects of haloperidol are relatively severe. In contrast to chlorpromazine, butyrophenones depress rather than increase appetite and produce hypothermia rather than poikilothermy. There are some indications that haloperidol has teratogenic effects. Like chlorpromazine, haloperidol predisposes to seizures, though to a lesser extent. The butyrophenones produce minimal early side effects.

Butyrophenones have been used experimentally to suppress withdrawal symptoms associated with chronic morphine use. Schizophrenia refractory to other neuroleptic medications may respond favorably to the more potent butyrophenones. Haloperidol is one of the best agents available for the treatment of acute mania. It is also the drug of choice in the rare Gilles de Tourette syndrome, a condition marked by the occurrence of multiple tics and outbursts of obscenity.

Thioxanthenes

The thioxanthenes resemble the phenothiazines structurally and pharmacologically. With respect to side effects, they are closest in pattern to the piperazine phenothiazines. Chlorprothixene (Taractan) has been reported to be effective in schizophrenias with a prominent depressive component. Although the overall responsiveness of schizophrenics to chlorprothixene is reportedly less than to chlorpromazine or haloperidol, some cases refractory to other drugs may respond to chlorprothixene. Thiothixene (Navane) has been used effectively in schizophrenia and in comparative studies appears to be the equal of the potent phenothiazines.

Atypical Neuroleptics

A few neuroleptics provide a dissociation of efficacy from extrapyramidal side effects and so have been designated *atypical* neuroleptics to distinguish them from *classic* neuroleptics, such as chlorpromazine and haloperidol, which produce marked extrapyramidal reactions. There are currently three drugs in the atypical group: thioridazine, which was discussed earlier as the prototypical piperadine phenothiazine, and two experimental drugs, clozapine and sulpiride, not available in the United States as of 1982. Sulpiride does not exhibit significant anticholinergic effects, yet is remarkably lacking in extrapyramidal effects. Experimental evidence indicates that the dissociation of antipsychotic efficacy from extrapyramidal effects noted with these drugs is due to their relative selectivity for dopamine receptors in the limbic system (nucleus accumbens, specifically) versus dopamine receptors in the corpus striatum.

Interactions of Neuroleptics

Although neuroleptics inhibit the effectiveness of antidepressants and may increase pathologic states, they are all too often used in combination with tricyclics. Etrafon and Triavil combine perphenazine and amitriptyline, a neuroleptic and an antidepressant respectively. Clinical trials have failed to document a value in this combination, even in the dubious schizoaffective classification. Some clinicians argue that the combination is rational for patients in this category. This approach amounts to hedging one's bets between alternative diagnoses: schizophrenia or major depression.

Combinations of two or more neuroleptics are frequently employed in particularly difficult cases, but controlled clinical trials have failed to indicate that such combinations enjoy any superiority over single-drug treatments [7]. This negative evidence, together with risks related to uncertainties concerning drug interactions and dosage parameters in drug combinations, would seem to argue against this approach.

Anxiolytics may be added adjunctively to the regimen of a psychotic patient. Again, there is no evidence that the addition of an anxiolytic improves the patient's fundamental condition. Anxiolytics do, however, serve to diminish akathisias and anxiety that may be present. The value of alleviating these symptoms must be weighed against the costs of complicating the drug regimen and additional drug side effects. The use of anxiolytics in psychotic patients should in any case be limited to short-term administration to alleviate akathisias or anxiety of intolerable dimensions.

The most common unplanned interaction of neuroleptics is additive CNS depression, which can occur with any two depressant drugs used concomitantly.

Matters of Strategy with Neuroleptics

The typical pattern of administration begins with a low daily dosage of one agent, which is gradually increased until a therapeutic response is obtained or significant side effects develop. Early administration may be intramuscular in noncooperative patients. Usually, oral administration can be effected later in the treatment sequence. The effective dose of neuroleptics varies considerably from patient to patient and even over time in the same patient. Therefore, dosage regimens need to be flexible and individualized in accordance with the response and side effects in each patient. Patients should be monitored closely, but judgments should not be made too hastily. Since a therapeutic response may not occur until after some weeks or months of treatment at an adequate dosage, a patient should not be prematurely judged refractory to pharmacotherapy. Moreover, a particular patient refractory to one agent may respond to another, although, as we stated earlier, there is little clinical evidence that any particular neuroleptic agent is superior to any other, overall. In the individual, then, substitution of one therapeutic agent for another may produce improvement.

Therapeutic effectiveness is judged in terms of amelioration of target symptoms. The various symptoms frequently accompanying schizophrenia respond differentially to neuroleptics, both as regards degree and time course. It has been noted that florid symptoms, such as combativeness or hallucinations, are more likely to respond than are negative symptoms, such as poor insight or memory. In general, symptoms such as hyperreactivity and hostility respond relatively quickly (in 1 to 2 weeks); affective changes occur with moderate rapidity (in 2 to 6 weeks); and cognitive and perceptual changes occur only slowly (in 2 to 3 months).

If the patient improves substantially in response to neuroleptic treatment, the question inevitably arises as to whether and when treatment should be curtailed or terminated. Relapse occurs with great frequency in both inpatients and outpatients who have been withdrawn from neuroleptic medication [11]; on the other hand, the side effects of these drugs are severe enough in many cases to encourage a reduction in dosage or cessation of drug treatment. For outpatients, the social environment is a critical factor in determining the likelihood of relapse and whether or not continued drug prescription is warranted [11]. Generally, a considerable reduction in dosage can be accomplished during the maintenance phase (to a level of about one-fifth or one-third of the dosage used during the acute phase). Some patients may be less subject to relapse and will make a better adjustment after discharge if never medicated with neuroleptics. When neuroleptic therapy is to be discontinued, or if a sharp dosage reduction is to be effected, dosage reduction should be gradual, to minimize the possibilities of recurrence of symptoms or development of tardive dyskinesias.

Maintenance drugs can and should be prescribed on a once-a-day basis. Many studies have indicated that outpatients frequently do not comply with medication instructions. The patient complies more readily if asked to take fewer different pills fewer times per day [1]. Arguments for divided doses are inadequate with reference to psychotropic drugs. Outpatients who repeatedly exhibit poor compliance can be placed on long-lasting dosage forms of fluphenazine, the enanthate and decanoate esters. These oil emulsions are injected intramuscularly or subcutaneously, in 1-ml volumes. The therapeutic effects last 1 to 3 weeks for fluphenazine enanthate and 4 weeks or longer for fluphenazine decanoate.

Maintenance treatment with neuroleptics generally continues no less than 6 months after an acute schizophrenic episode. Then, if conditions appear favorable, gradual withdrawal of drug treatment may be effected, with the understanding that resumption of treatment may be indicated later.

A specific contraindication for phenothiazines is in alcohol psychoses, since the likelihood of seizures is increased. Similarly, epilepsy may be aggravated by phenothiazines. The neuroleptics in general have not proved very useful in alcoholism, as initially hoped. Their use in elderly patients is fraught with special difficulties as well. Neuroleptics may increase cognitive impairment and confusion in elderly patients manifesting chronic organic brain syndrome. In addition, autonomic side effects such as hypotension may be more serious in elderly patients. On the other hand, the fact that neuroleptics interfere less with cognitive functioning gives them advantages over the sedative-hypnotics and favors their careful use in geriatric practice. Thioridazine may have special advantages in geriatric use because of its comparatively low extrapyramidal side effects.

Implications for Psychotherapy

Toxic delirium may accompany acute overdosage with phenothiazines and butyrophenones but has not been reported with thioxanthenes. Chronic administration of butyrophenones or phenothiazines, notably the aminoalkyl group, may precipitate depression and suicidal threats or attempts. Aminoalkyls and butyrophenones may precipitate epileptiform seizure activity.

Piperazine phenothiazines may induce feelings of anxiety with motor restlessness. Aminoalkyl phenothiazines may reduce initiative and produce feelings of apathy. Similarly, thioxanthines may elicit fatigue and drowsiness. Paradoxical insomnia is reported with all the major tranquilizers, particularly the piperazines and butyrophenones. The therapist should hesitate to dismiss somatic complaints, since they may be side effects of neuroleptic treatment. Impotence, a side effect seen most commonly with thioridazine, haloperidol, and thiothixene, may have an important psychological significance to the male patient.

Lack of generalization may occur in the undrugged state if therapy is conducted when the patient is on a neuroleptic of any type. On the other hand, tranquilization may increase receptiveness to psychotherapeutic intervention. Neuroleptics may blunt learning ability in the therapeutic setting, especially learning centering around affectual responses. Intervention that attempts to draw out affect in the therapeutic environment will be of diminished effectiveness.

The nonmedical psychotherapist is advised to consult with the patient's physician regarding the patient's use of a neuroleptic. It is certainly not too strong a statement to suggest that overlapping interest between the therapist and the prescribing physician would be the rule rather than the exception where neuroleptic treatment is involved.

Medically Important Neuroleptics

acetophenazine (Tindal), a piperazine phenothiazine neuroleptic: for psychotic disorders; low sedation favors use in withdrawn, apathetic schizophrenics. Usual: 60 to 120 mg. Extremes: 40 to 600 mg.

chlorpromazine (CPZ) (Thorazine, Largactil, Megaphen), an aminoalkyl phenothiazine neuroleptic: antipsychotic for chronic and acute schizophrenia, the manic phase of manic-depressive psychosis, and involutional, senile, organic, and toxic psychoses except delirium tremens; rarely, as an antiemetic. Antipsychotic: 300 to 800 mg usual. Extremes: 30 to 2,000 mg, 12.5 to 50 mg IV. Antiemetic: 25 mg.

chlorprothixene (Taractan), a thioxanthene neuroleptic: for psychotic disorders. Usual: 75 to 200 mg. Extremes: 45 to 600 mg.

fluphenazine (Prolixin, Permitil), a piperazine phenothiazine neuroleptic (see acetophenazine): available in long-acting injectable dosage forms (Prolixin enanthate, Prolixin decanoate). Usual: 2 to 10 mg. Extremes: 1 to 20 mg. Long-lasting: 25 mg.

haloperidol (Haldol), a butyrophenone neuroleptic: for psychotic disorders, possibly preferable in acute mania and Gilles de Tourette's syndrome. Usual: 6 to 9 mg. Extremes: 0.5 to 15 mg.

loxapine (Daxolin, Loxitane), a dibenzoxapine neuroleptic: for psychotic disorders. Usual: 60 to 100 mg. Extremes: 20 to 250 mg.

mesoridazine (Serentil), a piperidine phenothiazine neuroleptic: for schizophrenia, behavioral problems in retardation or chronic organic brain syndrome, withdrawal delirium, and severe behavioral problems in children. Usual: 75 to 300 mg. Extremes: 30 to 400 mg.

molindone (Lidone, Moban), an indolic neuroleptic: for psychotic disorders. Usual: 50 to 100 mg. Extremes: 15 to 225 mg.

perphenazine (Trilafon, Triavil [combined with amitriptyline], Etrafon [combined with amitriptyline]), a piperazine phenothiazine neuroleptic: see acetophenazine. Usual: 16 to 32 mg. Extremes: 6 to 64 mg.

piperacetazine (Quide), a piperazine phenothiazine neuroleptic: for psychotic disorders. Typical: 20 to 160 mg.

prochlorperazine (Compazine), a piperazine phenothiazine neuroleptic: for psychotic disorders; low sedation favors use in withdrawn, apathetic schizophrenics and in neurotic depression; useful in suppressing nausea. Usual: 75 to 100 mg. Extremes: 15 to 150 mg. Antiemetic: 2.5 to 15 mg.

reserpine (Serpasil and others, Rauzide [*Rauwolfia serpentina* extract combined with bendroflumenthiazide*]), a *Rauwolfia* antihypertensive and neuroleptic: discontinued as antipsychotic. Antihypertensive: 0.1 to 0.5 mg.

thioridazine (Mellaril), a piperidine neuroleptic: for psychotic conditions, dysthymic disorder, behavioral symptoms of organic brain syndrome, and severe behavioral problems in children, possibly preferable in autistic children and positive spike pattern syndrome. Usual: 100 to 500 mg. Extremes: 30 to 800 mg.

---

*Antihypertensive; no CNS effects.

thiothixene (Navane), a thioxanthene neuroleptic: for psychotic disorders. Typical: 10 to 20 mg. Extremes: 3 to 60 mg.

trifluoperazine (Stelazine), a piperazine phenothiazine neuroleptic: see acetaphenazine. Usual: 3 to 15 mg. Extremes: 2 to 64 mg.

triflupromazine (Vesprin), an aminoalkyl phenothiazine neuroleptic: similar to chlorpromazine. Usual: 30 to 150 mg. Extremes: 20 to 400 mg.

Selected References and Further Readings

1. Ayd, F. J., Jr. Once-a-day neuroleptic and tricyclic antidepressant therapy. *Int. Drug Ther. Newslett.* 7:33–40, 1972.
2. Cattabeni, F. et al. (Eds.). *Long-term Effects of Neuroleptics. Advanced Biochemical Psychopharmacology* Vol. 24. New York: Raven, 1980.
3. Committee on Nomenclature and Statistics of the American Psychiatric Association. *Diagnostic and Statistical Manual* (3rd ed.). Washington, D.C.: American Psychiatric Association, 1980.
4. Davis, J. M. Efficacy of tranquilizing and antidepressant drugs. *Arch. Gen. Psychiatry* 13:552–572, 1965.
5. Gilman, A. G., Goodman, L. S., and Gilman, A. *The Pharmacological Basis of Therapeutics* (6th ed.). New York: Macmillan, 1980.
6. Hanlon, T. E. et al. The comparative effectiveness of eight phenothiazines in chronic psychosis. *Psychopharmacologia* 7:89, 1965.
7. Hollister, L. E. Psychiatric Disorders. In K. L. Melmon and H. F. Morrelli (Eds.), *Clinical Pharmacology* (2nd ed.). New York: Macmillan, 1978.
8. Iversen, L. L. et al. (Eds.) Neuroleptics and Schizophrenia. *Handbook of Psychopharmacology,* Vol. 10. New York: Plenum, 1978.
9. Klein, D. F., and Gittelman-Klein, R. (Eds.). *Progress in Psychiatric Drug Treatment.* New York: Brunner/Mazel, 1975.
10. Lipton, M. A. et al. (Eds.). *Psychopharmacology: A Generation of Progress.* New York: Raven, 1978.
11. Wing, J. K., Leff, J., and Hirsch, S. Preventive Treatment of Schizophrenia: Some Theoretical and Methodological Issues. In J. O. Cole et al. (Eds.), *Psychopathology and Psychopharmacology.* Baltimore: Johns Hopkins University Press, 1973.

Anxiety and Anxiolytics

17

℞

Anxiety is a subjective feeling that does not readily lend itself to objective measurement. At the core of anxiety are feelings of heightened tension, apprehensiveness, and uneasiness. It is distinguished from fear on the basis of the absence of a specific object or circumstance generating the feeling.

Anxiety is remarkably fluid and pervasive, being capable of exerting powerful influences on all aspects of behavioral activity as well as on autonomic and motor tone (Table 17-1). Visceral concomitants of anxiety arise from the activation of the hypothalamic-pituitary axis. Motor symptoms, such as shakiness, tremor, and elevated muscle tension, involve the extrapyramidal motor system. So, anxiety, though in its essence a subjective feeling state, is closely associated with somatic symptoms. This mixed nature of anxiety provides a multiplicity of possible reasons for the patient to seek help. The complaint may relate directly to the subjective state or to one or more somatic symptoms that have become burdensome. Evaluation of the anxiety state, as well as clinical progression or improvement, can likewise center either on the subjective feeling or on the somatic manifestations. Anxiety can be operationally defined and quantified by means of subjective questionnaires, such as the Hopkins Symptom Checklist, the Hamilton Anxiety Scale, or the Physician Anxiety Questionnaire. Alternatively, treatment may center on alleviation of a somatic symptom, such as tension headaches, elevated blood pressure, gastrointestinal disturbances, tremor, or fatigability.

Since anxiety is a universal human experience, both as an independent feeling state and as a component of most psychiatric and medical problems, the first challenge facing the clinician is to determine whether or not a given instance of anxiety warrants treatment at all. Throughout history, the desire of humankind to find relief from anxiety through drugs has lured men and women along a course lined with profound dangers. The comfort found in suppressing anxiety often and thoroughly is a temptation that too often is not resisted. It is this temptation that lies at the root of most instances of drug dependence.

A certain amount of anxiety is a necessary corollary of need-fulfilling activity, coping, and personal growth. Adaptive neurochemical mechanisms of the brain tend to countermand, in the long run, furtive and futile efforts to be rid of the impetus of anxiety. There is no doubt that addiction can result from crude efforts at self-medication, usually in the form of alcohol, and it is equally certain that addiction can occur with the use of

Table 17-1. Symptoms of anxiety

Subjective

Worry, apprehensiveness, rumination, edginess, tension

Behavioral

Hypervigilance, distractability, insomnia, irritability, impatience, inability to relax, exaggerated self-consciousness, excessive need for reassurance

Motor

Shakiness, jumpiness, trembling, tremor, elevated tonus, fatigability, muscle aches, furrowed brow, fidgeting, restlessness, headaches

Autonomic

Increased heart rate, increased blood pressure, sweating, cold and moist palms, dizziness, upset stomach, diarrhea, frequent urination, flushing, pallor, dry mouth, headaches

---

any of the anxiolytic drugs. Dependence of both the psychological and physical varieties occurs along with abstinence phenomena. Addiction to minor tranquilizers ranks behind only abuse of alcohol, nicotine, and sedative-hypnotics in terms of numbers of persons involved.

Under what circumstances is anxiety maladaptive? Generally, anxiety is considered excessive when the patient is nonresponsive to psychotherapeutic interventions to alleviate hyperactivity, intense fearfulness, excessive inhibition, or withdrawal. Under such circumstances, drug treatment may reduce anxiety to tolerable levels and perhaps facilitate psychotherapy as well. On the other hand, it seems evident that the anxiolytics, like so many drugs of abuse, are often used indiscriminately and excessively as a means of escaping unwanted anxieties and as a substitute for coping behavior. Alternative treatments should not be neglected: psychotherapy aimed at improving the capacity to cope with anxiety; desensitization techniques for anxiety related to phobias; environmental manipulations aimed at reducing anxiety-provoking situations; and various forms of relaxation therapy.

Diagnostic Classification of Anxiety Disorders

Five broad categories comprising a total of thirteen specific diagnostic labels are defined in *DSM-III* [1] in relation to anxiety (Table 17-2). Antianxiety drugs are indicated for some of these categories, while antidepressants or nondrug modes of therapy are indicated for others. Anxiolytics are also employed for anxiety that accompanies other psychiatric conditions, such as personality disorders and adjustment disorders.

Phobic Neuroses, Panic Disorder, and Separation Anxiety

Phobic neuroses, panic disorder, and separation anxiety appear to be related disorders as regards etiology and drug responsiveness, although the clinical symptoms differ. Phobias and panic reactions are more common in women than men. Panic reactions may be triggered by phobic stimuli, as in agoraphobia with panic attacks, or they may occur episodically, independent of any circumscribed phobic stimulus, as in panic disorder. Panic reactions are characterized by discrete periods of apprehensiveness. The *DSM-III* criteria for panic disorder require at least three such episodes in a period of 3 weeks and at least four of the following associated symptoms: (1) dyspnea (irregular

Table 17-2. *Diagnostic categories of anxiety disorder*

Phobic disorders (or phobic neuroses)
  Agoraphobia with panic attacks
  Agoraphobia without panic attacks
  Social phobia
  Simple phobia
Anxiety states (or anxiety neuroses)
  Panic disorder
  Generalized anxiety disorder
  Obsessive compulsive disorder
Posttraumatic stress disorder
  Acute
  Chronic or delayed
Atypical anxiety disorder
Anxiety disorders of childhood or adolescence
  Separation anxiety disorder
  Avoidant disorder of childhood or adolescence
  Overanxious disorder

---

respiration); (2) palpitations; (3) chest pain; (4) sensations of choking or smothering; (5) dizziness; (6) feelings of unreality; (7) paresthesia (tingling in hands or feet); (8) hot or cold flashes; (9) sweating; (10) faintness; (11) trembling or shaking; and (12) fear of dying, going crazy, or losing control.

Panic reactions can be brought under control by treatment with imipramine, usually within a few weeks of administration. Imipramine is significantly better than placebo, neuroleptics, or anxiolytics in eliminating the occurrence of such panic episodes. Once a panic condition has been brought under control with imipramine, maintenance doses are effective in minimizing the risk of relapse. Supportive psychotherapy, or anxiolytic medication, or both may be useful in overcoming residual behavioral limitations.

A substantial percentage of patients experiencing panic reactions as adults are noted to have suffered separation anxiety as children. It thus seems likely that these two diagnostic categories are causally related, though affecting different age groups. Interestingly, imipramine is also highly effective and the drug of choice in separation anxiety disorder.

Phobic states without associated panic episodes are best treated with psychotherapy. These patients are not good candidates for anxiolytic or antidepressant treatment. A widely used mode of treatment for phobias has been desensitization therapy. Systematic desensitization is a technique of behavioral therapy that rests on the assumption that neurotic responses can be counterconditioned by eliminating the anxiety usually associated with the presence of the aversive stimuli. A patient is presented with graduated levels of the stimulus class (such as increasing altitude for an acrophobe), while relaxation is maintained through drug or nondrug techniques. Some therapists use muscle relaxation methods to maintain relaxation. Some utilize an anxiolytic or an ultrashort-acting or short-acting barbiturate, often methohexital. Methohexital produces a deep relaxation and facilitates counterconditioning. Good results have been reported with this procedure.

When a drug is used to maintain relaxation in conjunction with systematic desensitization, the problem of state dependency inevitably arises. The findings of several studies have suggested that carryover of counterconditioning does not readily occur in the nondrug state when drug treatment is abruptly terminated. On the other hand, carryover can be considerably enhanced if drug withdrawal is gradual. This suggests a possible means of avoiding state-dependency effects, not only as regards systematic desensitization but also as regards the broader issue of drugs and therapy in general.

Other Anxiety Disorders

Most of the remaining anxiety disorders are frequently treated with anxiolytic drugs, with greater or lesser success. Two factors are of prime importance in predicting responsiveness to anxiolytics: duration (chronic versus acute anxiety states) and etiology (reactive versus generalized). The chronic anxiety disorders such as generalized anxiety disorder, obsessive compulsive disorder, chronic posttraumatic stress disorder, and overanxious disorder of childhood and adolescence, are less effectively treated with anxiolytics than are acute posttraumatic stress reactions. For one thing, the effectiveness of most sedatives seems to be limited to less than 2 weeks of daily use. The benzodiazepines have a somewhat longer period of effectiveness, perhaps up to 2 months, but no controlled study has shown effectiveness for anxiolytics relative to placebos beyond 2 months on chronic use. Reactive anxiety is more readily treatable with anxiolytic medication than is generalized anxiety. Avoidant disorder of childhood or adolescence, the only diagnostic category listed in Table 17-2 that is a personality disorder rather than a neurotic disorder, is not appropriately treated with anxiolytics, since they will only serve to increase the shyness and social withdrawal that characterize this syndrome.

Considering the abuse potential of antianxiety drugs and sedatives, and allowing that there is a tendency to overmedicate anxiety, an attractive alternative to conventional drug therapy of anxiety is placebo or semi-placebo treatment. True placebo therapy involves the use of a tablet or capsule containing a pharmacologically inert substance such as lactose. Placebo responsiveness depends on the patient's expectation of benefit. In today's drug-sophisticated society, a sugar pill (the most commonly used placebo) is likely to be recognized for what it is, especially if the patient seeks information on the medication from a drug information resource. A physician who believes that drug treatment in a given case of anxiety is not warranted, but who suspects that it is expected and will be sought out until obtained, may wish to employ a more sophisticated variety of placebo therapy. Small, generally subeffective, doses of a neuroleptic are sometimes used in this way for anxiety. The identity of the drug as a "tranquilizer" will strengthen the patient's expectation of benefit. The use of hydroxyzine, an antihistamine of marginal effectiveness in anxiety, is an example of drug therapy that lies in the gray area between placebo therapy and pharmacologic treatment.

Anxiolytics

The spectrum of actions and the side effects of the group of drugs called anxiolytics, antianxiety drugs, or minor tranquilizers bear a closer resemblance to the sedative-hypnotics than to the major tranquilizers or neuroleptics. Indeed, anxiolytics may be considered daytime sedatives or sedative-hypnotics having greater-than-typical dosage separation between the dosage that will suppress anxiety and aggression and the dosage that will produce general depression.

Meprobamate

Meprobamate (Miltown, Equanil) was developed in the mid-1950s and caught on with unusual rapidity, being widely prescribed just 2 years after its introduction. It has both sedative and tranquilizing properties, so that some degree of sedation inevitably accompanies its use. It is difficult in practice to distinguish between the actions of meprobamate and a barbiturate. Like the sedative-hypnotics, withdrawal symptoms accompany acute withdrawal from chronic use of meprobamate. Moreover, meprobamate use may result not only in development of tolerance but also in physical and psychological dependence. Withdrawal resembles that following use of sedative-hypnotics and may involve convulsive seizures. Meprobamate is also an effective skeletal-muscle relaxant and is sometimes employed for this property.

Side effects with meprobamate are minimal. Drowsiness is the most frequent complaint, and ataxia may occur at high doses. Hypotension frequently occurs, and, in rare cases, skin rashes and gastrointestinal disturbances develop. Also rarely, headache, dizziness, or nausea may be reported.

Benzodiazepines

Several structurally related compounds belonging to the benzodiazepine group have been marketed as antianxiety drugs: chlordiazepoxide (e.g., Librium, A-Poxide), diazepam (Valium), oxazepam (Serax), clorazepate (Tranxene, Azene), lorazepam (Ativan), and prazepam (Verstran). They are effective antianxiety drugs that produce some sedation and are also effective skeletal-muscle relaxants. They are used extensively in psychoneuroses, petit mal epilepsy, and alcoholism. They also have a use in transient and chronic tic disorders and for parasomnias related to stage 4 of slow-wave sleep (i.e., sleepwalking and night terrors). Unlike the major tranquilizers, these compounds produce no extrapyramidal side effects. The benzodiazepines have several advantages: They produce very little change in normal sleep patterns, have a long duration of action, and are the only sedatives that cannot readily be used for suicide.

Approximately 100 million prescriptions per year are written for the treatment of anxiety (one in every six adults is involved), with about 80 percent of these calling for a benzodiazepine. Diazepam alone represents about 60 percent of the anxiolytic market.

There is no doubt that addiction can occur with the use of all the anxiolytic agents; most instances, however, involve either excessive doses or duration of use beyond 2 months. Dependence of both a psychological and a physical variety develops, and abstinence phenomena similar to those of alcohol and barbiturates ensue on withdrawal.

Neuroanatomic and Neurochemical Mechanisms of Benzodiazepine Action

The benzodiazepines produce an unusual and characteristic EEG effect in which both slow-wave and fast-wave activity are increased, while middle-range frequencies are diminished. Chlordiazepoxide reportedly slows the spontaneous EEG recorded from the septal region, amygdala, and hippocampus. Since EEG frequencies below the beta-wave range are generated by the diffuse thalamic projection system and its limbic inputs, it is likely that the loss of mid-range activity is related to depression of the limbic system (Figure 17-1).

The most striking behavioral effect of benzodiazepines is their ability to release punishment-suppressed behavior from inhibitory restraint. This effect is brought about

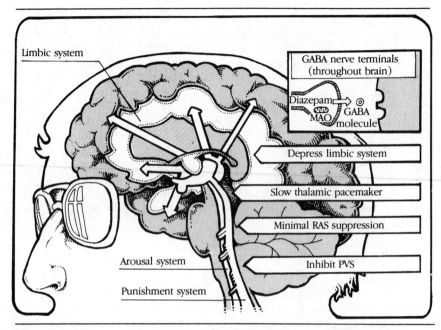

Fig. 17-1. Mechanisms of anxiolytics. GABA, gamma-aminobutyric acid; MAO, monoamine oxidase; PVS, periventricular system; RAS, reticular activating system. (Modified from A. K. Swonger. Nursing Pharmacology. Boston: Little, Brown, 1978.)

by their ability to suppress the activity of the periventricular punishment system, the brain system that produces behavioral suppression in relation to negative reinforcement. The punishment system is a brain region particularly vulnerable to the depressant action of any of the sedative-hypnotics, but especially the anxiolytics.

Some of the neurochemical alterations contributing to the action of benzodiazepines have become well established in recent years. Benzodiazepines facilitate gamma-aminobutyric acid (GABA) transmission by increasing GABA-binding to postsynaptic receptors (Fig. 17-2). The benzodiazepine receptor is a modulatory protein, closely associated with the GABA-receptor (or recognition protein). Several endogenous ligands for the benzodiazepine receptor have been found, including a protein called GABA-modulin, as well as inosine and hypoxanthine nucleotides. Activation of the benzodiazepine receptor by endogenous ligands has an inhibitory effect on GABA-binding. Benzodiazepines, on the other hand, act antagonistically to block the action of GABA-modulin or other endogenous ligands. Thus, benzodiazepines facilitate GABA-binding. The relationship between benzodiazepines and GABA is called positive cooperativity. Facilitation of GABA transmission results in a decreased turnover of several other transmitters because of the role of GABA as an inhibitory transmitter. Many of the behavioral effects result from the secondary neurochemical actions (Fig. 17-3).

Benzodiazepines also have an inhibitory effect on phosphodiesterase, the enzyme that destroys adenosine monophosphate (see Chap. 6). They mimic the effects of glycine and block dopamine reuptake.

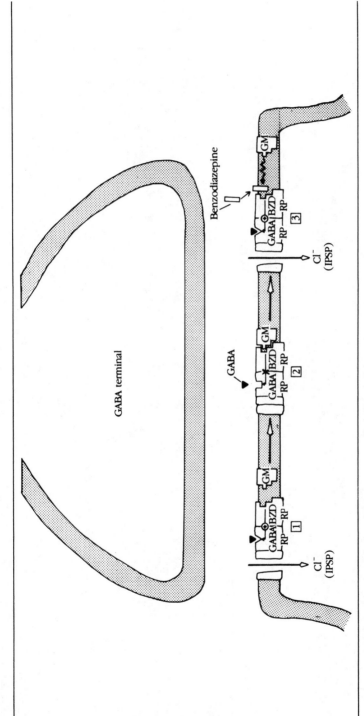

Fig. 17-2. *The neurochemical mechanism of benzodiazepine action. BZD RP, benzodiazepine recognition protein; GABA, gamma-aminobutyric acid; GABA RP, GABA recognition protein; GM, GABA-modulin; IPSP, inhibitory postsynaptic potential. [1] The benzodiazepine recognition protein is a modulator of GABA-binding to type 1 GABA-receptors. In the absence of GABA-modulin (an endogenous regulator of GABA-binding), the benzodiazepine receptor protein facilitates GABA-binding. [2] Introduction of GABA-modulin prevents this facilitation of GABA-binding by the benzodiazepine receptor protein. [3] Administration of a benzodiazepine blocks access of GABA-modulin to the modulatory protein, thus facilitating GABA-binding.*

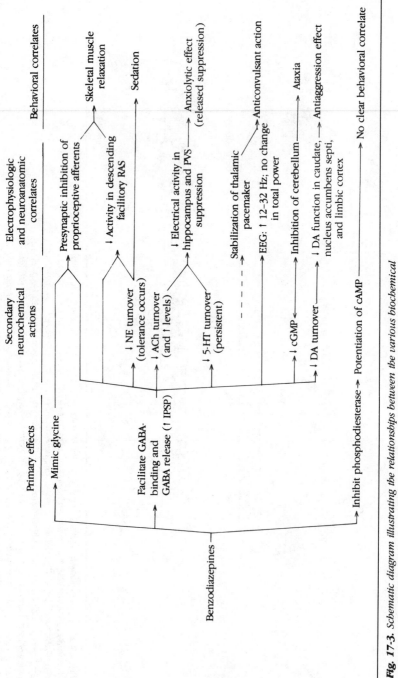

Fig. 17-3. *Schematic diagram illustrating the relationships between the various biochemical actions of benzodiazepines and electrophysiologic, neuroanatomic, and behavioral correlates. ACh, acetylcholine; 5-HT, 5-hydroxytryptamine; cAMP, cyclic adenosine monophosphate; cGMP, cyclic guanosine monophosphate; DA, dopamine; GABA, gammabutyric acid; IPSP, inhibitory postsynaptic potentials; PVS, periventricular system; RAS, reticular activating system.*

Table 17-3. Comparisons of anxiolytics

Drug	Equivalent dose	Plasma half-life* (hr)
Alprazolam	0.5	≈ 12
Chlordiazepoxide	10	8–28
Clorazepate	7	30–100
Diazepam	5	20–42
Halazepam	20	≈ 14
Lorazepam	1	12–15
Oxazepam	15	10–14
Prazepam	10	30–100

*For drug or active metabolite.

Adverse Effects of Benzodiazepines

Benzodiazepines may produce dependence and withdrawal symptoms similar in kind to those caused by sedative-hypnotics. Hypersensitivity reactions may occur. If a benzodiazepine is used during the first trimester of pregnancy, the risk of congenital defects is increased, and benzodiazepines are excreted in breast milk. Signs of excess depression include sedation, confusion, lethargy, ataxia, and disorientation. Paradoxical rage, agitation, nervousness, and insomnia also occur. Although rapid eye movement sleep suppression is absent, vivid dreams or nightmares may occur. Changes in libido and menstrual irregularities are fairly common, as are gastrointestinal disturbances.

Comparisons of the Various Benzodiazepines

By and large, differences within the benzodiazepine class are subtle. Diazepam is the most widely used, both within its class and among all prescription drugs. It is less sedative than chlordiazepoxide in most patients and has a fairly long half-life (20 to 42 hours) (Table 17-3). The antiepileptic properties of diazepam exceed those of other benzodiazepines except clonazepam, a benzodiazepine introduced expressly for use in epilepsy (see Chap. 28). One report based on a retrospective analysis suggests that diazepam may be preferable to chlordiazepoxide for dysthymic disorder and anxiety accompanied by insomnia or motor symptoms. Antianxiety properties of the two were found to be equivalent overall, while chlordiazepoxide was found more effective in reactive anxiety. These differences, if substantiated, can likely be attributed to the greater sedative properties of chlordiazepoxide.

Chlordiazepoxide has been found to be somewhat more effective than diazepam in treatment of alcohol withdrawal. It has a shorter plasma half-life (8 to 28 hours). Chlordiazepoxide is sometimes used in combination preparations for ulcers (e.g., Librax). Oxazepam is the shortest-acting of the benzodiazepine anxiolytics. Its half-life is only 10 to 14 hours. Two new benzodiazepines, approved for use in 1982, alprazolam (Xanax) and halazepam (Paxipam) are similarly short-acting. Clorazepate and prazepam have active metabolites with long half-lives, giving them extended durations of action.

Table 17-4. Correlates of responsiveness to benzodiazepines

Patient variables	Illness variables
Female	Acute
Older	Reactive
Married	Few previous drugs
More educated	Good previous drug response
Higher social class	High severity if generalized anxiety
Recognizes problem is emotional	Low severity if obsessive compulsive
Expects drug treatment	Many somatic symptoms
Physician variables	Treatment variables
Family practice	Occurrence of sedation
Predicts success	Short duration
Feels comfortable with patient	
Feels comfortable prescribing drugs	

Matters of Strategy in Using Benzodiazepines

A number of both controllable and uncontrollable variables have been found to correlate with responsiveness of anxiety to benzodiazepines (Table 17-4). These correlates of successful treatment are divided into patient variables, physician variables, illness variables, and treatment variables. The correlates support the notion that antianxiety medication should be used selectively for more severe cases of anxiety, particularly when acute and reactive.

The value of anxiolytics in the treatment of anxiety is constrained by abuse liability, lack of effectiveness beyond 2 to 3 months of daily use, and the purely symptomatic nature of the benefit. The decision to employ an anxiolytic should be limited to those cases where the degree of discomfort or dysfunction is considerable. In any case, the use of an anxiolytic should not take the place of psychotherapeutic efforts to get at the underlying causes or to provide improved means of coping with or dissipating anxiety.

Flexible dosage schedules are appropriate for antianxiety drugs provided the total recommended daily dose is not exceeded. Often, all, or a substantial part of, the daily dosage is taken in the evening, when sedative effects are least inconveniencing.

Hydroxyzine

Hydroxyzine (Atarax, Vistaril) has also found application as an anxiolytic. It is an antihistamine with sedative properties characteristic of that class. Its depressant effect is on subcortical centers, having little effect on the cerebrum. It is indicated for short-term alleviation of anxiety and stress, for example, in preoperative and postoperative applications. Side effects are minimal. Additive CNS depression occurs with other CNS depressants.

Implications for Psychotherapy

Rarely, toxic confusional states may occur following large doses of meprobamate or benzodiazepines. Outright depression is not reported, but drowsiness, sedation, and lethargy are frequent occurrences in early therapy. Paradoxical effects in which anxiolytics increase anxiety have been noted among people who are characterized as "jocks," extroverted and active in their approach to problem resolution, a characteristic that may be interfered with by anxiolytics. Although there is relatively little D-sleep suppression with anxiolytics, dream and sleep disturbances may occur. Oxazepam, a benzodiazepine, is said to cause increased incidence of nightmares. Paradoxical insomnia may result with any of the anxiolytics. Euphoric states resembling inebriation may occur. Ataxia (stumbling, clumsiness), headache, dizziness, and vertigo occur occasionally, while rare cases of slurring of speech may be noted. The therapist should take note of somatic side effects and hesitate to dismiss bodily complaints as psychosomatic or psychogenic. If the patient habitually uses anxiolytics, irritability and anxiety may reflect mild abstinence symptoms resulting from delayed or skipped medication. It is probable that some dissociation of learning occurs between the drugged and undrugged states with respect to anxiolytics. The therapist might wish to plan his therapeutic timetable around the patient's administration schedule or habits; or he might request the patient to refrain from taking a tranquilizer in the 4 to 6 hours preceding the session. On the other hand, if the patient's use is regular, the therapist might do better working with the patient in the drugged state, since this represents the patient's "normal" condition.

If abuse of tranquilizers is itself a therapeutic issue, the therapist is up against not only the withdrawal-postponing properties of the drug but the primary reinforcing properties as well. The anxiety-relieving capabilities of the tranquilizer may be perceived by the patient as preferable to what the therapist has to offer in the way of growth or change. The therapist should be alert to the possibility of personal and systemic dynamics in tranquilizer abuse which are analogs of those found in alcoholism.

Anxiety is, of course, related to life experience and, in many if not most cases, may even be regarded as a normal, even though dysphoric, experience which may be expected to wax and wane with the shifting influences of life circumstances. It is possible for drug therapy of anxiety to be a disservice. For many clients, psychotherapy, especially reality-oriented interventions into life-style and systemic interventions into familial and social networks, may be substantially more useful and to the point.

Medically Important Anxiolytics

alprazolam (Xanax), a benzodiazepine anxiolytic: antianxiety, short-acting, minimal D-sleep suppression. Anxiolytic: 0.75 to 1.5 mg.

chlordiazepoxide (Librium, A-Poxide, Libritabs, Librax [combined with clidinium*], SK-Lygen, Tenax), a benzodiazepine anxiolytic: antianxiety, management of alcohol withdrawal, centrally acting muscle relaxant, minimal D-sleep suppression. Anxiolytic: 15 to 100 mg.

clorazepate (chlorazepate) (Tranxene, Azene), a benzodiazepine anxiolytic: antianxiety, long-acting, minimal D-sleep suppression. Anxiolytic: 5 to 60 mg.

diazepam (Valium), a benzodiazepine anxiolytic: antianxiety, anticonvulsant, antiepileptic, skeletal-muscle relaxant, minimal D-sleep suppression. Anxiolytic: 6 to 40 mg.

halazepam (Paxipam), a benzodiazepine anxiolytic: antianxiety, short-acting, minimal D-sleep suppression. Anxiolytic: 60 to 120 mg.

hydroxyzine (Atarax, Vistaril, Marax [combined with ephedrine and theophylline]†), an antihistamine sedative. Sedative: 100 to 400 mg. Antianxiety: 50 to 400 mg.

---

*Peripheral anticholinergic effects with CNS side effects.
†Combination not prescribed for its CNS effects.

lorazepam (Ativan), a benzodiazepine anxiolytic: antianxiety, preanesthetic sedation. Anxiolytic: 1 to 10 mg.

meprobamate (Equanil, Miltown), a propanediol anxiolytic: antianxiety, skeletal-muscle relaxant. Anxiolytic: 1,200 to 1,600 mg.

oxazepam (Serax), a benzodiazepine anxiolytic: antianxiety, antispasmodic, minimal D-sleep suppression. Anxiolytic: 30 to 120 mg.

prazepam (Verstran), a benzodiazepine anxiolytic: antianxiety, minimal D-sleep suppression. Anxiolytic: 20 to 60 mg.

tybamate (Tybatran), a propanediol anxiolytic. Antianxiety: 750 to 2,000 mg.

Selected References and Further Readings

1. Committee on Nomenclature and Statistics of the American Psychiatric Association. *Diagnostic and Statistical Manual* (3rd ed.). Washington, D.C.: American Psychiatric Association, 1980.
2. Costa, E., and Greengard, P. (Eds.). Mechanism of Action of Benzodiazepines. *Advances in Biochemical Psychopharmacology,* Vol. 14. New York: Raven, 1975.
3. Costa, E., Guidotti, A., Mao, C. C., and Suria, A. New concepts of the mechanism of action of benzodiazepine. *Life Sci.* 17:167–186, 1975.
4. Gilman, A. G., Goodman, L. S., and Gilman, A. *The Pharmacological Basis of Therapeutics* (6th ed.). New York: Macmillan, 1980.
5. Hollister, L. E. Psychiatric Disorders. In K. L. Melmon and H. F. Morrelli (Eds.), *Clinical Pharmacology* (2nd ed.). New York: Macmillan, 1978.
6. Klein, D. F., and Gittelman-Klein, R. (Eds.). *Progress in Psychiatric Drug Treatment.* New York: Brunner/Mazel, 1975.
7. Lipton, M. A., DiMascio, A., and Killam, K. F. (Eds.). *Psychopharmacology: A Generation of Progress.* New York: Raven, 1978.
8. Rickels, K., Downing, R. W., and Winokur, A. Antianxiety Drugs: Clinical Use in Psychiatry. In L. L. Iversen et al. (Eds.), *Handbook of Psychopharmacology.* New York: Plenum, 1978. Vol. 13.

Depression and Antidepressants
18

Diagnostic Classifications of Depression

Depression, like anxiety, occurs both as a normal component of psychological processes and as a pathologic condition. As a normal, functional process, depression provides a means of protecting the nervous system for a better day, when the individual is confronted with adverse circumstances for which there is no effective coping response. The grief reaction one experiences following loss of a loved one is an example of a normal depressive reaction that generally follows predictable stages (protest, despair, detachment) with respect to severity and other features. As a pathologic condition, depression may occur as a primary affective disorder, as a drug reaction, or as an element in a wide variety of medical problems. The line between normal and pathologic depression is drawn only with difficulty, with attention to the etiology, severity, and duration of the condition. As with the treatment of anxiety, one choice that should be made carefully is whether drug treatment is warranted at all. "Benign neglect" is arguably the treatment of choice in mild, reactive depression.

Dichotomous Concepts of Depression

It is common practice to characterize a given case of depression further by additional descriptors. Seven pairs of adjectives that are widely used to describe depression warrant consideration. These adjective pairs may be called dichotomous concepts of depression, since each pair divides depression into two categories: unipolar versus bipolar, primary versus secondary, psychotic versus neurotic, endogenous versus reactive, major depression with or without melancholia, typical versus atypical, and agitated versus retarded. The unipolar versus bipolar is a well established (Table 18-1) and widely accepted distinction that we have acknowledged by choosing to treat these two categories of affective disorders in separate chapters. Bipolar disorders are taken up in the next chapter, while unipolar affective disorders occupy our attention in this chapter.

Primary versus Secondary Depression

The distinction between primary and secondary depression is clear in theory if not always in practice. Depression is primary when it occurs independent of other disorders or when the affective disturbance is the major presenting symptom. Depression is

Table 18-1. *Unipolar versus bipolar affective disorders*

	Unipolar	Bipolar
Essential features	Depressive mood; pervasive loss of interest or pleasure	Alternating episodes of manic and depressive moods
Incidence		
Frequency	Common	Much less common
Sex ratio	F > M	F = M
Familial history	Sometimes present	Often present
Physiological correlates		
Nocturnal EEG (usual)	↓ Sleep time ↓ REM % ↓ REM latency	Manic phase: ↓ Sleep time, ↓ REM %, ↑ REM latency, ↑ MHPG Depressive phase: ↓ Sleep time, ↑ REM %, ↓ REM latency, ↓ MHPG
Transmitter metabolites	↓ MHPG or 5-HIAA	↑ MHPG
Prognosis		
Spontaneous remission	Likely	Unlikely
Recurrent episodes	Second episode: 75% Third episode: 50%	Almost always many episodes
Drug effectiveness	Tricyclics >> lithium	Lithium >> tricyclics
Subtypes	Major depression vs dysthymic disorder Endogenous vs reactive With or without melancholia Atypical depression Serotonin vs norepinephrine type	Manic-depressive disorder vs cyclothymic personality Bipolar I vs bipolar II Acute or recurrent mania (rare) Atypical bipolar disorder (includes bipolar II)

Table 18-2. *Conditions to which depression is often secondary*

Psychiatric
  Organic brain syndrome
  Schizophrenia
  Obsessive compulsive disorder
  Generalized anxiety disorder
  Panic disorder
  Drug dependence
  Sexual deviances
Organic
  Metabolic: hypoglycemia, potassium or calcium depletion, elevated blood urea nitrogen, hepatic dysfunction
  Endocrine: hypothyroidism, diabetes, hyperthyroidism, Addison's disease, hypoglycemia
  CNS: mental retardation, tumors, Parkinson's disease, multiple sclerosis, Alzheimer's disease, cerebral vascular insufficiency
  Miscellaneous: anemia, carcinoma, systemic lupus erythematosus, infectious diseases, congestive heart failure, porphyria
Drug-induced
  Alcohol
  Other sedative-hypnotics
  Antipsychotics
  Anxiolytics
  Antihistamines
  Antiepileptics
  Narcotic analgesics
  Anticholinergics
  Antihypertensives
  Digitalis
  Corticosteroids (withdrawal)
  Estrogen preparations
  Immunosuppressives

secondary when it is related to another psychiatric disorder outside the affective category, an organic disorder, or drug utilization. There are many such conditions with which depression is associated (Table 18-2). The psychotherapist should be continuously alert to the possibility that complaints of depression stem from one of these causes. It is also possible for conditions such as those listed in Table 18-2 to exacerbate primary depression, compounding the difficulty of treating the primary disorder. For that reason, the possibility of such contributing factors should not be ignored, even when the primary affective disorder preexisted.

Major Depression versus Dysthymic Disorder

A third dichotomous concept of depression is psychotic versus neurotic. This distinction has been discarded in *DSM-III* [1]. Affective disorders are now catalogued separately from the psychoses and from the anxiety disorders. Three categories are offered for unipolar affective disorders: major depression, dysthymic disorder (or depressive neurosis), and atypical depression. The last category is generally utilized as a catchall for those cases of depression not fitting either of the other two specifically defined classifications. It is discussed below. Of the two specifically defined classifications, the latter, dysthymic disorder, is defined in DSM-III as equivalent to the older designation of depressive neurosis. Thus, it may be assumed that the label *major depression* replaces the former depressive psychosis. It would appear that the essence of the change is to dissociate major depression from psychotic conditions such as schizophrenia and paranoia, a change that we applaud.

Unfortunately, it is apparent from examination of the diagnostic criteria for major affective disorder and dysthymic disorder in DSM-III that something has been lost sight of in the new scheme: The two specifically defined types of unipolar depression are differentiated largely on the basis of severity, but numerous studies over the years support the notion that the conditions formerly called psychotic and neurotic depression differ not only in degree but also in terms of several measurable physiologic correlates. In psychotic depression, patients are insulin-resistant, have depressed sympathetic and corticosteroid stress responses, and have lowered barbiturate-induced sleep thresholds, all relative to normals. In neurotic depression, however, insulin and stress responses are not altered, and barbiturate sleep thresholds are higher even than in normals! Also, the two conditions exhibit markedly different pharmacotherapeutic responsiveness, with antidepressants clearly indicated in major depression, but less effective than either anxiolytics or neuroleptics in dysthymic disorder. For these reasons, we view the two conditions as differing qualitatively, not merely quantitatively. We hope that subsequent editions of the DSM will strengthen the distinction between major depression and dysthymic disorder, with emphasis on objectively measurable physiologic variables.

In any case, the current criteria for a major depressive episode focus on two matters: the dysphoric mood itself and the circumstantial symptom cluster (Table 18-3). Dysphoric mood is characterized by feelings of sadness, depression, hopelessness, irritability, or loss of interest or pleasure in most activities. The mood disturbance must be prominent, but not necessarily the dominant symptom. And the mood disturbance must be persistent, not shifting frequently to anxiety or anger. The second criterion requires the presence of at least four of the following circumstantial symptoms, nearly every day for at least 2 weeks: (1) significant appetite or weight changes; (2) insomnia or hypersomnia; (3) psychomotor agitation or retardation (we will return to this feature); (4) apathy and loss of interest or pleasure in usual activities; (5) lethargy and fatigue; (6) feelings of worthlessness, guilt, or self-reproach; (7) cognitive impairment (e.g., slowed thinking, poor concentration, indecisiveness), without marked incoherence; (8) recurrent thoughts of death or suicide, or suicide attempts.

The operational distinction separating dysthymic disorder from major depression is that the severity is not sufficient to meet the criteria for a major depressive episode. In addition, the limits on duration and persistence are redefined: Depressive symptoms must have been present most or all the time for 2 years, but manifestations of depression may be separated by periods of normal mood lasting days, weeks, or even a few months. The list of circumstantial symptoms is expanded to include the following, in addition to the eight just listed: (1) decreased effectiveness or productivity, (2) social withdrawal, (3) irritability, (4) nonresponsiveness to praise or rewards, (5) pessimism or brooding, and (6) frequent crying.

Susceptibility to major depression and dysthymic disorder is correlated with sex and age. Among the adult population in the United States and Europe, 18 to 23 percent of

Table 18-3. *Major depression versus dysthymic disorder*

Criteria	Major depression	Dysthymic disorder
Dysphoric mood		
Severity	Great	Less severe
Duration	At least 2 weeks	At least 2 years
Persistence	Nearly continuous	May be intermittent
Circumstantial symptoms	*At least four:*	*At least three:*
	Appetite or weight changes	Any of those listed under Major Depression *or*
	Sleep disturbances	Decreased effectiveness
	Psychomotor agitation or retardation	Social withdrawal
	Apathy	Irritability
	Lethargy	Nonresponsiveness to rewards
	Low self-esteem	Pessimism or brooding
	Cognitive impairment	Frequent crying
	Thoughts of death or suicide, or suicide attempts	
Physiologic correlates		
Barbiturate sleep threshold	Lowered	Elevated
Insulin responsiveness	Resistant	Normal
Stress response	Depressed	Normal
Pharmacologic responsiveness	Antidepressants clearly superior to other choices	No consistently effective drug treatment; anxiolytics $\simeq$ neuroleptics $>$ antidepressants

females and 8 to 11 percent of males have experienced at least one major depressive episode. Hospitalization for major depression has been required in 6 percent of adult females, and 3 percent of adult males. Dysthymic disorder is also more common in adult women than in adult men, but, interestingly, equally common in girls and boys, suggesting that either sex hormone differences or societal sex-role stereotyping may be a factor in predisposing to depression.

Endogenous versus Exogenous (Reactive) Depression

A fourth dichotomous concept of depression is the endogenous versus exogenous (or reactive) distinction. This distinction relates to etiology and characteristic symptoms and carries implications for prognosis. Endogenous depression is depression arising from within the individual, presumably at the organic level of organization, while reactive depression is triggered by an obvious, identifiable precipitant at the psychological or interpersonal level of organization. The presence of a precipitant does not, however, exclude the possibility of an endogenous contribution or "predisposition." And even when the etiology in a given case can be clearly ascribed to one level or another, one

Table 18-4. Endogenous versus reactive depression

Characteristic	Endogenous	Reactive
Etiology		
Onset	Gradual	Sudden
Precipitant	No or yes	Yes
Manifestations		
Somatic symptoms	Many	Few
Subjective impression	Not appropriate	Appropriate
Impairment of functioning	Great	Mild
Responsiveness		
Duration	Prolonged	Often brief
Spontaneous remission	Low	High
Environmental responsiveness	Low	High
Tricyclic responsiveness	High	Low-moderate

can rest assured that the manifestations of depression will ramify to each of the three levels of organization that contribute to psychological health: the organic, psychological, and interpersonal systemic. Nevertheless, the distinction between endogenous and exogenous depression provides some useful specifications (Table 18-4).

Endogenous depression is more likely than the exogenous type to entail significant somatic symptoms, such as appetite changes, altered psychomotor activity levels, and depressed stress responses. Reactive depression is usually experienced by the patient as comprehensible and appropriate in view of the precipitating circumstances. The patient knows why he or she is depressed. In endogenous depression, the patient does not understand the cause of the depression and feels helpless to correct it. The level of functional impairment is generally greater in endogenous depression.

As regards prognosis, exogenous depression is more responsive to serendipidous improvements in life circumstances and exhibits a fairly high rate of spontaneous remission. It is also more responsive to psychotherapeutic intervention, especially to supportive therapy. On the other hand, endogenous depression exhibits greater responsiveness to tricyclic antidepressant treatment, although exogenous depression also often responds. About 20 percent of cases of depression are endogenous and about 80 percent are exogenous. These are only estimates, since there is considerable variation in the application of these terms in practice.

Major Depression, with or without Melancholia

Some cases of major depression also meet the more restrictive set of criteria for melancholia. In this form of major depression, there is a marked anhedonia (loss of pleasure in all or most activities and a lack of responsiveness to rewarding or pleasurable stimuli). In addition, at least three of the following characteristics must be present: a quality of depressed mood distinct from a normal grief reaction; worsening of the depressed mood in the morning; early morning awakenings; marked psychomotor agitation or retardation; weight loss and anorexia; and excessive or inappropriate feelings of guilt. Melancholia lies at the severe end of the spectrum of depressive states. Whether it differs from other cases of major depression qualitatively or quantitatively is a matter of dispute.

Typical versus Atypical Depression

Although most patients suffering unipolar depression meet the criteria for either major depression or dysthymic disorder, some patients are not so readily classified. DSM-III provides a category for such residual cases, designated "Atypical Depression." This label can be employed for patients who deviate from the criteria for the two specific classifications of unipolar disorders, because, for example, the symptomatic criteria of major depression are absent or because the intermittent periods of normal mood exceed two months in a patient otherwise manifesting dysthymic disorder. These examples of atypical depression are varied and, by definition, lack a unitary pattern of presentation.

Another use of the term "atypical depression" is the designation of a distinctive form of depression characterized by recurrent short-lived depressive episodes resulting from personal rejection or loss of romantic attachment, and marked by lethargy, fatigue, hypersomnia, chronic anxiety, overeating and weight gain, and phobias. There is some evidence that MAO inhibitors may be of preferential value in this form of depression.

Agitated versus Retarded Depression

One last dichotomous concept of depression is the distinction between patients exhibiting psychomotor agitation and those experiencing psychomotor retardation. This characterization is highly specific, focusing on a particular symptom. The value of this distinction relates to drug selection. Since many of the antidepressants show approximately equivalent overall efficacy in depression, the selection of a particular drug is often based on matching it with the patient's psychomotor activity level. Antidepressants with significant sedative potential are utilized in agitated patients, while nonsedative drugs are selected for patients exhibiting pronounced psychomotor retardation or marked withdrawal.

Neurochemical Theories of Depression

Norepinephrine Hypothesis of Affective Disorders

The norepinephrine hypothesis asserts that affective disorders are related to an imbalance in the concentration of norepinephrine available to its postsynaptic receptors (Table 18-5). In depression, the concentrations are postulated to be subnormal, while in mania, the opposite of depression, it is supposed that levels of norepinephrine in the synapse are excessive. Cerebrospinal fluid (CSF) levels of the norepinephrine metabolite 3-methoxy-4-hydroxyphenylglycoaldehyde (MHPG) are considered to be a good index of norepinephrine activity (turnover) in the brain. The CSF levels of MHPG are frequently low in depressed patients, but increase after spontaneous or drug-induced recovery. The CSF levels of MHPG are high during mania and low during depression in manic-depressive disorder. Perhaps the strongest evidence in support of the norepinephrine hypothesis, however, is what is known about the neurochemical interactions of antidepressants with norepinephrine-containing neurons. The reader is advised to review that portion of Chapter 6 dealing with norepinephrine.

If, indeed, depression is related to a deficiency of free norepinephrine, an effective therapy would lead to an increase in free norepinephrine, one way or another. Each of the subgroups of antidepressant agents does, in fact, accomplish an increase in free norepinephrine concentrations, although the specific mechanism involved differs between groups. Both the MAO inhibitors and the tricyclic antidepressants act by slowing the inactivation process. The MAO inhibitors retard the metabolic degradation of

Table 18-5. *Neurochemical theories of depression*

Theory	Depression	Mania
Norepinephrine	Low	High
Permissive	Low 5-HT and low NE	Low 5-HT and high NE
Two-disease	NE type: low NE 5-HT type: low 5-HT	No specification
Down-regulation	Supersensitive NE receptors	Subsensitive NE receptors

NE, norepinephrine; 5-HT, 5-hydroxytryptamine (serotonin).

catecholamines, while the tricyclic antidepressants slow the reuptake of released norepinephrine back into the presynaptic nerve terminals. Some of the new generation of atypical antidepressants block presynaptic receptors, reducing feedback regulation of norepinephrine synthesis and release, thus allowing synaptic concentrations of the transmitter to increase. The CNS stimulants, such as amphetamine, sometimes used for short periods as antidepressants, act by releasing stored catecholamines, norepinephrine and dopamine, from storage vesicles. The norepinephrine hypothesis is also supported by the fact that drugs that deplete norepinephrine, such as reserpine and α-methylparatyrosine, cause depression. Thus, at first blush, the neuropharmacology of drugs that cause depression or are used to treat it appears to be uniformly supportive of the norepinephrine theory.

On the other hand, a number of observations seem to run counter to the norepinephrine hypothesis. (1) Both the tricyclic antidepressants and the MAO inhibitors require about 10 days to 2 weeks of administration before clinical effectiveness is observed, but the respective biochemical alterations in norepinephrine reuptake or degradation occur immediately in laboratory animals. (2) Some drugs in the new breed of atypical antidepressants do not alter either degradation or reuptake of norepinephrine. (3) The relative efficacy of a series of tricyclic antidepressants does not correlate well with potency in blocking reuptake. (4) Long-term use of tricyclic antidepressants leads to down-regulation, or subsensitivity, of postsynaptic norepinephrine receptors.

These apparently contradictory observations will be addressed later in the chapter in relation to the mechanism of action of tricyclic antidepressants. These contradictions have forced development of a more sophisticated understanding of how the various antidepressants bring about clinical improvement in depression, but the norepinephrine hypothesis itself survives the challenge, for the time being at least.

Permissive Theory

At about the same time that the norepinephrine hypothesis began to emerge, other researchers focused attention on another neurotransmitter, serotonin. A serotonin theory of depression was advanced that postulated that depression is related to low serotonin and mania is related to high serotonin. The serotonin hypothesis in this early form has not stood the test of time or experimentation. In fact, elevated serotonin levels are now known to be related to depression of CNS activity and onset of sleep (see Chap. 10), a flat contradiction of the serotonin hypothesis of depression. Also, drugs that deplete serotonin by blocking its synthesis (e.g., PCPA) cause hyperexcitability, not depression. Nevertheless, another, more useful theory, the permissive theory, has arisen from the ashes of the serotonin theory, and it combines elements of both the norepinephrine and serotonin theories.

According to the permissive theory, low-serotonin functional activity is a prerequisite for both depression and mania (Table 18-5). Insufficient serotonin activity is seen as having a destabilizing effect on mood, predisposing to either depression or mania. The actual outcome, mania or depression, is determined, in this view, by the norepinephrine functional state. Thus, depression occurs when serotonin is low and norepinephrine is also low; mania occurs when serotonin is low and norepinephrine is high.

This theory is useful in explaining why some depressed patients respond to the serotonin precursor 5-hydroxytryptophan (5-HTP). It also helps to explain the effectiveness of certain tricyclic antidepressants that act almost exclusively to block serotonin rather than norepinephrine reuptake. And it has been observed that about half of depressed patients exhibit a significantly reduced serotonin turnover rate in the brain, as measured by accumulation of the serotonin metabolite 5-hydroxyindoleacetic acid (5-HIAA) in the CSF following probenecid treatment. The permissive theory also opens up possibilities for defining the mechanism of lithium by relating it to the serotonin system. But the theory falls short in its failure to account for why so few depressed patients respond to 5-HTP. The two-disease theory attempts to rectify this shortcoming.

Two-Disease Theory

The two-disease theory postulates that depression occurs as a result of either low norepinephrine *or* low serotonin, and that there are therefore two types of depression, the norepinephrine type and the serotonin type (see Table 18-5). This theory is designed to explain the variable responsiveness to 5-HTP. Considerable effort has been directed toward trying to define clinical distinctions or diagnostic predictors of 5-HTP responsiveness that would support the idea of two neurochemical types of depression. Thus far, the only supporting evidence comes from studies indicating that patients with low serotonin turnover (determined by measurement of 5-HIAA levels in the CSF after probenecid) respond better to tricyclics that are potent in blocking the reuptake of serotonin. Unfortunately, the probenecid method for determining serotonin turnover in the brain does not lend itself to routine application in the evaluation of patients.

Antidepressants

The group of agents known as antidepressants began their clinical history in the late 1950s with the nearly simultaneous entrance of the MAO inhibitors and the tricyclic antidepressants. The former group is now generally considered too toxic, at least by American clinicians, while the latter group is still widely applied to clinical practice. Antidepressants are employed in major depression and are superior to other drug treatments in that condition. Antidepressants also find use in dysthymic disorder, but with less success overall than alternative drug treatments. In severe depression, chemotherapy may be adjunctive to electroconvulsant shock. The greatest success has been with endogenous depression. Reactive and episodic depressions are less appropriately and less successfully treated with drugs.

Tricyclic Antidepressants

The foremost class of drugs used for depression is the tricyclic antidepressant class. Ironically, the chemical structure and the spectrum of side effects of the tricyclic antidepressants closely resemble the phenothiazine tranquilizers (Table 18-6). Like the

Table 18-6. Various types of adverse reactions to tricyclic antidepressants

Clinical features	Anticholinergic	Cardiovascular	Allergies and dyscrasias	Psychiatric and neurologic	Endocrine
Symptoms	Blurred vision Mydriasis Acute glaucoma Dryness of mouth Sweating Constipation Urinary retention Paralytic ileus Tachycardia Dysmnesia Mental confusion	Orthostatic hypotension Heart block Arrhythmias	Cholestatic jaundice Skin rashes Agranulocytosis	Sedation (especially with tertiary amines) Drowsiness Excess stimulation Mood switch Tremors Epileptiform seizures Peripheral neuropathies Mild pseudoparkinsonism	Galactorrhea Amenorrhea Loss of libido Weight gain
Period of maximal risk	Common, early	Common, early	Early, rare	Persistent	Persistent
Clinical response options	Tolerance occurs	Tolerance occurs	Interrupt treatment; symptoms may or may not recur with resumption	Adjust dose	Adjust dose

phenothiazines, the tricyclics possess anticholinergic and antihistaminergic properties. The anticholinergic side effects include sedation, jaundice, mild parkinsonian symptoms, hypotension, dryness of the mouth, dizziness, constipation, tachycardia, palpitations, blurred vision, excessive sweating, and impotence. Such anticholinergic effects can be additive with those produced by other drugs (see Appendix B, *Anticholinergic Syndrome*). Both somnolence and insomnia occur during the early stages of therapy. Occasionally, manic reactions and toxic confusional states are reported. Fortunately, tolerance develops to the anticholinergic and antihistaminergic effects, so that only the jaundice and parkinsonism tend to persist or grow worse with continued drug treatment. There is no dependence with the tricyclic antidepressants. The effect on the EEG is an increase in both beta-wave and slow-wave activity, with diminished alpha-wave activity and no change in wave amplitude.

Mechanism of Action

The conventional view of the mechanism of action of tricyclic antidepressants attributed clinical efficacy to the ability of these drugs to block the reuptake of norepinephrine and perhaps of serotonin as well. Taken at face value, this interpretation of the mechanism of action of the tricyclics fits well with the norepinephrine hypothesis of depression. Blockade of reuptake would elevate the levels of free norepinephrine in the synapse, increasing postsynaptic receptor activation. The problem with this straightforward view is that there is a lack of correlation between the respective time courses for blockade of reuptake (which occurs acutely) and clinical efficacy (which requires 1 to 2 weeks). This and other discrepancies have led to a revised view that emphasizes the dynamic nature of adaptive neural mechanisms when a drug is used chronically (Figure 18-1). In this view, the immediate effect of tricyclics, blockade of reuptake, is largely offset by compensatory short-term adjustments in norepinephrine neurons, mediated by presynaptic receptors. With continued use of the antidepressant medication, the short-term compensatory adjustments undergo tolerance, but the primary effect, blockade of reuptake, does not undergo tolerance. Long-term adaptations begin to set in after 2 to 3 weeks of use, but these do not completely offset the direct effect of the drug on reuptake. Rather, the long-term adaptations are a reflection of the increased efficiency of norepinephrine transmission. The overall effect, after 3 weeks or so of treatment, is a more efficient neural system, stabilized against depression, with less sensitive postsynaptic receptors but more free norepinephrine to act on those receptors.

A competing hypothesis to explain the contrary observations regarding tricyclic action is called the down-regulation hypothesis. This view emphasizes the subsensitivity that develops at the postsynaptic noradrenergic receptors with long-term tricyclic administration. Accordingly, the hypothesis postulates that depression is related to the hypersensitivity of noradrenergic receptors; that is, excess, not insufficient, noradrenergic functional activity. Tricyclic therapy is seen as desensitizing the overactive postsynaptic receptors. This view is diametrically opposed to the norepinephrine hypothesis of depression.

The problem with the theory is that it cannot explain the depressive influence of norepinephrine-synthesis blockers and receptor blockers or the excitatory and antidepressant effect of catecholamine precursors, releasers, or degradation inhibitors. On the other hand, the observation that antidepressants decrease formation of cyclic adenosine monophosphate by adenyl cyclase associated with certain catecholamine receptors supports the down-regulation view and is contrary to the theory illustrated in Figure 18-1.

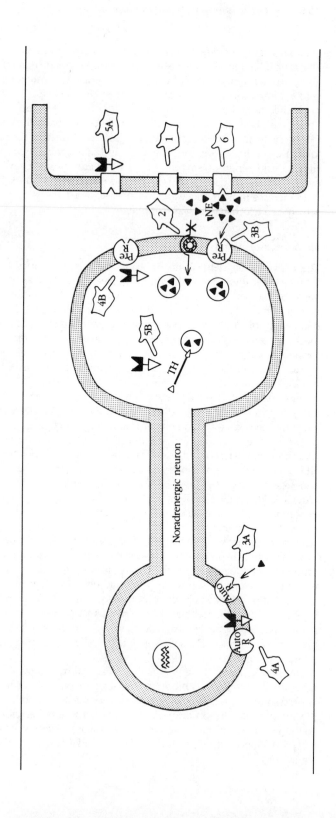

Clinical Effectiveness

Since 1957, when antidepressants first became available to medical practice, numerous studies of depression have been conducted to evaluate various antidepressants against each other and against electroconvulsant therapy, other psychotropic drugs, and placebos. Many of the studies have been hampered by the difficulties that compound the whole area of clinical studies. Moreover, the fact that close to half of depressed patients recover spontaneously further clouds evaluation of studies involving antidepressants.

With respect to general efficacy in depression, it can be said that imipramine, the most widely studied of the antidepressants, is significantly better than placebo or psychotherapy alone, although the margin of the difference is not great (approximately one-fourth of those not responsive to psychotherapy or placebo alone respond to the drug). In comparison with imipramine, amitriptyline is consistently found to be as good and sometimes better. Overall, about 65 to 70 percent of inpatients benefit from a well-planned trial with antidepressant medication as against the 50 percent spontaneous recovery rate. However, overall drug treatment benefits fewer patients than does electroconvulsant therapy, and the response to electroconvulsant therapy is considerably more rapid. However, it entails greater cost and the risk of debilitating effects on brain functioning. Other drug treatments of major depression, including neuroleptics, anxiolytics, and combinations of antidepressants with neuroleptics or anxiolytics, are no more effective than antidepressant medication alone and, in fact, are usually less effective.

Three classes of drugs have been employed in dysthymic disorder, partly because no one class has proved to be consistently effective. Tricyclic antidepressants, neuroleptics (usually thioridazine, acetophenazine, or thiothixene), and anxiolytics (e.g., diazepam or chlordiazepoxide) are all commonly used. Anxiolytics are perhaps the most effective medication for dysthymic disorder, especially if the treatment period is to be brief and the condition has been long-term but relatively mild, which is the usual case. Neuroleptics appear most effective when depressive neurosis is severe and of recent origin.

Fig. 18-1. *Mechanism of action of tricyclic antidepressants. Depression is associated with diminished functional activity at norepinephrine (NE) synapses [1]. (Serotonin may also be involved in some instances.) The problem may be of biochemical origin or a reaction to personal crisis. The primary and immediate biochemical action of tricyclic antidepressants is blockade of reuptake of NE [2] and/or serotonin, which prolongs the presence of released transmitter in the synapse. This potentially beneficial acute effect is largely offset in the short run by compensatory adjustments in the NE transmission process. Free NE acts on autoreceptors (Auto R) [3A] to slow neuronal firing rate (autoinhibition) and on presynaptic receptors (Pre R) [3B] to reduce transmitter synthesis and release. The result is a reduction in turnover that negates the reuptake blockade. With chronic administration of tricyclics, adaptation occurs in the compensatory mechanisms but not to the primary effect of tricyclic drugs on reuptake. Subsensitivity is exhibited by both the autoreceptors [4A] and the presynaptic receptors [4B], developing over about 2–3 weeks of daily tricyclic administration. As a result, feedback suppression of firing rate and turnover after a given dose in a chronic regimen offsets the primary action less completely than was the case acutely. Other adaptive changes (down-regulation of postsynaptic receptors [5A] and decreases in the activity of the synthetic enzyme, tyrosine hydroxylase [5B]) are reflective of, rather than the cause of, increased efficiency of the transmission process. Clinical efficacy correlates with occurrence of the long-term adaptive changes. The net effect is more postsynaptic receptor activity [6] and a more efficient neural system, less taxing on metabolic capacity for renewal and more resilient to suppression by neural inputs related to adverse experiences.*

Tricyclic antidepressants are the least effective of the three classes of drugs in dysthymic disorder.

The findings with respect to efficacy of maintenance antidepressant therapy for major depression are less clear than are the data on acute treatment of depression. A study of 72 depressed female patients [8] showed that relapse rates were substantially lower in amitriptyline-treated patients than in those receiving placebo or no medication.

Although therapeutic effectiveness is delayed with the tricyclic antidepressants, side effects begin to develop immediately on initiation of treatment. The influence of the therapist's attitude on the outcome of therapy may be especially critical during this early period. The patient may become discouraged because of side effects and the absence of therapeutic benefits and may discontinue taking the medication. Adequate forewarning and reassurance during the initial stages of treatment will help to prevent this. Suicide liability is elevated during the initial period of drug treatment, so patient monitoring and supportive psychotherapy should be intensified.

Variations Within the Class

Selection of a particular tricyclic antidepressant is seldom based on efficacy, since the available drugs are generally comparable in generating a clinical response. The main consideration, then, is the extent of sedation produced by a particular drug. The more sedative antidepressants are utilized in agitated patients, while the nonsedative drugs are used in patients who exhibit psychomotor retardation (Table 18-7).

The tricyclic antidepressants can be usefully divided into two subgroups: the tertiary amines and the secondary amines. The tertiary amines include amitriptyline (Elavil), imipramine (Tofranil, Presamine, Janimine), doxepine (Sinequan, Adapin), and trimipramine (Surmontil). The secondary amines include nortriptyline (Aventyl), desipramine (Norpramine, Pertofrane), protriptyline (Vivactil), and amoxapine (Ascendin). The tertiary amines have a relatively greater effect on serotonin than on norepinephrine reuptake, while the reverse is true of the secondary amines. Consequently, the tertiary amines are more sedative. Maprotiline (Ludiomil) is a tetracyclic compound and resembles the secondary amines.

Variables Predicting Responsiveness to Tricyclic Antidepressants

The general finding from studies of the influence of patient variables on the response to tricyclic therapy can be summarized as follows: Patients with more adequate personal and social resources and patients with realistic attitudes toward their condition respond better. Other disorder-related variables of significance, alluded to earlier in the chapter, are the observations that acute and endogenous forms of depression respond well to tricyclic therapy, and chronic and exogenous respond less well. As regards selection of a particular tricyclic drug, an interesting observation is that patients responding to serotonin-blocking tricyclics (notably amitriptyline) had significantly lower pretreatment CSF concentrations of 5-HIAA and higher urinary concentrations of the norepinephrine metabolite MHPG than did nonresponders. On the other hand, patients responding to tricyclics that significantly block norepinephrine reuptake show high pretreatment levels of 5-HIAA in the CSF but low urinary MHPG. Tests of biogenic amine metabolites, especially those requiring CSF sampling, are far from routine, however.

Dosage and Dosage Schedules

Tricyclic antidepressants show considerable variability in dosage requirements from patient to patient. We noted in an earlier chapter a similar variability in dosage require-

Table 18-7. *Comparison of tertiary and secondary amines*

Drug	Effect on		Side effects	
	NE	5-HT	Sedative	Anticholinergic
Tertiary amines				
Amitriptyline	0	++++	+++	++++
Imipramine	++	+++	++	+++
Doxepin	0	+++	+++	+++
Secondary amines				
Nortriptyline	++	++	+	+++
Desipramine	++++	0	0	++
Protriptyline	++	0	0	+++

0, no effect; one to four plusses, weakest to strongest effect.

ments for neuroleptics, but the reasons and implications are dissimilar. In the case of tricyclic antidepressants, the variability is largely due to differences in pharmacokinetic factors, namely, absorption and metabolism. Once the dosage is adjusted to produce plasma levels in the established therapeutic range, clinical effectiveness occurs with reasonable predictability. So, while neuroleptic doses are titrated against alleviation of symptoms or occurrence of adverse effects, tricyclic doses can be and should be titrated against plasma concentrations to produce a plasma level within the therapeutic "window." Typical dosages for young adults are listed for various tricyclics in the final section of the chapter. Elderly patients should receive substantially lower doses: one-fourth the dosage at the lower end of the dosage range and half the dosage at the upper end.

Initially, doses are usually small and divided, typically three times daily. The dosage is gradually increased based on plasma levels (ideally) or on efficacy and side effects (the actual practice in many facilities). If sedation poses a problem, all or most of the daily allotment can be given at bedtime. A single nighttime dose is usually given in maintenance applications.

Additional Uses of Imipramine

A psychopathologic condition that frequently responds dramatically to treatment with imipramine is the episodic panic disorder. Indeed, responsiveness to imipramine can be an important aid in identifying patients in this group and in defining the nosologic grouping itself. Imipramine has been found to be similarly effective in blocking separation panic in school-phobic children.

Imipramine has also been used in treating functional enuresis. Relatively small doses are used (15 to 50 mg daily), so the incidence of side effects is low. Imipramine is highly effective in reducing the number of episodes during the period of its use, but recidivism is high when the drug is discontinued. Psychotherapeutic approaches should be considered preferentially in the treatment of enuresis.

Monoamine Oxidase Inhibitors

Although many MAO inhibitors have been synthesized and examined, only three are currently marketed as antidepressants, and a fourth is available as an antihypertensive.

The three antidepressant MAO inhibitors currently available are isocarboxazid (Marplan), phenelzine (Nardil), and tranylcypromine (Parnate). Tranylcypromine, the most widely used member of this class, has been employed successfully in reactive and psychoneurotic depressions as well as in involutional melancholia. Phenelzine has been employed alone or with chlordiazepoxide in various psychoneuroses with favorable results.

The EEG effect of MAO inhibition is a general decrease in wave amplitude with no shifting in frequency distribution or production of epilepsy-related electrical phenomena. The MAO inhibitors are one of the most toxic groups of psychoactive drugs. Side effects that occur most frequently include convulsions brought on by excess stimulation, orthostatic hypotension, liver toxicity, and weight gain.

In part, MAO-inhibitor toxicity is a result of the lack of specificity inherent in the mechanism of action. Monoamine oxidase is an important enzyme that metabolizes many endogenous as well as exogenous substances. Inhibition of MAO increases the concentrations of all the substances, not just the catecholamines. Many foods prepared by a fermentation process, such as beer, cheese, and wine, contain an amine (tyramine) that elevates blood pressure and is broken down by MAO. In the normal person, the effect of tyramine is slight and transient because it is rapidly metabolized by liver and platelet MAO. In the patient taking an MAO inhibitor, the effect of tyramine on blood pressure is greatly exacerbated, and the patient may suffer a hypertensive crisis if such foods are eaten indiscriminately. This interaction of MAO inhibitors with certain foods is one of the most important examples of interactions between drugs and diet.

Many drugs are metabolized by MAO, including barbiturates, cocaine, meperidine, and aminopyrine. Any drug metabolized by MAO will have a prolonged and intensified activity in the presence of MAO inhibition. Thus, the drug regimen of a patient on an MAO inhibitor must be carefully reviewed for drug interactions.

There is a delay of days or weeks after the initiation of MAO-inhibitor treatment before therapeutic efficacy is attained. A stimulant may be prescribed during this period if immediate improvement is deemed necessary, but the risk of excessive stimulation is exceedingly great with such a combination. One MAO inhibitor tranylcypromine uniquely combines inhibition of MAO with a direct stimulatory effect and therefore has a more rapid onset of therapeutic effectiveness.

The problems and toxicity involved with MAO inhibitors have curtailed their use in recent years. They are now generally considered inferior to the tricyclics. Some investigators have suggested that MAO inhibitors are especially effective in atypical depressions marked by brief recurrent depressive reactions and a constellation of somatic symptomatology including lethargy, fatigue, hypersomnia, overeating, and chronic anxiety.

Atypical Antidepressants

A new generation of atypical antidepressants is currently in various stages of development. These drugs are structurally unrelated to the tricyclics and differ from them in one or more pharmacologic actions. Some, such as nisoxetine and viloxazine, block reuptake of norepinephrine with no effect on serotonin reuptake. Some, such as amoxapine, trazodone (Desyrel), and nomifensine, though similar to tricyclics in blocking the reuptake of norepinephrine or serotonin (or both), possess no anticholinergic properties. Fluoxetine is specific in blocking the reuptake of serotonin. Mianserin lacks anticholinergic properties and does not block the reuptake of any of the biogenic amines. It appears to act on presynaptic (α-2) noradrenergic receptors. Initial clinical trials have shown mianserin to be effective in depression and devoid of adverse effects. Caroxazone is a newly developed MAO inhibitor that is much shorter-acting than conventional MAO inhibitors. It is devoid of anticholinergic, antihistaminergic, and antiserotonergic effects. Trozodone was approved for use in 1982. Amoxapine and caroxazone are into advanced stages of clinical testing; several of the others are in an early phase of clinical trials in the United States.

Stimulants Used as Antidepressants

Catecholamine-releasing stimulants, discussed in detail in Chapter 13, occasionally find application as antidepressants, although there are several disadvantages to their use. The most obvious problem is that rebound depression invariably follows their use as a result of the exhaustion of amine stores. A second serious concern is the risk of the development of dependence with chronic use. Because of these limitations, use of amphetamine and similar drugs is confined to interim treatment or short-term treatment of mild reactive depression when an immediate response is deemed necessary.

Implications for Psychotherapy

Psychotherapists must develop an awareness of the frequent involvement of depressant drugs, especially alcohol, in producing or aggravating depression. Significant consumption of alcohol or the use of depressant drugs commonly leads to increased depression. A person suffering depression should decrease or eliminate drinking or ad lib use of hypnotics or daytime sedatives, whether or not there is unequivocal evidence of a history of problems with the drug. The therapist might suggest elimination of, or sharp reduction in, consumption as an experiment for a period of several weeks. More often than not, patients will experience noticeable improvement in depressive symptoms.

Any of the antidepressants, particularly in combinations, can produce excess stimulation. On the other hand, toxic doses of tricyclic antidepressants may produce sedation, depression, or even coma. The MAO inhibitors and stimulants may trigger recurrence of schizophrenic symptoms. The tricyclics can precipitate either manic or hypomanic responses, fatigue, or somnolence.

Side effects of drugs in the antidepressant class may appear to be psychiatric symptoms. Headaches and dizziness may occur with tricyclics or MAO inhibitors. Muscle twitches, weakness, tremors, or outright convulsions may occur with the tricyclics. Mild tremors are observed in 10 percent of patients, but more severe motor impairments are rare. Other psychiatric side effects of tricyclics include mood switches, confusion and dysmnesia, and loss of libido. Various autonomic and gastrointestinal effects, including impotence, are related to the anticholinergic properties of the tricyclics. Impotence may have an important psychological significance to the patient.

During the early stages of treatment with either tricyclics or MAO inhibitors, annoying side effects may appear before the onset of therapeutic effectiveness. The patient may become discouraged and discontinue taking the medication. Also, suicide liability rises during initial drug therapy. The therapist can be instrumental in assuring that the patient is adequately forewarned and provided with supportive therapy during the early phase of treatment.

State dependency has not been reported to occur with antidepressants other than such stimulants as amphetamine. The antidepressants other than the stimulants are not potent primary reinforcers in spite of their interaction with catecholamine nerve terminals. They are, in fact, seldom abused and probably do not interact in any adverse way with psychotherapeutic efforts.

Consultation with the prescribing physician is in order when dealing with a patient taking an antidepressant.

Medically Important Antidepressant Agents

amitriptyline (Elavil, Triavil [combined with perphenazine], Etrafon [combined with perphenazine]), a tricyclic antidepressant, tertiary amine. Typical: 100 to 200 mg. Extremes: 40 to 300 mg.

amoxapine (Ascendin), a tricyclic antidepressant, secondary amine. Typical: 75 to 300 mg.

amphetamine (Benzedrine), a stimulant: primarily used for narcolepsy and hyperkinesis; largely superseded by other agents as an anorectic and antidepressant. Narcolepsy: 20 to 100 mg. Hyperkinesis (children over 5): 10 to 30 mg.

desipramine (desmethylimipramine) (Norpramin, Pertofrane), a tricyclic antidepressant, secondary amine. Typical: 75 to 200 mg. Extremes: 50 to 300 mg.

dextroamphetamine (Dexedrine), a D-isomer of amphetamine: see amphetamine.

doxepin (Sinequan, Adapin), a tricyclic antidepressant, tertiary amine. Typical: 75 to 150 mg. Extremes: 25 to 300 mg.

imipramine (Tofranil, Presamine, Janimine), a tricyclic antidepressant, tertiary amine. Typical: 100 to 250 mg. Extremes: 30 to 300 mg.

isocarboxazid (Marplan), a MAO-inhibitor antidepressant. Typical: 20 to 30 mg. Extremes: 10 to 30 mg.

maprotiline (Ludiomil), a tetracyclic antidepressant. Typical: 75 to 225 mg. Extremes: 50 to 300 mg.

methylphenidate (Ritalin), an amphetamine-like stimulant: used in mild depression (but see text), hyperkinesis, and narcolepsy. Hyperkinesis and narcolepsy: 10 to 60 mg.

nortriptyline (Aventyl), a tricyclic antidepressant, secondary amine. Typical: 75 to 100 mg. Extremes: 20 to 150 mg.

phenelzine (Nardil), an MAO inhibitor. Typical: 30 to 60 mg. Extremes: 15 to 75 mg.

protriptyline (Vivactil), a tricyclic antidepressant, secondary amine: psychomotor-stimulating properties. Typical: 30 to 60 mg. Extremes: 10 to 120 mg.

tranylcypromine (Parnate), an MAO-inhibitor antidepressant: some amphetamine-like stimulant properties. Typical: 20 to 30 mg. Extremes: 10 to 60 mg.

trazodone (Desyrel), an atypical antidepressant. Typical: 150 mg.

trimipramine (Surmontil), a tricyclic antidepressant, tertiary amine. Typical: 75 to 150 mg. Extremes: 50 to 300 mg.

Selected References and Further Readings

1. Committee on Nomenclature and Statistics of the American Psychiatric Association. *Diagnostic and Statistical Manual* (3rd ed.). Washington, D.C.: American Psychiatric Association, 1980.
2. Enna, S. J., Malick, J. B., and Richelson, E. *Antidepressants: Neurochemical, Behavioral and Clinical Perspectives.* New York: Raven, 1981.
3. Gilman, A. G., Goodman, L. S., and Gilman, A. *The Pharmacological Basis of Therapeutics* (6th ed.). New York: Macmillan, 1980.
4. Hollister, L. E. Psychiatric Disorders. In K. L. Melmon and H. F. Morrelli (Eds.), *Clinical Pharmacology* (2nd ed.). New York: Macmillan, 1978.

5. Klein, D. F., and Gittelman-Klein, R. (Eds.). *Progress in Psychiatric Drug Treatment.* New York: Brunner/Mazel, 1975.
6. Kupfer, D. J., and Detre, T. P. Tricyclic and Monoamine-Oxidase Inhibitor Antidepressants: Clinical Use. In L. L. Iversen et al. (Eds.), *Handbook of Psychopharmacology.* New York: Plenum, 1978. Vol. 14.
7. Lipton, M. A., DiMascio, A., and Killam, K. F. (Eds.). *Psychopharmacology: A Generation of Progress.* New York: Raven, 1978.
8. Paykel, E. S., Klerman, G. L., DiMascio, A., Weissman, M. M., and Prusoff, B. A. Maintenance Antidepressants, Psychotherapy, Symptoms, and Social Function. In J. O. Cole et al. (Eds.), *Psychopathology and Psychopharmacology.* Baltimore: Johns Hopkins University Press, 1973.
9. van Praag, H. M. Amine Hypotheses of Affective Disorders. In L. L. Iversen et al. (Eds.), *Handbook of Psychopharmacology.* New York: Plenum, 1978. Vol. 13.

Manic-Depressive Disorder and Lithium

19

Manic-Depressive Disorder

The *sine qua non* of manic-depressive disorder is the occurrence of one or more manic episodes. The depressive component is secondary and need not be present. Therefore, a good starting point in examining this disorder is to review the characteristics of a manic episode [1].

There are four fundamental sets of criteria (Table 19-1): the mood disturbance itself, associated behavioral manifestations, duration, and exclusions. The mood itself is elevated and energetic. The patient may feel irritable or euphoric. The high energy level is reflected in behavioral changes such as talkativeness, continuous activity, and racing from one idea and one project to another. The duration of these behaviors must exceed 1 week, and the symptoms must not be attributable to other disorders, such as schizophrenia, intoxication, or organic brain syndrome.

When a patient has one or more such episodes, five diagnostic categories may be employed in defining the condition: bipolar, mixed; bipolar, manic; bipolar, depressed; atypical bipolar (bipolar II); and cyclothymic personality. The first three are similar in severity. The term following *bipolar* in each case describes the current state of the patient. *Mixed* is used when manic and depressive episodes are intermixed or rapidly alternating every few days. A typical bipolar disorder is characterized by recurrent major depressive episodes with intervening manic periods of only modest intensity (called hypomanic episodes). This type of bipolar syndrome is easily mistaken for (unipolar) major depression. The designation *cyclothymic personality* is used when a person has frequent periods of manic and depressive symptoms, but not of sufficient severity to warrant the designation of bipolar disorder. Unlike the relationship between dysthymic disorder and major depression, the relationship between cyclothymic disorder and bipolar disorder is clearly a matter of degree of severity only. Symptoms typical of cyclothymic personality disorder are listed in Table 19-2. Cyclothymic personality disorder is diagnosed more commonly in women than in men. By contrast, bipolar disorder is equally common in men and women, occurring in about 0.4 to 1.2 percent of the adult population.

Lithium

Lithium salts have been used successfully in mania and in manic-depressive disorder since 1954 and appear to be superior to the phenothiazines in these conditions. Before

Table 19-1. *Criteria for a manic episode*

Mood disturbance
  Elevated, expansive, or irritable mood
Behavioral symptoms (at least three):
  Increased activity (e.g., physical, social, occupational, sexual)
  Pressure to keep talking
  Flight of ideas
  Grandiosity
  Decreased need for sleep
  Distractability
  Risk-seeking behaviors (e.g., reckless driving, buying sprees, sexual indiscretions)
Duration
  At least 1 week
Exclusions
  Does not meet criteria for schizophrenia:
    No mood-incongruent delusions of hallucinations
    No bizarre behavior
  Not superimposed on schizophrenia, paranoia, or schizophreniform disorder
  Not secondary to organic brain syndrome
  Not secondary to substance intoxication

Table 19-2. *Symptoms characteristic of cyclothymic personality disorder*

Depressive periods	Hypomanic periods
Insomnia or hypersomnia	Decreased need for sleep
Lethargy or fatigue	Increased energy
Feelings of inadequacy	Inflated self-esteem
Ineffectiveness	Increased productivity
Poor concentration, attention, and cognition	Sharpened thinking
Social isolation and quietness	Gregariousness and garulousness
Loss of libido	Hypersexuality
Anhedonia	Reckless pleasure-seeking
Pessimism	Overoptimism
Crying	Laughing and joking

the spread of lithium therapy, chlorpromazine, reserpine, and haloperidol were the primary antimanic agents. Thus far, the most clearly established use of lithium is in manic episodes. Lithium carbonate is the lithium compound most commonly employed. A half-dozen studies have reported amelioration of symptoms of mania in from 54 to 100 percent of patients. A number of studies have also indicated that lithium salts are an effective prophylactic treatment in manic-depressive disorder, sometimes preventing the recurrence of manic-depressive cycles after the drug has been discontinued, but usually only during the period of drug maintenance. The principal effect of lithium is during the manic phase; however, amelioration of the manic phase leads secondarily to a less severe depression. Used chronically, lithium causes a leveling-out of mood, and further manic-depressive cycles are aborted. It is this prophylactic effect of lithium that gives it a unique place in psychopharmacology.

Clinical Indications

Lithium has also been tried in depression and schizoaffective disorders. Neither application has been established by clinical tests as yet, although the latter use has been described as promising. One reason that lithium is sometimes thought to be effective in depression is because some instances of bipolar disorder consist principally of recurrent depressions with only rare hypomanic episodes. In such cases, the disorder (referred to as bipolar II, or atypical bipolar disorder) may be initially misdiagnosed as unipolar depression, and lithium will be effective in these apparent instances of major depression.

Lithium may be useful in treating character disorders (chronic maladaptive behavioral patterns marked by exaggerated resistance to authority, truancy, poor work history) when secondary to depressive and hypomanic mood swings. Other conditions for which lithium has been employed but with variable results include hysterical personality, narcissistic personality disorder, hyperkinetic syndrome, alcoholism and other forms of drug abuse, aggressive psychopathology, and premenstrual tension syndrome.

Mechanism of Action

The mechanism of action of lithium is not known with certainty. It appears to stabilize nerve cells, and four hypothetical mechanisms have been advanced. One notion is that lithium accelerates reuptake of norepinephrine, causing a shift toward intraneuronal degradation. A second is that lithium inhibits adenyl cyclase–mediated responses to catecholamine release (see Chap. 6). A third hypothesis emphasizes the similarities between lithium and 5-hydroxytryptophan effects, invoking the permissive theory of affective disorders discussed in Chapter 17. The fourth and most widely accepted theory relates to ion distribution (Fig. 19-1). Lithium ions can substitute for sodium ions during an action potential, but once inside the cell, lithium is not pumped out by the sodium pump. Instead, it exchanges with sodium via the countertransport mechanism. The sodium that enters into this exchange stimulates the electrogenic sodium-potassium pump, causing the cell to become hyperpolarized.

Lithium is rapidly absorbed from the gastrointestinal tract, but the onset of therapeutic effectiveness is nevertheless slow. It has been suggested that this delay is related to its slow rate of passage across cellular membranes into intracellular spaces.

Matters of Strategy with Lithium

In considering lithium treatment for a patient, laboratory evaluation serves two purposes: It serves to rule out underlying organic disorders to which mania or depression might be secondary and to assess the patient's ability to tolerate lithium therapy. In the first respect, tests of CNS and endocrine function are paramount. Evaluation of CNS function may include EEG analysis, a brain scan, a computed tomographic scan, a brain biopsy, or a lumbar puncture (to measure transmitter metabolites). Endocrine evaluation is important because disorders of the thyroid, adrenal cortex, or pancreas may produce symptoms that mimic or aggravate mania or depression; also, in the case of the thyroid, because lithium may have a significant impact on thyroid function. Other tissues frequently adversely affected by lithium (see Table 19-3) are the cardiovascular system, kidney, liver, and gastrointestinal tract. Examination of these systems prior to

Extracellular fluid

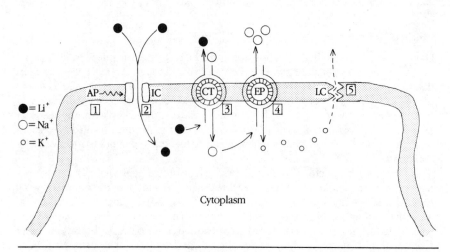

Cytoplasm

Fig. 19-1. *The ion distribution theory of lithium action. AP, action potential; CT, countertransport mechanism; EP, Na⁺-K⁺ exchange pump; IC, ion channel; LC, leakage channel. The arrival of an action potential [1], allows the influx of ions, such as lithium and sodium, that have an electrochemical gradient toward the inside of the cell. The influx occurs through ion channels [2] that open up in response to arrival of the action potential. Lithium cannot substitute for sodium in the exchange pump, but it can substitute for sodium in the countertransport mechanism [3], which ordinarily exchanges sodium for sodium, but now exchanges lithium for sodium. The sodium that enters the cell by countertransport in exchange for lithium is subsequently expelled from the cell by the exchange pump [4] in exchange for a potassium ion. The exchange pump is electrogenic, because some of the potassium brought in is able to leak back out [5]; but sodium expelled cannot leak back in because of its larger hydrated radius. Therefore, stimulation of the sodium pump leads to hyperpolarization of the cell.*

initiation of lithium treatment provides both a means of predicting susceptibility to lithium toxicity and a baseline for later quantification of such toxicity. A standard workup would include an electrocardiogram, blood pressures, and a complete blood count for assessment of cardiovascular function; serum enzyme measurement for evaluation of liver function; and blood urea nitrogen, electrolytes, urinanalysis, creatine clearance, and urine osmolarity for kidney function evaluation.

Because the onset of lithium's action is delayed until a threshold tissue concentration is reached, lithium therapy is generally combined with other agents. From five to ten doses may be needed to reach effective lithium levels, during which time a neuroleptic is administered for symptom control. Haloperidol or molindone is preferred for this purpose because these drugs both exhibit substantial efficacy and have less effect on lithium distribution and toxicity than do the phenothiazines. Some phenothiazines double the ratio of distribution of lithium between red blood cells and plasma. Electroconvulsive therapy has been used in the past as an interim adjunctive treatment, but its use is declining.

The delay in onset of lithium effectiveness can be reduced somewhat by proper dosing procedures. High loading doses are used initially. A typical first order might be

Table 19-3. Adverse effects of lithium

Type of effect	Symptoms	Frequency and period of maximal risk	Clinical responses
Neurologic and psychiatric	Somnolence, fatigue, lethargy, slurred speech, aphasia, anesthesia of skin, blurred vision, tinnitus, dizziness, ataxia, giddiness, confusion, blackouts, stupor, convulsions, coma	Common, late	Reduce dose Spread medication
Neuromuscular	Tremor, weakness, fasciculations, twitching, clonic movements, choreoathetotic movements, dysarthria	Common, late	Reduce dose Spread medication Propranolol for tremor
Gastrointestinal	Nausea, vomiting, diarrhea, abdominal pain, anorexia, weight loss	Common, early	Adaptation may occur Spread medication
Cardiovascular	T wave abnormality in ECG, arrhythmias, hypotension, circulatory collapse	Common, persistent	Avoid drugs with additive cardio-vascular effects (e.g., quinidine, tricyclics, neuroleptics)
Renal	Nephrogenic diabetes insipidus, polyuria, dehydration, xerostomia, thirst or (conversely) edema	Common early; rarely, late	Thiazide diuretic (paradoxical use in diabetes insipidus)
Endocrine	Hypothyroidism	Early or late	Reversible; lower dose or treat with thyroid hormone
Skin	Acneiform eruptions, folliculitis	Early	Interrupt treatment, then resume; skin reactions may or may not recur

900 mg per day, adjusted thereafter to 900 to 3600 mg per day until the condition is under control. A plasma concentration range of 0.9 to 1.4 mEq per liter of blood is sought during this initial phase. After the condition is stabilized, lower maintenance doses are utilized to achieve a plasma concentration in the range of 0.5 to 0.8 mEq per liter.

In contrast to what has been said about the advantages of once-a-day dosing for other psychotropics, division of doses is essential in lithium administration. Lithium is absorbed rapidly into the bloodstream, serum concentrations peaking in 2 to 4 hours. Toxic reactions set in at blood concentrations above a certain level (approximately 2 mEq per liter). Lithium is also excreted rapidly; serum levels may halve in only a day. To maintain effective tissue concentrations without excessive serum levels, several daily doses are needed.

Adverse Reactions

Lithium produces a large number of side effects (Table 19-3), and even fatalities may result from lithium toxicity. The side effects are frequently divided into two types, early side effects, which dissipate after a few days, and persistent side effects. Early side effects include tremor, nausea, vomiting, diarrhea, and dry mouth. Persistent central side effects include blackouts, stupor, vertigo, ataxia, fatigue, headache, and slurred speech. Other persistent side effects are weight change, hypotension, and cardiac arrhythmias. Lithium does not have significant overall sedative or excitatory effects on arousal state.

Tremor is a common side effect of lithium at the usual therapeutic levels and can be controlled with propranolol. Tremor and other motor symptoms, such as hyperactivity, ataxia, and aphasia, can often be reduced by spreading medication over the full 24 hours or by dosage reduction. Hypersensitivity reactions may occur early in treatment and may or may not recur when treatment is interrupted and resumed.

Lithium intoxication is characterized by drowsiness, slurred speech, and muscle spasms, which may persist for several days of elevated lithium levels before more serious symptoms set in. Eventually, coma and death result. Treatment of lithium intoxication consists of administration of quantities of sodium chloride (sodium antagonizes the action of lithium) and supportive measures as in barbiturate poisoning.

Maintenance medication with lithium appears actually to prevent recurrence of either manic or depressive episodes rather than simply modifying symptoms. Medication, however, must continue indefinitely. Even after years of use, a single missed dose may precipitate a recurrence. For this reason, and because toxic levels are very close to therapeutic levels, close adherence to dosage regimens and close medical supervision are required.

Lithium interacts in an important way with the patient's diet. Sodium competes with lithium, reducing both its effectiveness and its toxicity. Sodium depletion has the opposite effect. Patients should avoid irregular sodium intake, maintaining instead a low, steady level of sodium chloride ingestion. Drugs that deplete body sodium, notably the diuretics, intensify lithium toxicity.

Implications for Psychotherapy

Although sedation is minimal with lithium, ataxia, slurred speech, stupor, and fatigue are side effects that can occur early in lithium treatment or later on. A common neurologic symptom of lithium is tremor. The psychotherapist must be cautious in interpreting the cause of tremor, recalling the range of possible causes.

Manic or hypomanic symptoms in the generally well-controlled lithium-treated patient may indicate a need to reevaluate the dose, failure to maintain a steady level of dietary sodium, or a missed dose.

Patients exhibiting personality disorders associated with emotional instability can be considered for lithium therapy. The psychotherapist can play a significant role in identifying such cases. Similarly, the psychotherapist should be attentive to signs indicating cyclothymic personality.

Lithium as a Medically Important Agent

lithium (Eskalith, Lithane, Lithonate), an antimanic: used in manic and hypomanic episodes and may be prophylactic in manic-depressive syndrome. Initial: 900 to 1,800 mg, maintenance individualized to 0.5 to 1.5 mEq per liter serum level.

Selected References and Further Readings

1. Committee on Nomenclature and Statistics of the American Psychiatric Association. *Diagnostic and Statistical Manual* (3rd ed.). Washington, D.C.: American Psychiatric Association, 1980.
2. Gerbino, L., Olesharsky, M., and Gershon, S. Clinical Use and Mode of Action of Lithium. In M. A. Lipton et al. (Eds.), *Psychopharmacology: A Generation of Progress.* New York: Raven, 1978.
3. Gilman, A. G., Goodman, L. S., and Gilman, A. *The Pharmacological Basis of Therapeutics* (6th ed.). New York: Macmillan, 1980.
4. Hendler, N. H. Lithium Pharmacology and Physiology. In L. L. Iversen et al. (Eds.), *Handbook of Psychopharmacology.* New York: Plenum, 1978. Vol. 14.
5. Hollister, L. E. Psychiatric Disorders. In K. L. Melman and H. F. Morrelli (Eds.), *Clinical Pharmacology* (2nd ed.). New York: Macmillan, 1978.
6. Klein, D. F., and Gittelman-Klein, R. (Eds.). *Progress in Psychiatric Drug Treatment.* New York: Brunner/Mazel, 1975.
7. Prien, R. F. Lithium in the treatment of affective disorders. *Clin. Neuropharmacol.* 3:113–131, 1978.
8. Shopsin, B., and Gershon, S. Lithium: Clinical Considerations. In L. L. Iversen et al. (Eds.), *Handbook of Psychopharmacology.* New York: Plenum, 1978. Vol. 14.

Motor Function
and Drugs
VI

Part VI examines motor function, first, in Chapter 20, from the point of view of normal process. The extrapyramidal system is reviewed with respect to neuroanatomic and neurochemical mechanisms. A dual-process theory is proposed to define the relationship between response selection and motivational aspects of response generation.

In Chapter 21, we turn our attention to dysfunctions of the extrapyramidal system, including organic, drug-induced, and functional disorders. Where applicable, drug treatments for these disorders are examined. Emphasis is placed on the need of the psychotherapist to be able to recognize the variety of possible causes of motor symptoms such as tremors and to determine the correct etiology. Psychiatric side effects of drugs used for extrapyramidal disorders are also emphasized.

The Extrapyramidal Motor System

20

The extrapyramidal motor system is a diffusely distributed network of brain regions and nuclei, richly interconnected, and organized toward maintenance of motor regulation. The components of the extrapyramidal system include two major brain regions, the cerebellum and the corpus striatum, and several nuclei and pathways of the subthalamus, midbrain, pons, and medulla—virtually all motor influences that lie outside the pyramidal system (Fig. 20-1). The pyramidal system is a well-defined fiber tract that originates out of cells in the cerebral cortex and extends without break through the midbrain and brainstem and on down to the α-motor neurons of the spinal cord (Chap. 26). By contrast, the extrapyramidal system is not a discrete, monolithic system but rather a loose association of structures that compete for and cooperate in control of certain aspects of motor activity. In general, the pyramidal system is involved in volitional, conscious motor behavior, whereas the extrapyramidal system is concerned with subconscious, automatic, and associated motor activity. How absolute these distinctions are is open to conjecture. For example, when one has focused attention on his or her own body posture or "body language," is this consciousness extending into the extrapyramidal system, or is the appropriate information being passed from the extrapyramidal system into the cortex and consciousness? The balance between pyramidal and extrapyramidal control of motor activity appears to be regulated by the corpus striatum.

Corpus Striatum

The corpus striatum, a nuclear group that lies just interior to the inner surface of the cerebral cortex, constitutes the highest level of organization of the extrapyramidal motor system. The corpus striatum consists of three bilateral nuclear pairs: the caudate, globus pallidus, and putamen. These three, together with the amygdala, which belongs to the limbic system, are frequently referred to as the basal ganglia because of their location deep in the base of the telencephalon. The term *corpus striatum* refers to the striated appearance of this nuclear group, which is due to the fact that whitish myelinated fibers traveling from the cortex to the brainstem and beyond pass through and interdigitate with the grayish neurons of the corpus striatum.

Acetylcholine synthesis and degradation are unusually high in the caudate. Moreover, direct, local application of acetylcholine to the caudate causes stimulation of a sizable number of nerve cells in this area. For these reasons, it is apparent that acetylcholine is

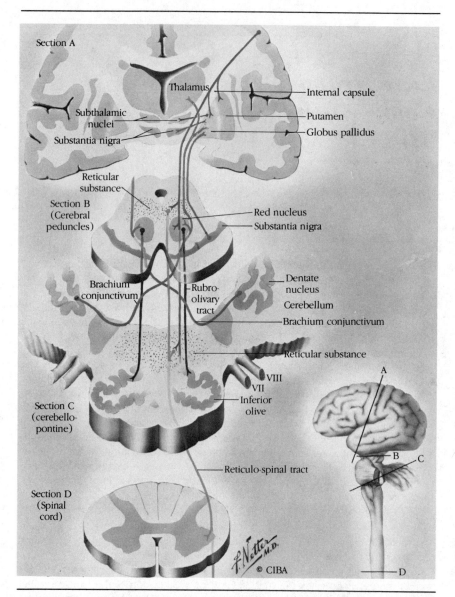

Section A

Thalamus

Internal capsule

Subthalamic nuclei

Putamen

Substantia nigra

Globus pallidus

Reticular substance

Section B (Cerebral peduncles)

Red nucleus

Substantia nigra

Brachium conjunctivum

Rubro-olivary tract

Dentate nucleus

Cerebellum

Brachium conjunctivum

Reticular substance

VIII

VII

Inferior olive

Section C (cerebello-pontine)

Reticulo-spinal tract

Section D (Spinal cord)

A

B

C

D

© CIBA

Fig. 20-1. *The extrapyramidal system at various levels of the central nervous system. (© Copyright 1965 CIBA Pharmaceutical Company, Division of CIBA-GEIGY Corporation. Reproduced, with permission, from The CIBA Collection of Medical Illustrations by Frank H. Netter, M.D. All rights reserved.)*

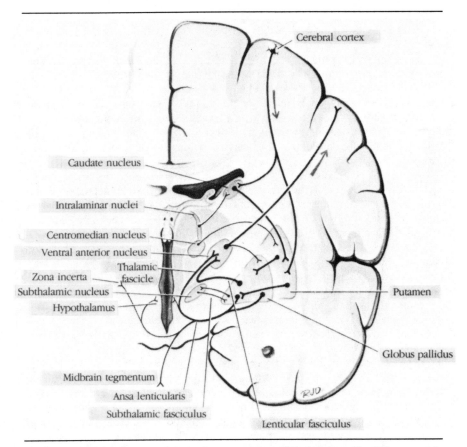

Fig. 20-2. *The subthalamus and major interconnections of the basal ganglia, thalamus, and cerebral cortex. From S. R. Noback.* The Human Nervous System. *New York: McGraw-Hill, 1974. © 1974 by McGraw-Hill Book Company, New York. Used with permission.*

an important transmitter in the caudate. Parkinsonism, as will be shown later, is related to dysfunctioning of the corpus striatum and is treatable with cholinergic-blocking drugs.

The corpus striatum is also rich in dopamine and serotonin. Most of the dopamine is found in nerve terminals of cells originating in the substantia nigra of the midbrain. The serotonin is found in nerve terminals of cells arising in the raphé nuclei of the pons. Both dopamine and serotonin contribute to the input side of corpus striatal activity. Drugs that block dopaminergic receptors frequently produce parkinsonian symptoms. The corpus striatum receives inputs chiefly from the vestibular system and proprioceptive receptors of the muscles, joints, and tendons and uses these in regulation of body posture, stabilization of movement, and production of certain automatic, and associated movements, such as the swinging of arms that accompanies walking. There are many interconnections between the corpus striatum, cerebellum, and the vestibular system, some of these utilizing important extrapyramidal, relay nuclei of the brainstem (Fig. 20-1) and subthalamus (Fig. 20-2) as way stations.

Cerebellum

The cerebellum lies at the back of the brainstem. Its role is the organization of muscle contractions into useful sequences. It generates rapid patterns of muscle activity that constitute skilled movements. The inputs to the cerebellum come most immediately from the brainstem and spinal cord, by way of three bridges, called the cerebellar peduncles, which connect the cerebellum to the remainder of the brainstem. The afferents to the cerebellum are mainly proprioceptive signals. Some of these reach the cerebellum directly from the secondary cell bodies in the spinal cord at the level of signal entry. Other signals relay first in the brainstem before continuing on to the cerebellum. The inferior olive of the medulla is a prominent afferent relay nucleus of the extrapyramidal system.

The cerebellar cortex is more homogeneous in its cellular structure than most brain regions. The Purkinje cell is the focal point of organization. Purkinje's cell axons project to the output nuclei of the cerebellum, deep in the cerebellar white matter. Inhibitory stellate and basket cells intertwine with Purkinje's cell dendrites and soma, while deeply-lying granule cells produce excitation of Purkinje's cells through a system of parallel fibers. Afferent axons from cells outside the cerebellum are called mossy fibers and climbing fibers. The inputs to the cerebellum include cholinergic, noradrenergic, serotonergic, and aspartate-releasing axons.

Outputs from the cerebellum travel to the midbrain reticular formation, especially the cuneiform nucleus, and to the red nucleus, thalamus, dorsal raphé nucleus, vestibular nucleus, and descending reticular formation of the medulla.

With the exception of a few direct pathways from the cerebellum to the spinal cord, all outputs of the extrapyramidal motor system are ultimately exerted on the descending reticular formation, the caudalmost portion of the brainstem reticular formation. Although the mesodiencephalic portion of the reticular formation is important in control of cortical arousal, the caudalmost portion of the reticular formation is a critically important region, integrating and relaying descending, extrapyramidal signals.

From the reticular formation, extrapyramidal discharges proceed via spinal pathways (rubrotegmental-spinal tracts) to innervate principally gamma motor neurons of the somatic nervous system. The gamma motor neurons differ in function from the alpha motor neurons. Whereas the latter elicit muscle activity directly, the former control muscle tone or excitability by altering the functional parameters of the proprioceptive receptors in the muscles and tendons. It is appropriate, given the tonic nature of functional control carried out by the extrapyramidal system, that its influences are exerted primarily on the gamma motor neurons.

Summary of Functions of the Extrapyramidal System

It is well established that the extrapyramidal system has a regulatory role over movement: stabilization of simple movements, control of muscle tone in relation to posture, and generation of rapid sequences. The outputs of the corpus striatum are inhibitory and are directed toward both the cortex and brainstem nuclei. It has been suggested that the corpus striatum is important in mediating motor and cortical inhibition.

In recent years, it has been suggested that the corpus striatum may also be involved in regulating brain operations that underlie cognitive capabilities. It seems clear from the pattern of connections, as well as from evolutionary considerations, that the neostriatum must be considered a functional part of the neocortical system rather than of more primitive limbic or brainstem systems. The inputs to the corpus striatum come almost entirely from the thalamus and cortex, while its outputs serve to complete circuits back to the cortex or to provide discharge through the globus pallidus to brainstem centers. The circuits involving the cortex, neostriatum, and thalamus are now thought to provide a cognitive regulatory function, while the discharge pathways to the brainstem provide the stabilization and suppression of motor activity.

Dual-Process Theory of Response Execution

The dual-process theory is a conception of behavioral control that posits two distinct processes: a "response-selection" process (the selection between alternative active responses or "how to respond") and a "motivational" process (the choice between activity or passivity or "whether to respond"). The dual-process view developed simultaneously but independently in two branches of psychology—the learning and physiologic branches.

In the physiologic realm, the dual-process viewpoint grew out of the early theoretical formulations of Cannon and Hess. Cannon proposed in 1927 that there were present in the brainstem sympathetic and parasympathetic centers that controlled emotionality and arousal. Since it was already known at that time that specific, though then unidentified, hormones were released by the two autonomic branches, Cannon was implying that particular neurotransmitter substances mediated broad functional activities within the CNS as well. About a decade later, Hess coined the terms *ergotropic* and *trophotropic* to designate, respectively, similarly conceived system-wide excitatory and inhibitory subsystems. Increasing information about the function of particular brain regions led to some shifting of the anatomic loci to which these concepts were attached. The discovery of the reticular arousal system in 1949 by Magoun and Moruzzi opened up interest in the reticular formation as a possible anatomic substrate of the motivational or ergotropic process.

The descending reticulum modulates behavior not by altering the probabilities relating various response choices but rather by shifting the likelihood that any response whatsoever will occur, i.e., motivational state. The reticular system is stimulated by adrenergic stimulants such as amphetamine and is depressed by sedative-hypnotics, tranquilizers, and adrenergic-blocking drugs. The effectiveness of drugs that alter the functioning of adrenergic neurons is so consistent that the reticular system can be described as a noradrenoceptive system.

The answering of the "how to respond" question or response-shaping process presumably resides diffusely in many portions of the brain—throughout the limbic system, portions of the cerebral cortex, and in the extrapyramidal structures. Response selection results from selective and differentiated suppressive and facilitory influences exerted by these areas on the descending reticular pathways. Carlton's proposal concerning hippocampal function (Chap. 15), postulated such a relationship to the reticular formation for one of these brain regions.

Balance and interaction between the motivation-shaping and response-shaping processing centers is regulated by ascending monoamine pathways, especially the dopaminergic fibers arising from the midbrain, serotonergic fibers arising from the raphé nuclei, and noradrenergic fibers of the median forebrain bundle. These pathways regulate the level of activity of the response-shaping brain areas in response to influences from the motivational processing region, the reticular formation.

Selected References and Further Readings

1. Angevine, J. R., Jr., and Cotman, C. W. *Principles of Neuroanatomy.* New York: Oxford University Press, 1981.
2. Carpenter, M. B. *Human Neuroanatomy* (7th ed.). Baltimore: Williams & Wilkins, 1976.
3. Divac, I., and Öberg, R. G. E. (Eds.). *The Neostriatum.* New York: Pergamon, 1979.

Disorders of the Extrapyramidal System

21

In this chapter, we will examine disorders of the extrapyramidal system and the corresponding drug treatments. Extrapyramidal disorders can arise from organic, drug-induced, or functional causes.

Organic Extrapyramidal Disorders

Parkinsonism and Antiparkinsonian Agents

Parkinsonism is a clinical syndrome related to dysfunction of the corpus striatum and characterized by disturbances of muscle tone, derangement in movements, and loss of automatic associated movements. The triad of symptoms in parkinsonism consists of rigidity, tremors, and akinesias. The muscular rigidity is caused by the loss of inhibitory control exerted by the corpus striatum on tonic cerebellar discharge to the reticular formation. Rigidity and akinesias of the facial muscles result in the characteristic "diplomat's expression." Another sign of muscle rigidity is the "cogwheel motion" observed when the patient is asked to bend the arm. Movement abnormalities include involuntary tremor, pill-rolling motions of the hands, abnormalities of gait, and trembling of the voluntary muscles. The muscles gradually weaken, and akinesias may develop. Akinesias may take several forms: loss of expressiveness; loss of associated movements (such as arm swinging while walking); disturbances of gait or voluntary movements; and postural distortions. The senses and intellect are not usually impaired until the condition is well advanced.

The neurochemical basis of parkinsonism is understood in part (Fig. 21-1). Deficiency of dopamine in the corpus striatum is found in the brains of parkinsonian patients at autopsy. The disease is relatively rare in people born after 1930, and it is now believed that many cases resulted from a β encephalitis virus that was prevalent in the United States in the late 1920s. Parkinsonism developed in some patients at the time of the infection; in others, it developed much later. Other causes for parkinsonism include carbon monoxide or heavy metal neurotoxicity; neurosyphilis; cerebrovascular disorders (arteriosclerosis, thrombosis, embolism, or hemorrhage); tumors; and degenerative disease of the corpus striatum (paralysis agitans, or idiopathic parkinsonism).

Two pharmacologic approaches have proved effective in parkinsonism. The first, discovered some 100 years ago by Ordenstein, is the use of anticholinergic drugs of the

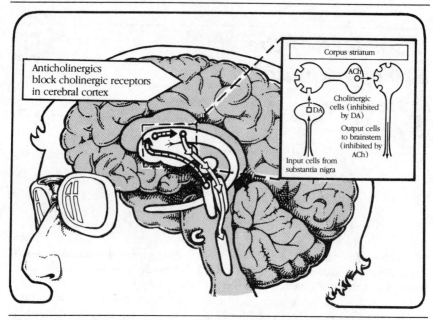

Fig. 21-1. *Mechanisms of antiparkinsonian agents. ACh, acetylcholine; DA, dopamine.*
(1) Cholinergic cells in the corpus striatum are overactive in parkinsonism, leading to insufficient
corpus striatum impulses to the brainstem. One agent, levodopa (2), alleviates this by elevating DA
levels, increasing inhibition of the cholinergic cells. A second class of agents—anticholinergics,
such as benztropine (3)—are thought to alleviate this overactivity by blocking the overstimulated
cholinergic receptors that inhibit the output cells. Anticholinergics also produce sedation by
blocking cholinergic receptors in the cerebral cortex (4). (Modified from A. K. Swonger. Nursing
Pharmacology. *Boston: Little, Brown, 1978.)*

belladonna type, which leads to about a 20 percent improvement in about 70 percent of patients. Atropine-like compounds (belladonna alkaloids) are widely used, especially benztropine (Cogentin) and trihexyphenidyl (Artane). Benztropine combines anticholinergic and antihistaminergic properties and is relatively effective. Other anticholinergics in use for parkinsonism include procyclidine (Kemadrin), cycrimine (Pagitane), biperiden (Akineton), and ethopropazine (Parsidol). Other antihistamines employed in combination regimens for parkinsonism include diphenhydramine (Benadryl, etc.), chlorphenoxamine (Phenoxene), and orphenadrine (Disipal). Numerous toxic effects are associated with the belladonna alkaloids and other anticholinergics. The most common and least surprising are anticholinergic side effects: dryness of the mouth, confusion, headaches, hallucinations, urinary retention, constipation, glaucoma, blurred vision, and tachycardia. These effects derive from the widespread CNS-blocking and parasympathetic-blocking actions of these agents at muscarinic-type cholinergic receptors. The EEG is markedly slowed by atropine-like drugs, with a concomitant clouding of consciousness.

The second, and newer, treatment, dating from 1961, is levodopa (L-dopa) (Dopar, Larodopa), a drug that is converted in the brain to dopamine. Levodopa is, in a sense, a replacement therapy, since most parkinsonian patients are deficient in brain dopamine. The drug is dramatically effective in blocking akinesias and resting tremor, but less effective in blocking action tremors and rigidity. Antihistamine or anticholinergic

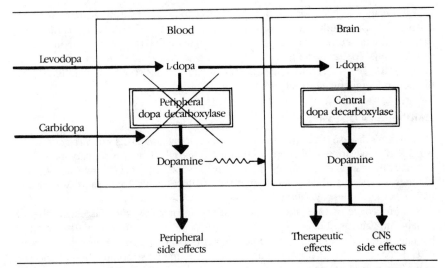

Fig. 21-2. Schema illustrating the rationale for use of a peripheral decarboxylase inhibitor with levodopa to reduce peripheral side effects and increase accumulation of the levodopa by the brain.

therapy, by contrast, is more effective in reducing action tremors and rigidity, but ineffective in alleviating muscle weakness and akinesias. Therefore, a typical regimen for parkinsonism includes both levodopa and an anticholinergic or antihistamine. Patients with advanced parkinsonism are less likely to respond to levodopa therapy than are patients in earlier stages. Adverse effects of levodopa include postural hypotension, granulocytopenia, vomiting, abnormal movements, and a wide range of psychic manifestations.

Levodopa, rather than dopamine itself, is used in parkinsonism because dopamine does not cross the blood-brain barrier to any appreciable extent. Systemic administration of dopamine will not elevate brain levels of dopamine sufficiently. Levodopa is converted to dopamine both outside the CNS (peripherally) and inside the CNS (centrally) (Fig. 21-2). Insofar as the conversion occurs peripherally, the value of the drug treatment is lessened because (1) the dopamine synthesized peripherally cannot enter the brain, and (2) the dopamine in the periphery produces side effects such as postural hypotension.

The enzyme responsible for conversion of levodopa to dopamine is dopa decarboxylase, found both in the brain and in peripheral neural structures. One strategy for reducing peripheral conversion of levodopa to dopamine is simultaneous administration of an inhibitor of the decarboxylase enzyme, which is itself unable to cross the blood-brain barrier—that is, a peripheral decarboxylase inhibitor. A preparation that combines levodopa with a peripheral decarboxylase inhibitor (carbidopa) is available under the trade name Sinemet.

Anticholinergics and antihistamines may produce noticeable sedation, with feelings of apathy, lethargy, or depression. Levodopa, in contrast, may elicit psychic disturbances in the form of acute anxiety, agitation, delirium, depression, or increased cognitive impairment. Levodopa and anticholinergics are each liable to precipitate tardive dyskinesias. Levodopa is a potent suppressor of dreaming sleep, a fact that may be related to the psychic disturbances.

The therapeutic effect of levodopa is subject to antagonism by vitamin B_6 (pyridoxine). Most probably, the basis of this antagonism is the role of pyridoxine in the synthesis of the neurotransmitter gamma-aminobutyric acid (GABA). Pyridoxine serves as an essential coenzyme for glutamic acid decarboxylase (GAD), the enzyme that produces GABA. The GABA-releasing striatonigral pathway has an inhibitory influence on the dopaminergic nigrostriatal pathway.

Huntington's Disease

Huntington's disease is another type of organic extrapyramidal disorder. The condition is marked by occurrence of choreiform movements, which are involuntary motor tics. The first motor sign of the condition is usually the appearance of facial twitches. Among the most dangerous of the motor symptoms is difficulty in speaking and swallowing, which can lead to asphyxiation.

In terms of age of onset, there are two modal age groups. In the largest number of patients, the disease begins between the ages of 37 and 47. In about 10 percent of patients, it begins prior to age 15. Dementia occurs in most patients, more often in cases of early onset. Behavioral symptoms may precede motor symptoms by a decade or more. The behavioral symptoms include increased libido, catatonia, paranoia, and aggression. The condition is easily mistaken for schizophrenia, and there is an etiologic relationship to the extent that both conditions involve elevated dopaminergic activity in the brain. Huntington's disease, however, is genetically linked, being an autosomal dominant inherited disorder.

The neuroanatomic basis of Huntington's disease is established up to a point. There is a loss of neurons in the caudate and putamen nuclei; atrophy is present throughout the brain, but is most pronounced in these regions. The loss of neurons is associated with degeneration of a GABA pathway that runs from the caudate nucleus to the zona reticulata of the substantia nigra. This leads to a decrease in GABA in the corpus striatum and substantia nigra. This GABA pathway in the normally functioning brain maintains an inhibitory control over the nigrostriatal dopamine pathway, which is the pathway implicated in parkinsonism. The release of the nigrostriatal dopamine pathway from the inhibitory influence of GABA results in excessive dopamine turnover in the corpus striatum. Thus, Huntington's disease, from a neurochemical point of view, is directly opposite to parkinsonism. Huntington's disease involves excess dopamine activity, while parkinsonism entails a dopamine deficiency.

One would have reason to suppose that gabamimetic drugs might be useful in Huntington's disease, but they are not. Apparently, when the GABA pathway degenerates, the GABA receptors in substantia nigra also degenerate.

Drug approaches in current clinical use for Huntington's disease involve depletion of dopamine or blockade of dopamine receptors. The current drug of choice is a drug called tetrabenazine (Nitoman), a rapid-acting, reserpine-like drug. It blocks storage of dopamine, leading to depletion of the transmitter. Dosages that eliminate choreiform movements completely (25 mg three times a day) often cause depression. Frequently, it is necessary to accept incomplete symptom suppression to lessen side effects. The alternative to tetrabenazine is the use of neuroleptics; thioridazine or haloperidol is most often selected. Neuroleptic therapy should be reserved for patients who are dangerously aggressive or severely ataxic.

Other Organic Causes of Motor Dysfunction

Tremor may arise from a variety of organic causes other than parkinsonism, notably, the following: paresis (a fine, rapid tremor that is an early symptom of neurosyphilis);

Table 21-1. *Drug management of motor disorder symptoms*

Symptom	Origin	Drug treatments
Hyperkinesias		
Choreas	EP	Neuroleptics, tetrabenazine; sedatives and anti-
Athetosis	EP	inflammatory drugs (if due to infection)
Ballismus	EP	Neuroleptics, tetrabenazine
Tardive dyskinesias	EP	Neuroleptics, tetrabenazine, α-methylparatyrosine
Dystonic movements	EP	Spasmolytics
Tremor		
At rest	EP	L-dopa
Action	EP	Propranolol, anticholinergics
Intention	CB	None
Myoclonus	SC, EP, C	Clonazepam, L-5-hydroxytryptophan
Akathisias	EP	Benzodiazepines
Tics, habit rhythmias,	C	Haloperidol for Gilles de la Tourette's syndrome;
hysterical movements		benzodiazepines for other tics
Fasciculations	SC	None
Hypokinesias		
Akinesias	EP	L-dopa for parkinsonian akinesias
Ataxias	CB	None
Weakness or paralysis	Various	Neostigmine for myasthenia gravis
Dystonias		
Hypertonias		
Myotonia	M	Quinine, quinidine, procaine, or phenytoin
Rigidity	EP	Spasmolytics, anticholinergics, antiepileptics
Spasticity	C	Spasmolytics, antiepileptics
Hypotonia	Various	None

C, cortical; CB, cerebellar; EP, extrapyramidal; M, muscle; SC, spinal cord.

multiple sclerosis; degenerative diseases of the cerebellum; senility; hyperthyroidism (a rapid, fine tremor of the hands and fingers); and Wilson's disease.

Wilson's disease (hepatolenticular degeneration) is a hereditary disease involving an error in copper metabolism and leading to copper deposits in many organs and tissues. In the CNS, this leads to degeneration of the corpus striatum, with the occurrence of tremors and choreas (especially "wing-beating"). Treatment involves chelating copper with penicillamine to enhance its excretion, and a diet low in copper. Pyridoxine (vitamin B$_6$) is given as well.

Other symptoms of organic motor hyperfunction besides tremor (Table 21-1) include choreas, athetosis, and ballismus. All three are extrapyramidal symptoms best con-trolled with neuroleptics or tetrabenazine. Choreas are involuntary, purposeless move-ments, but they are subject to voluntary modification. Athetosis consists of slower, writhing movements, usually confined to the distal muscles of the limbs. Ballismus is a rare symptom marked by violent extensions of a limb or limbs, usually limited to one side of the body (hemiballismus). Most cases derive from damage to the contralateral subthalamic nucleus. These symptoms can occur in a variety of pathologic conditions (Table 21-2).

Dystonic movements (such as torticollis) often develop into full-fledged dystonias, suggesting they may be intermittent dystonic states. The various hypertonic states that

Table 21-2. *Clinical symptoms of motor disorder syndromes*

Pathologic syndromes

Clinical symptoms	*Infections* / Encephalitis	Neurosyphilis	Chorea gravidarum	Sydenham's chorea (St. Vitus' Dance)	Cerebrovascular lesions	CNS tumors	*Metabolic disorders* / Tay-Sachs disease	Hypoglycemia, hyperthyroidism, or elevated sympathetic tone	*Drug-induced disorders* / Heavy-metal or gas toxicities	Neuroleptic side effects	Stimulants, sympathomimetics, tricyclics, and lithium	Hypnotic or opiate intoxication	Hypnotic or opiate withdrawal
Hyperkinesias													
Choreas	•		•	•	•								
Athetosis	•	•			•			•					
Ballismus	•				•								
Tardive dyskinesias										•			
Dystonic movements	•	•			•								
Tremor													
Alternating	•	•			•	•		•	•	•	•		•
Intention													
Myoclonus	•	•			•	•							
Akathisias	•									•			
Tics, habit rhythmias, hysterical movements													
Fasciculations													
Hypokinesias													
Akinesias	•									•			
Ataxias		•										•	
Weakness or paralysis								•					•
Dystonias													
Hypertonias													
Myotonia													
Rigidity	•	•			•					•			
Spasticity					•	•							
Hypotonia													

originate within the CNS (see Table 21-1) are responsive to spasmolytics, such as diazepam, clonazepam, baclofen (Lioresal), and dantrolene (Dantrium).

Encephalitis is usually of viral origin. Idoxuridine can be used successfully if the infecting virus is herpes simplex, while adenine arabinoside is of value for treating herpes zoster encephalitis.

Drug-Induced Extrapyramidal Disorders

Extrapyramidal symptoms occur as side effects of drugs and as a component of withdrawal from sedative-hypnotics and narcotics. In alcoholism, a rapid, coarse tremor

Pathologic syndromes

Degenerative disorders → Huntington's chorea	Wilson's disease	Double athetosis	Torsion dystonia	Spasmodic torticollis	Parkinsonism	Creutzfeldt's disease	Essential myoclonias	Myoclonic epilepsy	Cerebellar disorders	*Functional disorders*	*Multiple sclerosis*	*Peripheral neuromuscular disorders*	Muscular atrophies	Myasthenia gravis	Muscular dystrophies	Myotonic syndromes	Clinical symptoms
																	Hyperkinesias
•	•																Choreas
	•	•															Athetosis
																	Ballismus
																	Tardive dyskinesias
	•	•	•	•													Dystonic movements
																	Tremor
	•				•												Alternating
									•		•						Intention
•	•		•	•		•	•	•			•						Myoclonus
										•							Akathisias
										•							Tics, habit rhythmias, hysterical movements
												•					Fasciculations
																	Hypokinesias
•					•	•											Akinesias
									•		•						Ataxias
											•		•	•	•	•	Weakness or paralysis
																	Dystonias
																	Hypertonias
																•	Myotonia
•	•	•	•	•	•	•											Rigidity
											•						Spasticity
									•				•	•	•		Hypotonia

develops involving the fingers, tongue, limbs, and head, most evident in the morning prior to alcohol ingestion and particularly severe in delirium tremens.

Extrapyramidal side effects are associated with two classes of psychotropic drugs: the neuroleptics and tricyclic antidepressants. The frequency and severity of such side effects are greatest for the neuroleptics. These extrapyramidal side effects are of four types: pseudoparkinsonism, tardive dyskinesias, acute dystonias, and akathisias.

Pseudoparkinsonism

Pseudoparkinsonism, or drug-induced parkinsonism, bears a considerable resemblance to the organic extrapyramidal disorder parkinsonism, hence the name pseudoparkinsonism. (For a complete description of the symptoms, see Parkinsonism and Antiparkinsonian Agents.) Pseudoparkinsonism is a common consequence of therapy involving dopamine-blocking drugs. The period of maximal risk is generally 5 to 30 days following the initiation of drug therapy. There is a positive correlation between the likelihood and severity of pseudoparkinsonian symptoms and the dosage and anti-dopaminergic potency of the neuroleptic employed.

When pseudoparkinsonism develops, there are several possible therapeutic responses. The first choice when feasible is to lower the dose of the offending drug. This may not be possible without recurrence of symptoms if the dosage was carefully titrated to the minimal level sufficient to control the symptoms for which the drug is being employed. The second option is to switch drug selection to a neuroleptic that produces fewer extrapyramidal reactions, for example, thioridazine. This may also prove not to be feasible if the severity of the psychotic condition is great, since the neuroleptics producing the fewest extrapyramidal symptoms are also generally the least efficacious. The third option is the addition of an antiparkinsonian agent. This is the least satisfactory option in that antiparkinsonian agents serve only to mask the overt manifestation of drug-induced parkinsonism and do not prevent development of the underlying neural damage.

Antiparkinsonian drugs should never be added to a neuroleptic regimen *prophylactically* in anticipation of pseudoparkinsonian symptoms, because this practice will interfere with the ability to monitor the development of symptoms as they occur and will preclude alternative responses. When an antiparkinsonian drug is to be added to a neuroleptic regimen as a last resort, levodopa is not used, since it would aggravate schizophrenia or other psychotic states. The usual choice is an anticholinergic drug such as benztropine.

Tardive Dyskinesias

A second type of drug-induced extrapyramidal disorder consists of tardive dyskinesias, which are late-occurring motor defects. Although they usually occur late, in rare cases they occur after a single administration of a neuroleptic. The risk of tardive dyskinesias continues to grow as the duration of treatment increases.

The symptoms of tardive dyskinesias are reminiscent of Huntington's disease. Motor tics develop, most commonly involving the muscles of the tongue and face. The earliest sign is usually a forward-backward or lateral movement of the tongue. Later, the tongue will protrude obviously or press against the inside of the cheek, in twisting, curling movements. Gnawing movements of the jaw are common. Eye-blinking and spasmodic grimacing are frequently observed.

The relationship of tardive dyskinesias to neuroleptic administration is akin to the relationship of delirium tremens to alcohol use. It is a form of withdrawal and is believed to be related to the development of supersensitivity in dopamine receptors. Tardive dyskinesias are likely to develop if a patient is abruptly withdrawn from neuroleptic therapy, or a sharp dosage reduction is instituted. But tardive dyskinesia (and here the analogy to delirium tremens breaks down) may develop even without a reduction in dosage. Those that develop in the absence of dosage reduction are for the most part irreversible, while those accompanying neuroleptic withdrawal are generally transient, in the mode of the symptoms of sedative-hypnotic withdrawal. Tardive dyskinesias may also be triggered by use of antiparkinsonian drugs such as benztropine and levodopa.

Tardive dyskinesias associated with abrupt neuroleptic withdrawal can be minimized by gradual weaning instead of sudden elimination of the drug. When tardive dyskinesias develop in the absence of a change in dosing, the therapeutic response options are limited to two choices, neither of which is good. If tardive dyskinesias are recognized early, discontinuation of the neuroleptic must be considered, even though the symptoms will temporarily worsen with drug withdrawal, and even though the manifestations of schizophrenia will worsen. If the neuroleptic is withdrawn, the tardive dyskinesias will generally be permanent but nonprogressive. The second option is to increase the dosage of the neuroleptic. This will suppress, at least temporarily, the manifestations of tardive dyskinesias, in the same sense that a drink will suppress the alcohol abstinence syndrome in a person in alcohol withdrawal. This is a makeshift treatment, since the tardive dyskinesias will ultimately progress to the point of breaking through at the higher dosage.

Akathisias and Acute Dystonic Reactions

Akathisias and acute dystonic reactions are two other forms of extrapyramidal reactions to neuroleptics. Akathisias are symptoms of motor restlessness. The patient cannot sit or stand still and jumps about continuously. Somatic discomfort is another component; the patient complains of "feeling bugs" or being on "pins and needles." The importance of recognizing akathisias is that these symptoms are easily mistaken for worsening symptoms of schizophrenia. The therapeutic response in the two circumstances should be, of course, diametrically opposite, akathisias indicating a need for dosage reduction and recurrence of schizoid symptoms suggesting dosage elevation. Akathisias are most common during the first 2 months of neuroleptic treatment. A benzodiazepine may be useful in alleviating akathisias.

Acute dystonic reactions occur early in treatment, most commonly in the first 5 days, and consist of a grimacing that is due to distortions in facial-muscle tone. Acute dystonic reactions respond to anticholinergic drug treatment.

Functional Motor Disorders

It should be kept in mind that both tremor and motor tics may arise in relation to functional disorders. Most people experience tremor at one time or another when faced with a challenging or threatening situation. Tremor of a more common or persistent nature occurs in generalized anxiety disorder. Usually, tremor related to anxiety is coarse and irregular. Hysteria often entails tremor, which may be fine or coarse, limited or generalized, constant or paroxysmal.

About 75 percent of motor tics are classified as functional rather than organic, though it is possible that the distinction here between organic and functional will blur as our understanding of etiology increases. A common form of functional tic is a burst of eye blinks. Other tics usually involve muscles of the face, especially the eyes and mouth, sometimes spreading to the trunk. Three-fourths of functional tics develop prior to age 30; the peak period of onset is ages 6 to 12.

Five categories of "stereotyped movement disorders" are designated in the DSM-III: transient tic disorder, chronic motor tic disorder, Gilles de la Tourette's disorder, atypical tic disorder, and atypical stereotyped movement disorder. The use of the neuroleptic haloperidol in Gilles de la Tourette's disorder was discussed in Chapter 16.

Implications for Psychotherapy

Movement disorders may be organic, drug-induced, or functional in origin. The psychotherapist needs to recognize the variety of causes of such disorders, so that erroneous assumptions as to etiology are avoided. Some movement disorders are treatable with drugs, but these drugs may cause psychiatric side effects or other motor problems. The psychotherapist should be aware of the psychiatric side effects of extrapyramidal drugs, so that their impact on the overall psychological state of the patient and on therapy can be evaluated.

Medically Important Antiparkinsonian Agents

baclofen (Lioresal), an antispastic and muscle relaxant. Usual: 40 to 80 mg. Maximum: 80 mg.

benztropine (Cogentin), an anticholinergic and antihistaminic: used as an antiparkinsonian agent. Initial: 0.5 to 1.0 mg, increasing to 4 to 8 mg.

carbidopa (Sinemet [with levodopa]), a peripheral decarboxylase inhibitor: used to enhance action and reduce the side effects of levodopa. Maximum: 200 mg.

chlorzoxazone (Paraflex; Parafon and Saroflex [with acetaminophen]), a centrally acting skeletal-muscle relaxant. Usual: 750 to 2,000 mg. Maximum: 3,000 mg.

dantrolene (Dantrium), an antispastic. Maximum: 400 mg.

diphenhydramine (Benadryl), an antihistamine: sedative, antiparkinsonian, allergies, cold-pill combination. Antihistaminic: 25 to 50 mg. Antiparkinsonian: 75 to 200 mg.

L-dopa (levodopa) (Bendopa, Dopar, Larodopa), a dopamine precursor: antiparkinsonian. Initial: 300 to 1,000, increasing to 4,000 to 8,000 maximum.

penicillamine (Cuprimine), a heavy metal chelator: used in Wilson's disease. Usual: 1 to 4 gm.

tetrabenazine (Nitoman), a depletor of biogenic amines: used in the management of choreas, athetosis, and ballismus. Usual: 75 to 300 mg.

trihexyphenidyl (Artane, Pipanol, Tremin), an anticholinergic antiparkinsonian: commonly used as adjunct to levodopa. Initial: 2 to 6 mg, increasing to 15 to 30 mg.

Selected References and Further Readings

1. Bardeau, A., and McDowell, F. H. L-Dopa and Parkinsonism. Philadelphia: Davis, 1970.
2. Bird, E. D. Chemical pathology of Huntington's disease. *Annu. Rev. Pharmacol. Toxicol.* 20: 533–551, 1980.
3. Gilman, A. G., Goodman, L. S., and Gilman, A. *The Pharmacological Basis of Therapeutics* (6th ed.). New York: Macmillan, 1980.
4. Klawans, H. L., Jr. The pharmacology of parkinsonism. *Dis. Nerv. Syst.* 29:805–816, 1968.
5. Klein, D. F., and Gittelman-Klein, R. (Eds.). *Progress in Psychiatric Drug Treatment.* New York: Brunner/Mazel, 1975.
6. Weiner, W. J., and Bergen, D. Prevention and management of the side effects of levodopa. *Clin. Neuropharmacol.* 2:1–24, 1977.

Pain and Its Drug Management

VII

Pain, especially chronic pain and its management, play an important role in a person's psychological status. Chronic pain can have a debilitating impact on one's composure, feeling of well-being, and even one's sense of self-worth. The drugs that are used to manage pain may have dramatic effects on psychological functioning as well. This is especially true of the narcotic analgesics, because their action is largely within the CNS and in substantial measure is exerted on limbic centers that give an affective quality to pain. The narcotic analgesics are also important in their role as classic drugs of abuse. Nonnarcotic analgesics, though less frequently relevant to psychotherapy, may produce neurologic side effects. And a person's general attitudes toward drug-taking are bound to be reflected in his or her use of nonnarcotic analgesics, given their ready availability.

Chapter 22 outlines the neurophysiologic mechanisms of pain transmission and temperature regulation. Chapters 23 and 24 take up the two major classes of pain-killers, the narcotics and nonnarcotics respectively. The final chapter in this section, Chapter 25, examines a specific kind of pain, headaches.

Neurophysiology of Pain and Temperature

22

Neurophysiology of Pain

Pain Receptors

The classic view is that there are four basic modalities of cutaneous sensation, subserved by four specific types of receptors: pain, served by fine nerve endings; cold, by bulbs of Krause; warmth, by Ruffini's corpuscles; and touch, by Pacini's and Meissner's corpuscles and nerve endings on hair follicles. Some receptors appear to respond to appropriate stimuli in more than one modality, but most are tuned to a single modality.

In addition to the cutaneous senses, there are sensory afferents, called proprioceptive afferents, arising from receptors associated with the skeletal musculature. These receptors provide information regarding the degree and rate of contraction of each striated muscle. The receptors involved are spindle organs embedded in the muscle fibers and Golgi tendon organs.

Cutaneous and proprioceptive afferents flow into the nervous system along two projection systems called the epicritic (or lemniscal) and the protopathic (spinothalamic) systems. The latter system is further divided into the neospinothalamic and paleospinothalamic branches (Fig. 22-1).

The epicritic system carries signals related to light (or discriminative) touch and proprioception. The fibers of this system are well myelinated and thick; both of these characteristics promote rapid conduction.

The protopathic system carries signals related to pain, temperature, and crude touch. The protopathic system, because of its relationship to pain sensations, will be our main focus of attention, as we prepare to examine the antinociceptive effect of narcotic and nonnarcotic analgesics.

A pain signal originates at a free nerve ending in the periphery. These receptors act as transducers, converting physical or chemical stimuli into electrical impulses. For example, pain receptors can be stimulated by a substance called bradykinin, an autocoid that is released by injured cells. Another chemical involved in pain sensitivity is prostaglandin E (PgE). This substance sensitizes pain receptors to bradykinin, and it is implicated in the mechanism of nonnarcotic analgesics. Pain receptors may exhibit a decrease in sensitivity when stimulated intensely over a period of time, a phenomenon called *adaptation*.

Gating of Pain Signals

When a sensory receptor is stimulated, it produces a generator potential that triggers an action potential in the associated nerve fiber. If the pain receptor is located below the cranium, this fiber is a long, extended dendrite from a bipolar cell located in the dorsal root ganglion of the spinal cord (see Fig. 22-1). Bipolar cell dendrites are functionally more akin to axons in that they exhibit the capacity of propagation. Thus, the action potential arising at the level of the receptor travels into and past the bipolar cell body, to reach the gray matter of the cord. The primary-cell axon terminates in a portion of the gray called the substantia gelatinosa. If the pain receptor is located in the cranium, the nerve impulse will enter the brainstem along the 5th, 7th, or 9th cranial nerves to synapse in the spinal root and nucleus of the 5th cranial nerve, the brainstem analogue of the substantia gelatinosa. These two regions, the substantia gelatinosa and the spinal root and nucleus of the 5th cranial nerve, are the "lower gates" for pain sensations from the body and head respectively. These regions act as gates in that the flow of pain signals can be attenuated at these sites by endogenous control mechanisms.

Secondary cell bodies located in the substantia gelatinosa or in the spinal root and nucleus of the 5th cranial nerve project upward to reach the thalamus. Axons from cells in the spinal root and nucleus of the 5th cranial nerve travel in a pathway called the trigeminal lemniscus; fibers from the substantia gelatinosa travel in the neospinothalamic or paleospinothalamic pathways. The latter pathway is multisynaptic, synapsing at several levels in the periaqueductal gray, an area rich in enkephalins. Activity along this branch of the spinothalamic system is experienced as dull, aching pain. The neospinothalamic system, on the other hand, reaches the thalamus without synapsing in the brainstem. This branch of the spinothalamic system conveys sharp, burning pain sensations. The multisynaptic paleospinothalamic branch offers more possibilities for drug-induced suppression of pain because analgesics, like most centrally active drugs, work on the chemical transmission process at synapses.

The thalamus is a second or "upper" gate in the projection of pain sensations. Some, but not all, pain signals reaching the thalamus are relayed upward to the somatosensory cortex of the parietal lobe. When pain signals are persistent, the proportion of impulses allowed to pass through the gates gradually declines. This phenomenon, called *habituation,* should not be confused with adaptation, which occurs at the receptor level.

Peptide and amine transmitters are involved in regulating the gates of the pain pathways (Fig. 22-1). The lower gate for somatic pain sensations, the substantia gelatinosa, is controlled by the peptide enkephalin and the amine serotonin. Bipolar cells carrying pain signals release a peptide called substance P to activate secondary cell bodies in the substantia gelatinosa. The release of substance P can be inhibited by enkephalin, perhaps through an axoaxonal synapse. Descending serotonin fibers from medullary raphé nuclei control enkephalin release.

The lower gate for cranial pain signals is controlled by norepinephrine terminals. It has long been known that both norepinephrine and serotonin are involved in mediating the action of narcotics. The upper gate for both cranial and somatic pain signals, the thalamus, is controlled by serotonergic inputs from the medial raphé nucleus.

Implications for Psychotherapy

The interplay of the organic, functional, and interpersonal systemic facets of psychological processes is nowhere more profound or complex than in relationship to the

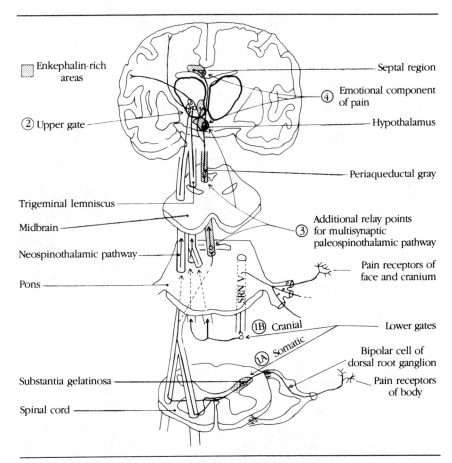

Fig. 22-1. *The pain pathways, illustrating the lower [1A and 1B] and upper [2] gates, where pain impulses are subject to modulation; additional relay points [3] of the paleospinothalamic pathway; and brain centers that contribute the affective quality to pain [4].*

experience of pain. The presence of physical pain may be an antecedent of depression (the functional level) or feelings of intensive guilt (the interpersonal systemic level). The presence of chronic pain has been observed to lead to hypochondria or to patients' being labeled hypochondriacs. On the other hand, psychological and interpersonal processes may influence the occurrence and experience of pain. Migraine and tension headaches, lower back pain, pelvic pain, facial pain, arthritic pain, and even susceptibility to neoplasms have been correlated to various degrees with the psychological state. The presence of psychiatric illness, including anxiety, schizophrenia, and depression, can increase sensitivity to pain or may be the cause of pain, as in the conversion of hysterical pain. And socioeconomic factors influence exposure to occupational hazards or impoverished living conditions that may lead to illness and pain. Many of these same factors also influence responsiveness to treatment for pain. The full meaning of the use of an analgesic by a client can only be appreciated when the psychological significance of the pain and pain relief have been thoroughly explored.

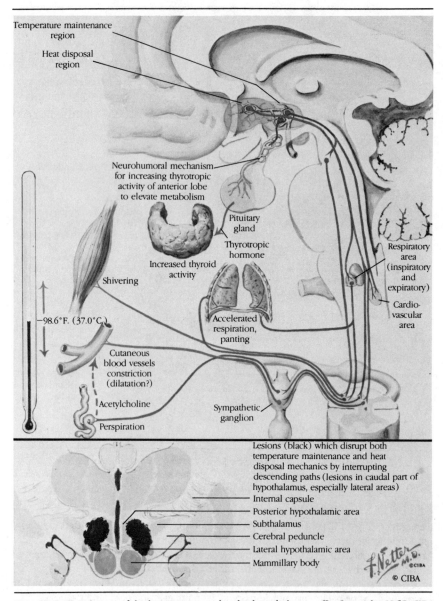

Temperature maintenance region

Heat disposal region

Neurohumoral mechanism for increasing thyrotropic activity of anterior lobe to elevate metabolism

Pituitary gland

Thyrotropic hormone

Increased thyroid activity

Shivering

Respiratory area (inspiratory and expiratory)

Cardio-vascular area

—98.6°F. (37.0°C.)

Accelerated respiration, panting

Cutaneous blood vessels constriction (dilatation?)

Acetylcholine

Perspiration

Sympathetic ganglion

Lesions (black) which disrupt both temperature maintenance and heat disposal mechanics by interrupting descending paths (lesions in caudal part of hypothalamus, especially lateral areas)

Internal capsule

Posterior hypothalamic area

Subthalamus

Cerebral peduncle

Lateral hypothalamic area

Mammillary body

© CIBA

Fig. 22-2. *Regulation of body temperature by the hypothalamus.* (© *Copyright 1965 CIBA Pharmaceutical Company, Division of CIBA-GEIGY Corporation. Reproduced, with permission, from the CIBA Collection of Medical Illustrations by Frank H. Netter, M.D. All rights reserved.*)

Neurophysiology of Temperature
The human is a homeothermic animal in that human body temperature is maintained within narrow limits despite wide fluctuations of environmental temperature. Maintenance of body temperature involves control of both heat production and heat loss. Body temperature is normally between 36° and 38°C (96.8° and 100.4°F). An increase of only 5° brings one to the edge of a zone in which brain damage and heat stroke may occur and the temperature-regulating function itself lost. This results in further elevation of temperature into the lethal range. The upper limit for survival is less than 10° above normal.

A drop of 5° also leads to impairment of the temperature-regulating function, and a 10° drop results in loss of control. At this temperature, human beings are highly susceptible to fatal disturbances of cardiac rhythm. Otherwise, tissues other than the heart would be able to tolerate a further reduction, provided artificial means were available for rewarming. Heat production involves control of cutaneous vasoconstriction; metabolism of carbohydrate, fat, and protein; and shivering, muscle tension, and exercise or activity. Heat loss involves control of cutaneous vasodilatation, sweating, panting, fur-licking, and body position.

Peripheral cold receptors discharge continuously even at normal skin temperature, but increase their degree and rate of firing when the skin is cooled. The sensation of warmth appears sometimes to involve increased firing of "warmth receptors," but in other instances, to be due to a decreased firing of cold receptors.

Various neurons in the anterior hypothalamus (about 20 percent of all neurons in this region) are sensitive to temperature changes (Fig. 22-2). Most respond to increases in temperature; about one-fourth respond to cooling. No markedly temperature-sensitive neurons have been found in other parts of the brain.

The anterior hypothalamus acts as a thermostat. The "set point" undergoes diurnal variations and may be displaced, for example, by pathogens, to produce fever. Prostaglandin production is involved in the elevation of the set point. The anterior hypothalamus also controls heat loss. Stimulation results in panting, sweating, and vasodilatation. Destruction of the anterior hypothalamus results in hyperthermia.

The posterior hypothalamic region controls heat conservation. Stimulation provokes shivering and peripheral vasoconstriction. Destruction of the posterior hypothalamus results in poikilothermy (not hypothermia as one might expect), owing to interruption of fiber tracts from the anterior hypothalamus as well as to local neuronal damage.

Injection of serotonin into the cerebral ventricles of cats or dogs, or microinjections into the anterior hypothalamus of cats, has been shown to produce shivering and an increase in rectal temperature. However, more recent work has indicated that the effect in the cat is biphasic—hypothermia at low doses, hyperthermia at higher doses. Intraventricular injection of serotonin produces hypothermia in rats, mice, and rabbits. Thus, the significance of serotonin in temperature regulation appears to be species-dependent. In cats and dogs, intraventricular epinephrine or norepinephrine produces a reduction in rectal temperature.

The most that can be stated with certainty at this time is that temperature regulation by the hypothalamus seems to involve the interaction of the various amines.

Selected References and Further Readings
1. Angevine, J. B., Jr., and Cotman, C. W. *Principles of Neuroanatomy.* New York: Oxford University Press, 1981.
2. Carpenter, M. B. *Human Neuroanatomy* (7th ed.). Baltimore: Williams & Wilkins, 1976.
3. Cox, B., and Lomax, P. Pharmacological control of temperature regulation. *Annu. Rev. Pharmacol. Toxicol.* 17:341–353, 1977.

Narcotic Analgesics

23

R⃝

History

Opium is one of the oldest drugs known to human beings. Until the nineteenth century, only crude preparations of the extract were available. Opium derives from the poppy plant, which is cultivated in many regions of the world, particularly in Turkey and southeastern Asia.

Morphine, the first alkaloid ever isolated in purified form, was extracted from opium in 1803. Synthesis of morphine was not achieved until 1952. The term *morphine* comes from Morpheus, the Greek god of dreams. Although the actions of morphine on the body are diverse, its use in medicine is largely related to its analgesic potency.

In addition to morphine, codeine is a naturally occurring narcotic alkaloid derived from opium. Dozens of other drugs of more or less similar structure have been synthesized. As with other classes of drugs, we will discuss the pharmacology of the drug-class prototype—morphine in this case—in some detail and then compare it with other drugs of this class.

Actions on the Central Nervous System

The effect of narcotic drugs is known as narcosis and is manifested by analgesia, a change in mood, mental clouding, impairment of mental and physical performance, especially in recently acquired and complex learning. The mood change effected by narcotics is variable, being dependent on the physical condition and drug experience of the patient. Patients in severe pain generally experience euphoria, simply as a result of the pain relief. The addict experiences euphoria, especially if the narcotic is taken intravenously rather than orally. Frequently, however, the naive patient may experience discomfiture and dysphoria related in part to the annoying gastrointestinal effects of the narcotic.

The analgesic effect of narcotics is related to an ability to suppress the affective component of pain. Narcotics act on relay centers along the pain pathway, including the substantia gelatinosa in the spinal cord and limbic centers in the paleospinothalamic pathway, which relays dull pain, especially from the viscera. The actual sensory threshold is unaffected, but the emotional component is diminished. Analgesia produced by narcotics is additive with that produced by nonnarcotic analgesics. Narcotics act centrally, while the nonnarcotic drugs act largely at the level of the peripheral pain receptors.

Two important centers located in the brainstem are sensitive to narcotics. The cough center is depressed by narcotics, and it is this action that has resulted in the use of codeine and other narcotics in cough suppressants. A synthetic derivative, dextromethorphan, is an effective cough suppressant that has no narcotic or addicting properties and is now widely used in cough suppressants. The respiratory center is a second significant center depressed by morphine. Narcotics depress the brain's responsivity to elevated carbon dioxide levels more than its response to low oxygen or the basic rhythmicity of the respiratory neurons. Respiratory depression is the usual cause of death in cases of narcotic overdose. It may be treated by artificially maintaining respiration, by a specific narcotic antagonist such as naloxone, or with analeptics such as doxapram. Use of a narcotic antagonist in an addict risks precipitation of a severe withdrawal syndrome, while use of an analeptic risks producing convulsions.

The chemoreceptor trigger zone located in the medulla is stimulated by many narcotics. This zone is part of a reflex system that regulates vomiting. Narcotic stimulation of the chemoreceptor trigger zone results in vomiting or feelings of nausea and dizziness, depending on the dosage and potency of the particular agent. Narcotics slow the EEG and, in particular, increase theta activity and the integrated amplitude.

Endogenous Morphine-Like Substances

The mechanism of action of narcotic analgesics relates to an interaction with receptors, called opiate receptors, normally acted on by endogenous morphine-like substances. The endogenous opiate receptor ligands include two pentapeptides called met-enkephalin and leu-enkephalin and a protein called beta-endorphin. The peptides are heavily concentrated along the pain pathways and in the substantia gelatinosa, periaqueductal gray, hypothalamus, and limbic system (refer to Fig. 22-1). Beta-endorphin is localized in a descending pathway that influences the reward and punishment systems. Morphine and other narcotic agonists bind to and activate opiate receptors, while narcotic antagonists, such as naloxone, merely bind.

Opiate receptors exist in three interconvertible affinity states, designated μ, κ, and σ. The affinity state is determined by the relation of the receptor site, or recognition protein, to modulatory and coupling proteins. The nature of the effector protein for opiate receptors is not known, but in some brain regions it may be the coupling protein of the D_1 type of dopamine receptor. At these sites, narcotics decrease the effect of dopamine action on D_1-receptors, producing a "functional blockade" of dopamine receptors. At certain other receptor sites, narcotics are noted to inhibit prostaglandin stimulation of adenyl cyclase. Morphine affinity for opiate receptors is greatest for the μ state and least for the σ state.

Opiate receptors exhibit adaptability. Chronic administration of opiate agonists such as morphine leads to down-regulation, brought about by reduced receptor-effector coupling, not by a reduced number of receptor sites. Narcotic antagonists, on the other hand, cause up-regulation when administered chronically. This up-regulation is associated with an increase in the number of receptor sites.

Peripheral Actions of Morphine

Narcotics produce orthostatic hypotension primarily because of release of histamine. Certain smooth muscles are directly contracted by morphine, such as the smooth muscle of the gut and the pupils. The former effect leads to constipation; the latter effect produces the characteristic constricted pupil of the addict. Narcotics produce a flushing and warming of the skin that is related to dilatation of cutaneous blood vessels.

Intoxication, Tolerance, and Dependence

Narcotic intoxication (the narcotic stupor) is defined in the DSM-III based on five criteria: (1) recent use of an opioid; (2) pupillary constriction; (3) one or more psychological signs (euphoria, dysphoria, apathy, or psychomotor retardation); (4) one or more neurologic signs (drowsiness, slurred speech, or impaired memory or attention; and (5) absence of an organic or psychiatric cause.

Tolerance develops to all the effects of narcotics except those related to a direct action on smooth muscle, such as pupillary constriction and constipation. Tolerance does not necessarily develop uniformly to all actions at the same time, however. Although an increase in the rate of metabolism of narcotics (drug disposition) may account for a small part of the tolerance, most of the tolerance appears to be of the pharmacodynamic variety.

During the initial stages of tolerance development, there is an increase in the turnover of dopamine in the corpus striatum. Since morphine is believed to produce a functional blockade of dopamine receptors, this may account for the early development of tolerance. After a few days of chronic morphine treatment, however, dopamine turnover returns to normal. Thus, a second mechanism appears to account for long-term tolerance. During this long-term phase of tolerance, opiate receptors exhibit subsensitivity, and dopamine receptors become supersensitive.

Both psychological and physical dependence occur with chronic narcotic use. In fact, dependence is such a characteristic occurrence with narcotics that the term *narcotic* as used by the legal profession has come to include many drugs that are unrelated to morphine but produce dependence. There is considerable range in the degree of abuse potential within the narcotic group. The abuse potential is related to the intensity of the euphoria produced by the agent, the intensity of withdrawal symptoms that follow its use, and its efficacy in suppressing withdrawal symptoms.

Withdrawal from narcotics, while distinctly unpleasant, is less life-threatening than withdrawal from a sedative-hypnotic. The syndrome is characterized by anxiety, body aches, insomnia, yawning, lacrimation, runny nose, perspiration, pupillary dilation, tachycardia, "goose bumps," nausea, diarrhea, vomiting, and anorexia.

Narcotic Abuse

It is estimated that in 1969 there were about 200,000 heroin addicts. Two years later there was an estimated 250,000. In the early and mid-1970s, according to United States government reports, the number essentially leveled off because of the agreements reached with Turkey, which at one time supplied about 80 percent of the illegal opiates found in the United States.

The average age of abusers has steadily declined over the years; by 1969, it had declined to 22 years; by 1978 the modal age group for onset of narcotic addiction was 11 to 20 years of age. There has also been a spread of the use of opium to areas outside the traditional opiate center, New York City. Numerically, the heroin problem is not so great as that of alcohol, tranquilizers, or several other drugs. On the other hand, an estimated 1 to 2 percent of the addict population die yearly from overdosage. Chronic use of narcotics is less likely to produce tissue damage than is chronic use of stimulants or alcohol, but neurologic complications occur in about 3 percent of long-term addicts.

Morphine Analogues

Codeine is similar to morphine in all its actions but less potent (Table 23-1). It is about one-fifth to one-tenth as potent as an analgesic, about one-tenth as potent as a respira-

Table 23-1. Comparison of narcotic analgesics

Drug	Source	Potency	Special features
Morphine	Natural	Strong	Poor oral effectiveness; releases histamine
Codeine	Natural	Intermediate	Orally effective; good antitussive
Heroin	Semisynthetic	Strong	Favorable ratio of central to peripheral actions; high abuse liability
Meperidine	Synthetic	Strong	Orally effective; less constipating; more orthostatic hypotension
Dihydromorphinone	Synthetic	Strong	More respiratory depression; less emesis and less pupillary constriction
Methadone	Synthetic	Strong	Long-acting; orally effective
Propoxyphene	Synthetic	Weak	Less abuse liability
Pentazocine	Synthetic	Weak	Mixed agonist-antagonist; least abuse liability; more side effects than propoxyphene

tory depressant and emetic, but about one-half as potent as a cough suppressant. This greater *relative* potency with respect to cough suppression made codeine the drug of choice for cough preparations until the introduction of dextromethorphan. Codeine is marketed in a number of combination preparations. It is combined with acetaminophen (Tylenol with Codeine) or aspirin (Emperin with Codeine) for analgesia; with phenergan, an antihistamine (Phenergan VC Expectorant with Codeine) or with phenergan and phenacetin (Phenaphen) for use as an expectorant; or with Fiorinal, a barbiturate, for tension headache. Tylenol with Codeine is among the most widely prescribed drugs. A great advantage of codeine over morphine is its greater oral effectiveness. Note in Table 23-2 that the oral equivalent dose of codeine is only about 1.5 times its intramuscular dose, while the corresponding ratio for morphine is sixfold.

Heroin is diacetylmorphine and is prepared from morphine by a simple chemical reaction. Since it is deacetylated in the brain, heroin acts simply as a carrier of morphine into the brain, and, indeed, heroin does cross the blood-brain barrier more readily than does morphine. Because of this increased delivery to the brain, heroin produces less peripheral effect for a given level of central action. On a weight basis, it is two to three times more potent than morphine. It is a severe respiratory depressant.

Dihydromorphinone (Dilaudid) is some 5 to 10 times more potent than morphine as an analgesic and a respiratory depressant. It has less action on the pupil and is less emetic. Meperidine (Demerol) is, next to morphine, the most widely used potent analgesic. It is well absorbed orally and about equal to morphine as an analgesic. It produces less gastrointestinal stimulation and is preferred for this reason in elderly patients. Other meperidine-like cogenors are diphenoxylate (Colonil, Lomotil), loperamide (Imodium), and ethoheptazine (Zactane). Methadone (Dolophine) is similar to morphine in action and is well absorbed orally. Its principal use is in methadone-maintenance programs, where its prolonged duration is especially advantageous. Propoxyphene (Darvon) is less potent than codeine and has less addiction liability. It is

Table 23-2. *Pharmacokinetic parameters for various narcotics*

Drug	Typical onset (min)	Typical peak effect (min)	Typical duration (hr)	Half-life (hr)	Equivalent dose (mg)	
					IM	Oral
Morphine	20	60	7	2–3	10	60
Codeine	25	60	5	3–4	130	200
Meperidine	15	45	3	3–4	75	300
Dihydromorphinone	25	60	5	3–4	1.5	8
Methadone	15	120	5	22–25	10	20

marketed in combinations such as Darvocet (with acetaminophen) and Darvon Compound (with aspirin). Pentazocine (Talwin) has mixed antagonist and agonist properties. It has little or no abuse potential, but its side effects are greater than those of meperidine. Oxycodone is a narcotic used in analgesic mixtures and with APCs (aspirin, phenacetin, and caffeine), for example, Percodan. Fentanyl is used largely in combination with droperidol, a neuroleptic, for preanesthetic tranquilization.

Naloxone (Narcan) is a specific narcotic antagonist that can reverse the effects of any narcotic or precipitate withdrawal in an addict minutes after injection, but it is ineffective in reversing nonnarcotic CNS depressants. It is an effective treatment in cases of accidental opiate poisoning.

Methadone Treatment Programs

Methadone has been employed both to wean and to maintain narcotic addicts. In the first procedure, an appropriate dose of methadone is given to the addict, the amount being determined by the intensity of the habit. One difficulty is the highly variable quality of street drugs. Such factors as the frequency of use, the age of the habit, the cost of the habit, and the quality of illicit material generally found in the locale are taken into account. Once the habit has been stabilized for about 48 hours, the dose is reduced by 5 to 10 mg per day until withdrawal is complete. Methadone withdrawal symptoms are considerably milder than those accompanying morphine or heroin abstinence, although the symptoms may be more drawn out.

In a methadone maintenance program, stabilization of the habit occurs in the manner described. One factor in determining dosage in this type of program is whether it is felt necessary to preclude the potential for getting a "rush" from surreptitious use of street drugs. Higher doses of methadone (50 to 100 mg) will prevent the addict from obtaining a "rush" from street drugs. Lower doses (30 to 50 mg) do not block the action of street drugs, but they do eliminate drug craving. The maintenance program differs from the weaning program in that the dosage is not reduced after the habit is stabilized.

Methadone maintenance programs have both advocates and detractors. On the plus side, methadone does not produce the mood swings associated with heroin, because it is long-acting and has a prolonged plasma half-life (Fig. 23-1). The duration of action of methadone when used acutely is about 4 to 6 hours, but it increases with daily use because of a cumulative effect due to the very long plasma half-life of 22 to 25 hours (Table 23-2). Thus, the addict adhering to a maintenance schedule of daily high-dose

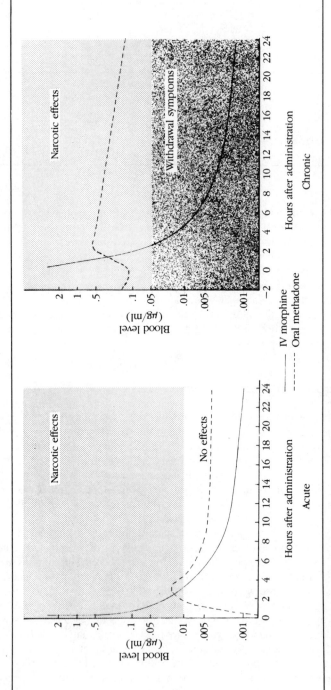

Fig. 23-1. *Narcotic blood levels of morphine and methadone. Acutely, oral methadone is slower to take effect and only slightly longer-acting than morphine. With chronic daily administration of 50- to 100-mg doses, methadone blood levels build up to produce a continuous, nearly stable level of narcotic effect.*

methadone administration cannot get the "rush" usually obtained by "shooting" heroin and is protected somewhat from the temptation to return to the use of "street stuff." And in the optimal case, some addicts may be ready for detoxification after a period on methadone maintenance has provided them with the opportunity to reconstruct support systems, such as family ties and stable employment, which may have been destroyed in the addiction cycle.

On the negative side, the risk of overdosage with methadone has proved to be substantial, and methadone maintenance leaves the addict completely dependent on continued drug usage with the attendant risks that are discussed throughout this book.

Typical criteria utilized in accepting applicants into a methadone maintenance program are (1) a minimal age of 18, or if the candidate is 16 to 18 years of age, guardian consent and at least two prior failures in a detoxification program; and (2) no history of dropping out of a maintenance program within the last 2 years (time period varies). During the first few months of participation in a program, the addict takes each dose under observation. After several months in the program, this requirement might be relaxed to allow four or five of the seven weekly doses to be taken at home. Among the variables found to predict successful retention in a methadone maintenance program (as opposed to relapse to street drugs) are being older, better educated, employed, white, married, and having had few or no criminal convictions.

Implications for Psychotherapy

The regular use of narcotics, especially those having short durations of action, impairs the ability of the user to function in a social context. The CNS effects of potent narcotics on mood, cognitive and motor functioning, and arousal level are profound. Narcotics are powerful primary reinforcers, produce physical as well as psychological dependence, suppress dreaming sleep, and presumably produce state-dependent learning in humans as they are known to do in animals. Narcotic dependence is a profound problem that is all too often resistant to even our best treatment programs.

Medically Important Narcotic Analgesics

codeine, a narcotic analgesic: moderate analgesia, lasting 4 to 6 hours, used in many cough suppressant and analgesic combinations. Typical: 30 to 60 mg per administration.

ethoheptazine (Zactane), a narcotic analgesic: strong, related to meperidine. Typical: 75 to 150 mg per administration.

fentanyl (Sublimaze, Innovar [combined with droperidol]), a narcotic analgesic: strong, often combined with droperidol for anesthetic premedication and postmedication. Typical: 0.05 to 0.1 mg per administration.

hydrocodone (Codone, Dicodid; Vicodin and Norcet [combined with acetaminophen]), a narcotic analgesic: strong. Typical: 5 to 10 mg per administration.

hydromorphone (dihydromorphinone) (Dilaudid), a narcotic analgesic: strong, lasting 4 to 5 hours. Typical: 2 to 4 mg per administration.

levorphanol (Levo-Dromoran), a narcotic analgesic: strong. Typical: 2 to 3 mg per administration PO or SQ.

meperidine (pethidine) (Demerol), a narcotic analgesic: strong, lasting 2 to 4 hours, less gastrointestinal stimulation, more orthostatic hypotension. Typical: 50 to 150 mg per administration.

methadone (Dolophine), a narcotic analgesic: strong, with its principal use in withdrawal from morphine-like drugs and in maintenance of addicts; acute duration 3 to 5 hours, but its cumulative effect extends duration to about 24 hours when used daily. Typical: 2.5 to 15 mg per administration.

morphine, a narcotic analgesic: strong, lasting 4 to 5 hours. Typical: 2.5 to 15 mg IV per administration.

naloxone (Narcan), a narcotic antagonist: closest to being a pure antagonist. Typical: 0.4 mg IV, IM, or SQ.

opium (Brown mixture, Pantopon, opium tincture, paregoric [combined with aspirin, phenacetin, and caffeine]; Atoka [combined with aspirin and phenacetin]), a narcotic analgesic and antidiarrheal agent. Typical antidiarrheal: 20 to 40 mg per administration.

oxycodone (Percodan [combined with aspirin]), a narcotic analgesic: mild to moderate analgesia, lasting 4 to 5 hours. Typical: 5 mg per administration.

oxymorphone (Numorphan), a narcotic analgesic: strong. Typical: 0.5 mg IV or 1.0 to 1.5 mg per administration SQ or IM.

pentazocine (Talwin), a narcotic analgesic: mixed narcotic agonist and antagonist, weak as analgesic, lasting 2 to 3 hours, with little abuse potential. Typical: 50 to 100 mg per administration.

propoxyphene (Darvon, Darvon-N [napsylate salt], Darvon Compound [combined with aspirin, phenacetin, and caffeine], Darvocet [combined with acetaminophen], Dolene, Pargesic, Proxagesic, Proxene, SK-65), a narcotic analgesic: weak analgesic, low abuse liability. Typical: 65 to 100 mg per administration.

Selected References and Further Readings

1. Gilman, A. G., Goodman, L. S., and Gilman, A. *The Pharmacological Basis of Therapeutics* (6th ed.). New York: Macmillan, 1980.
2. Loh, H. H., and Ross, D. H. (Eds.), Neurochemical mechanisms of opiates and endorphins. *Adv. Biochem. Psychopharmacol.* 20, 1979.
3. Mansky, P. A. Opiates: Human Psychopharmacology. In L. L. Iversen et al. (Eds.), *Handbook of Psychopharmacology.* New York: Plenum, 1978. Vol. 12.
4. Snyder, S. H., and Childers, S. R. Opiate receptors and opiate peptides. *Annu. Rev. Neurosci.* 2:35–64, 1979.

Nonnarcotic Analgesics
24

A large selection of nonnarcotic drugs is available for alternative use in the treatment of pain. By and large, the nonnarcotic analgesics are less effective than the potent narcotics, but have the distinct advantage of being nonaddictive. Moreover, for certain types of pain, nonnarcotic analgesics may actually be more effective than narcotics. Nevertheless, neurologic side effects sometimes occur and may be relevant in neuropsychological assessment. Many of the agents discussed in this chapter share two pharmacologic actions in addition to ability to produce analgesia, namely, an antipyretic and an anti-inflammatory effect. The common thread in these three seemingly diverse effects is the relationship of each to the family of endogenous autocoids, the prostaglandin E series.

Shared Pharmacologic Properties of Aspirin-Like Drugs

Analgesic Effect

Aspirin-like drugs alleviate low-intensity pain, such as headaches, rheumatic pain, dysmenorrhea, and muscle aches. Aspirin-like drugs are less effective as an analgesic than morphine or even codeine and about on a par with low-potency narcotics such as pentazocine or propoxyphene. The type of pain is important in comparisons of aspirin-like drugs with narcotics. Basically, aspirin is highly effective in alleviating pain associated with synthesis and release of prostaglandins, often being even more effective than morphine in this respect. Prostaglandins are produced and released in tissue injury or inflammation (Fig. 24-1), being derived from a cellular membrane constituent, arachidonic acid. Prostaglandins are produced by a group of enzymes collectively called *prostaglandin synthetase*. The action of prostaglandins in promoting pain sensations is a sensitization of pain receptors. The sensitized receptors are then more readily activated by the autocoid bradykinin, also derived from cellular constituents released from ruptured cells. Aspirin-like drugs are effective in postoperative pain, for example, because in this situation pain derives from prostaglandin release from cells damaged during incision and stitching. Generally, dull, throbbing pain is prostaglandin-related and aspirin-sensitive, while sharp, stabbing pain is related to direct sensory receptor activation and is aspirin-insensitive.

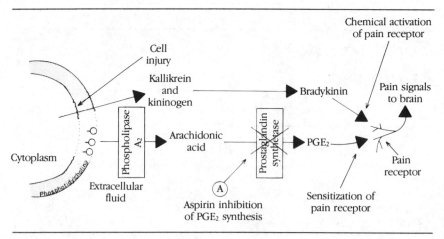

Fig. 24-1. *Mechanism of action of aspirin-like drugs. PgE₂, prostaglandin E₂.*

Antipyretic Effect

Aspirin-like drugs are effective in reducing elevated body temperature when it is due to an alteration in the "set point" established by the hypothalamus. On the other hand, aspirin does not lower normal body temperature or hyperthermia due to exposure to excessive environmental temperature, or excessive heat production from exercise, or both. Hyperthermia related to an alteration in set point is called fever. Fever may result from infection, inflammation, allergic reactions, tissue damage, malignancies, toxins, dehydration, or other disease states. These conditions cause fever by stimulating release of an endogenous pyrogen from neutrophils and other cells. This pyrogen travels through the circulation to the hypothalamus, where it triggers release of prostaglandins. Prostaglandins cause a shift in the set point. By blocking synthesis and release of prostaglandins, aspirin-like drugs bring about a resetting of the set point to the normal value (typically 98.6°F). Heat loss is then achieved by conventional mechanisms, most significantly, vasodilatation and sweating.

Anti-inflammatory Effect

The process of inflammation is critical to survival of the human organism and is a prelude to all reparative activities. The body is constantly being infiltrated by potentially dangerous microorganisms, such as viruses and bacteria. During the inflammatory process, the invading organisms are destroyed by phagocytosis—the engulfment and encapsulation of microorganisms or foreign particles by specialized phagocytic cells. Production of these cells and their delivery to the area of invasion is the function of the so-called reticuloendothelial system.

Two types of blood cells, monocytes and neutrophils, are of importance in inflammation. They are the phagocytic cells that engulf whole bacterial cells or cell debris. The inflammatory process consists of a sequence of three events called the triple response: redness, flare, and wheal. Redness occurs immediately in the area of injury, because autocoids, including histamine and serotonin, are released, causing dilatation of arterioles and constriction of venous capillaries. This fenestration of the microvasculature causes congestion of blood at the injured site. Bradykinins and prostaglandins are released in profusion, triggering pain impulses and advancing the inflammatory process. The initial phase of redness next activates autonomic compensatory reflex action that constricts vessels in the surrounding tissue, limiting the edema and redness to the region of injury. The third phase of the inflammatory process, wheal, involves the massing of leukocytes in the area of injury. These supplement the limited pool of tissue macrophages to help destroy the invading organism and clear away cellular debris. The massing of leukocytes is directed by chemotaxic chemicals released in the area of injury, including bradykinin and prostaglandin.

The anti-inflammatory action of aspirin-like drugs is related, of course, to its ability to counter the effects of prostaglandin. The vascular permeability and vasodilatation occurring in the redness phase is reduced, and sensitization of pain receptors throughout the inflammatory process is diminished.

Shared Side Effects of Nonnarcotic Analgesics

Although some side effects of drugs of the nonnarcotic group are unique to a given drug, some are common problems for the class as a whole. The most commonly shared adverse effect is an irritative effect on the gastrointestinal mucosa. The invariable result is an increase in gastrointestinal bleeding; a frequent result is outright ulceration and consequent anemia. Epigastric distress, as well as nausea and vomiting, may result from gastric irritation. The consistent association of this particular side effect with the many varied drugs in the nonnarcotic analgesic class suggests that it is related in some way to prostaglandins.

Another shared side effect is an anticoagulant action due to inhibition of platelet agglutination. This effect is definitely linked to prostaglandin synthetase inhibition. Platelet prostaglandin synthetase activity is required for production of a substance called thromboxane A_2, which promotes platelet aggregation. Another adverse effect related to prostaglandin is an antifertility effect in males. Many aspirin-like drugs are potentially nephrotoxic, especially when abused, an effect possibly related to prostaglandin.

Clinical Indications

The clinical applications of aspirin-like drugs are multitudinous. They find widespread use as an analgesic and antipyretic. Their anti-inflammatory applications include acute rheumatic fever, rheumatoid arthritis (often in combination with gold compounds), psoriatic arthritis, osteoarthritis, gouty arthritis, bursitis, and ankylosing spondylitis. A typical dose of aspirin for analgesic or antipyretic purposes is 650 mg, repeated in no less than 4 hours. For anti-inflammatory purposes, higher dosages are often required, for example, 8 g daily in 1-g doses. Thus, toxicity is most likely when aspirin is used for anti-inflammatory purposes.

Salicylates

Though the nonnarcotic analgesic class is now populated by a wealth of individual drugs, the oldest representatives, the salicylate family, are still most widely used and most thoroughly researched. Salicylates are derived from salicylic acid, a substance originally found in willow bark, but now synthesized from phenol. The parent compound, salicylic acid, was first prepared from oil of wintergreen in 1844, but it proved too irritating for internal use. Acetylsalicylic acid, or aspirin, is the most important salicylate, widely used in medicine and the prototype of the class.

Salicylate Poisoning

Aspirin is one of the top five drugs in terms of frequency of drug-induced fatalities (about 200 annually). The fatal dose range is 10 to 30 g. Salicylate poisoning is especially common in children, accounting for 15 percent of all fatal poisonings in children under five. About 50,000 cases of aspirin poisoning (accidental or associated with suicide attempts) occur yearly; a few instances occur when aspirin is used for inflammation. The critical symptoms of salicylate poisoning fall into four categories: (1) vomiting, dehydration, and hyperthermia (an immediate threat to life); (2) tinnitis, mental confusion, delirium, and convulsions (another potentially fatal component); (3) bleeding, anemia, and lung damage (all related to the inhibition of platelet aggregation); and (4) acid-base imbalance. The acid-base imbalance is initially triggered by stimulation of respiration (hyperpnea) due to an action of aspirin on the medullary respiratory center. Increased respiration causes excessive breathing off of carbon dioxide, which raises plasma pH. Usually, alkalosis is adequately compensated by increased kidney excretion of alkalis, but this reduces blood buffering capacity and leaves the individual vulnerable to further acid-base problems.

Treatment of salicylate toxicity is based on removal of the drug (by stomach lavage, induced vomiting, or intravenous fluid replacement) and symptomatic treatment (correcting the pH with bicarbonate and stimulating synthesis of clotting factors with intravenous vitamin K).

The mental disturbances that occur in salicylate toxicity are sometimes called the "salicylate jag." The syndrome may simulate alcohol inebriation and includes incoherent speech, delirium, hallucinations, garrulousness, lassitude, drowsiness, confusion, and apprehensiveness. Euphoria does not occur, however, and may aid in differentiating the two conditions.

Drug Interactions of Aspirin

Aspirin is highly bound to plasma albumin–binding sites. Consequently, it has an interaction of mutual potentiation with drugs such as phenytoin and penicillin. The anticoagulant effect of aspirin is additive with other anticoagulants. Analgesia produced by aspirin is additive with that produced by narcotics. Many combinations of narcotic and nonnarcotic analgesics are available commercially.

Other Salicylates

The great therapeutic value of aspirin, together with its less-than-ideal spectrum of side effects, has stimulated a search for better salicylate drugs or better delivery mechanisms that would reduce gastrointestinal ulceration. Next to aspirin, the most widely used salicylate is sodium salicylate, less effective than aspirin. Also less effective is salicylamide, no longer an official drug. Sodium thiosalicylate is marketed for intramuscular use in inflammatory conditions, particularly in acute gout and rheumatic fever. Two salicylates with fewer gastrointestinal effects than aspirin are choline salicylate and magnesium salicylate. Salsalate is a molecule that hydrolyzes into two acetylsalicylic acid molecules, but only in the intestine. It is free of irritant effects on the stomach, but the intestine is still vulnerable. Another salicylate derivative, diflunisal (Dolobid), first marketed in 1982, appears to be lower in toxicity than aspirin. Aspirin is often buffered, which reduces gastric irritation and hastens absorption, but may also speed excretion.

Table 24-1. *Effectiveness of nonnarcotic analgesic, antipyretic, anti-inflammatory drugs*

Drug class	Analgesic	Antipyretic	Anti-inflammatory
Salicylates	Yes	Yes	Yes
Para-aminophenols	Yes	Yes	No
Zomepirac	Yes	Yes	Yes

Other Aspirin-Like Drugs

Next to the salicylates, the para-aminophenol family is the most widely encountered group of aspirin-like drugs. Acetaminophen (e.g., Tylenol) is second only to aspirin in frequency of use among nonnarcotic analgesics. It is approximately equal to aspirin in analgesic and antipyretic effectiveness (Table 24-1) but has only weak anti-inflammatory effects. Side effects are less common with acetaminophen than with aspirin, but nephrotoxicity is somewhat more common than with aspirin. Acute overdose may cause fatal hepatic toxicity. Phenacetin, another para-aminophenol, is metabolized in the body to acetaminophen. It is more toxic, but no more effective than acetaminophen. It is often marketed in APC combinations of aspirin, phenacetin, and caffeine (APC).

In the fall of 1982, in a notorious case of drug tampering, seven deaths occurred in the Chicago area when victims ingested Tylenol capsules in which cyanide had been substituted for acetaminophen. In the aftermath, a wave of outrage and cautiousness toward medications swept briefly across the sensitivity of an alarmed public; yet one is tempted to note that annually, in the United States and Great Britain, some 5,000 hospitalizations occur from acetaminophen overdoses, 50 to 100 of these resulting in fatalities.

A newer aspirin-like analgesic is zomepirac (Zomax). It is a more potent prostaglandin inhibitor than aspirin and hence has greater effects. On a weight basis it is 13 times more potent than aspirin; a 50-mg dose is roughly comparable to 650 mg of aspirin.

Other aspirin-like drugs are marketed expressly for anti-inflammatory applications, although most or all produce analgesic and antipyretic effects as well. Proprionic acid derivatives used for arthritis and other anti-inflammatory purposes include ibuprofen (Motrin), fenoprofen (Nalfon), and naproxen (Naprosyn). The incidence of gastrointestinal irritation is lower with these drugs, and their therapeutic benefit is equivalent to aspirin's in rheumatoid arthritis and osteoarthritis (Table 24-2). Another family, the fenamates, differ slightly in mechanism from aspirin in that they appear to have some ability to antagonize prostaglandin action as well as inhibit prostaglandin synthesis and release. The fenamates include meclofenamate (Meclomen) and mefenamic acid (Ponstel). They are roughly equivalent to aspirin in both effectiveness and toxicity. Tolmetin (Tolectin) is a new anti-inflammatory drug that is often better tolerated than aspirin.

Two families of aspirin-like drugs are both more potent and more toxic than those that have been discussed and are reserved for patients not adequately responsive to other drugs. The methylated indole family includes indomethacin (Indocin) and sulindac (Clinoril). Neurologic symptoms, such as headache, vertigo, mental confusion, and light-headedness, are common with indomethacin. The pyrazolone family includes phenylbutazone (Butazolidin) and oxyphenbutazone (Tandearil). These drugs produce induction of liver enzymes and have been known to cause fatal blood dyscrasias.

Table 24-2. *Comparisons of non-steroidal anti-inflammatory drugs*

Drug	Daily maximum dosage (mg)	Anti-inflammatory effectiveness	Overall toxicity
Salicylates			
Aspirin	3,900	++	++
Diflunisal	1,500	++	+
Proprionic acid derivatives			
Ibuprofen	2,400	++	+
Fenoprofen	3,200	++	+
Naproxen	1,100	++	+
Fenamates			
Meclofenamate	400	++	++
Mefenamic acid	1,000	++	++
Parachlorobenzoic acid derivatives			
Indomethacin	50	+++	++++
Sulindac	400	+++	?
Tolmetin	1,800	++	+
Pyrazolone derivatives			
Phenylbutazone	600	+++	++++
Oxyphenbutazone	600	+++	++++

+, lowest degree of effectiveness or toxicity; ++++, highest degree of effectiveness or toxicity.

Implications for Psychotherapy

Aspirin, while not a drug of abuse in the strict sense of the word, is widely overused. The excessive use of aspirin in part reflects a mistaken belief that it is free of important side effects. And aspirin is readily available, giving an opportunity for a generally overmedicated society to throw caution to the wind once again. The psychotherapist should keep in mind that the person who shows a lack of appreciation for the potential hazards of frequent aspirin use is likely to generalize this attitude to other decisions about drugs.

The symptoms of salicylate toxicity may mimic alcohol intoxication. Differential diagnosis is critically important in deciding on the appropriate intervention.

Medically Important Nonnarcotic Analgesics, Antipyretics, and Nonsteroidal Anti-inflammatory Drugs

acetaminophen (Tylenol, Pedric, Phenaphen, many combinations), a nonnarcotic analgesic and antipyretic. Typical: 300 to 650 mg per administration. Maximum daily: 4,000 mg.

aspirin (Empirin, many others; Bufferin, many others [buffered]; many combinations), a nonnarcotic analgesic, antipyretic, and anti-inflammatory agent. Typical: 650 mg per administration. Maximum daily: 7,800 mg.

choline salicylate (Arthropan), a nonnarcotic analgesic, antipyretic, and anti-inflammatory agent: fewer gastrointestinal side effects than aspirin. Typical: 600 mg per administration. Maximum daily: 9,600 mg.

diflunisal (Dolobid), a nonsteroidal anti-inflammatory and nonnarcotic analgesic. Typical: 500 to 1,500 mg daily. Maximum: 2,000 mg daily.

fenoprofen (Nalfon), a nonsteroidal anti-inflammatory and nonnarcotic analgesic: fewer gastrointestinal side effects than aspirin. Typical: 300 to 600 mg per administration. Maximum daily: 3,200 mg.

ibuprofen (Motrin, Rufen), a nonsteroidal anti-inflammatory and nonnarcotic analgesic: fewer gastrointestinal side effects than aspirin. Typical: 300 to 600 mg per administration. Maximum daily: 2,400 mg.

indomethacin (Indocin), a nonsteroidal anti-inflammatory agent: reserved for refractory cases. Typical: 25 to 50 mg per administration. Maximum daily: 200 mg.

magnesium salicylate (Mobidin, Magan), a nonnarcotic analgesic, antipyretic, and anti-inflammatory agent: fewer gastrointestinal side effects than aspirin. Typical: 600 mg per administration. Maximum daily: 9,600 mg.

meclofenamate (Meclomen), a nonsteroidal anti-inflammatory agent: reserved for refractory cases. Typical: 50 to 100 mg per administration. Maximum daily: 400 mg.

naproxen (Anaprox, Naprosyn), a nonsteroidal anti-inflammatory agent: fewer gastrointestinal side effects. Typical: 250 to 375 mg per administration. Maximum daily: 1,000 mg.

oxyphenbutazone (Oxalid, Tandearil), a nonsteroidal anti-inflammatory agent: reserved for refractory cases. Typical: 100 to 150 mg per administration. Maximum daily: 600 mg.

phenacetin (many combinations, e.g., APC combinations), a nonnarcotic analgesic and antipyretic: more toxic than acetaminophen. Typical: 130 to 162 mg per administration. Maximum daily: 1,000 mg.

phenylbutazone (Azolid, Butazolidin), a nonsteroidal anti-inflammatory agent: reserved for refractory cases. Typical: 100 to 150 mg per administration. Maximum daily: 600 mg.

salicylamide, a nonnarcotic analgesic, antipyretic, and anti-inflammatory agent: poorly effective. Typical: 325 to 650 mg per administration. Maximum daily: 2,600 mg.

sodium salicylate (Parbocyl), a nonnarcotic analgesic, antipyretic, and anti-inflammatory agent: less effective than aspirin. Typical: 325 to 650 mg per administration. Maximum daily: 1,950 mg.

sodium thiosalicylate (Arthrolate, Asproject, Thiodyne), a nonnarcotic analgesic, antipyretic, and anti-inflammatory agent: for intramuscular administration. Initial: 400 to 900 mg daily, IM. Maintenance: 200 mg daily, IM.

sulindac (Clinoril), a nonsteroidal anti-inflammatory agent: reserved for refractory cases. Typical: 300 mg daily. Maximum: 400 mg daily.

tolmetin (Tolectin), a nonsteroidal anti-inflammatory agent: fewer gastrointestinal side effects. Typical: 600 to 1,800 mg daily. Maximum: 2,000 mg daily.

zomepirac (Zomax), a nonnarcotic analgesic, antipyretic, and anti-inflammatory agent: more potent than aspirin. Typical: 100 mg per administration. Maximum daily: 400 mg.

Selected References and Further Readings

1. Gilman, A. G., Goodman, L. S., and Gilman, A. *The Pharmacological Basis of Therapeutics* (6th ed.). New York: Macmillan, 1980.

2. Miller, R. L., Insel, P. A., and Melmon, K. L. Inflammatory Disorders. In K. L. Melmon and H. F. Morrelli (Eds.), *Clinical Pharmacology* (2nd ed.). New York: Macmillan, 1978.
3. Samuelsson, B., Goldyne, M., Granstrom, E., Hamberg, M., Hammarstrom, S., and Malmsten, C. Prostaglandins and thromboxans. *Annu. Rev. Biochem.* 47:997–1029, 1978.

Headaches
and Neuralgia
25

Headaches and face pains may arise from a wide variety of causes (Table 25-1). Consequently, therapy, whether with drugs or otherwise, takes many forms. Headaches may be associated secondarily with structural defects such as tumors, hemorrhage, head injuries, with common viral or bacterial infections, or with organic diseases such as syphilis, meningitis, Paget's disease, and others. In all these cases, the logical approach is the diagnosis and treatment of the underlying disease state by surgery, with antibiotics, nonnarcotics or narcotic analgesics, or by whatever treatment is specific for the particular pathologic state. Some headaches are allergic reactions to pollens, foods, or environmental allergens. Other headaches are referred pains, originating in the teeth, ears, sinuses, or eyes. Ophthalmic causes, such as glaucoma and eyestrain, are common causes. Sinus headaches are referred to the face, around the eyes, and the jaw and are treated with antihistamines and decongestants. In this chapter, another class of head and face pains will be considered—those that are not associated with obvious organic or structural pathologic conditions or infection, but do not appear to be wholly psychogenic in nature.

Migraine and Cluster Headaches

The term *migraine* is one that can be employed in either of two ways. In most English-language medical literature on the subject the term is used in a broad, inclusive sense to encompass both "classic" and "common" migraine. Non-English-language writers, on the other hand, generally employ *migraine* only for the classic variety and designate headaches of the common type as *nonmigrainous vascular headaches, cephalea vasomotoria,* or *common headache.* We will employ the term in the broader sense, differentiating between classic and common varieties as required.

Migraine is characterized by brief, recurring headaches. It is generally believed to be associated with stress, but psychotherapy has proved effective in only a limited number of cases. Often, there are associated neurologic and gastrointestinal symptoms. Any of the following symptoms may occur: blurred vision, arcs or waves of color, tunnel vision, partial or complete temporary blindness, double vision, partial aphasia or other verbal disturbances, deafness, ataxia, or vertigo.

The visual prodromata occur exclusively in classic migraine. Other prodromata occur in both classic and common migraine but are more prominent in the former. The head-

Table 25-1. *Headaches: Classifications, age and sex correlates, and treatments*

Headache classification	Type	Age or sex correlates	Treatments other than analgesics
Vascular headaches			
Migraine	PS	Postpuberty; F > M	Ergotamine, caffeine, methysergide, propranolol, rest, biofeedback (temperature)
Cluster	PS	> 25; M >> F	Methysergide, propranolol, activity
Drug-induced			
Caffeine withdrawal	OG	None	Caffeine or amphetamine
Alcohol "hangover"	OG	None	Oxygen
Vasodilators	OG	None	Adjust dose
Histamine	OG	None	Antihistamines
Other			
Allergies	OG	None	Antihistamines, pressors
Systemic infection	OG	None	Antihistamines, antibiotics
Hypoglycemia	OG	None	Dietary adjustments
Anoxia	OG	None	Oxygen
Postictal	OG	None	Oxygen
Hypertension*	OG	Adult	Antihypertensives, etc.
Muscle tension headaches	PS	None	Muscle relaxants, analgesics, rest, biofeedback (EMG)
Traction headaches			
Tumors	OG	None	Surgery, radiation
Hematoma or abscess	OG	Adults	Bed rest
Inflammatory headaches			
Meningitis	OG	None	Antibiotics
Subarachnoid hemorrhage	OG	Adults	Bed rest, hypotensives, surgery
Temporal arteritis	OG	> 60; M > F	Steroids
Referred head pains			
Sinus	OG	None	Antihistamines, decongestants, rest, wet heat
Ophthalmologic	OG	None	Antiglaucoma drugs, glasses, etc.
Dental, otologic	OG	None	Antibiotics, dental care, surgery, etc.
Neuralgias			
Trigeminal	OG	Aged; F > M	Carbamazepine, phenytoin
Glossopharyngeal	OG	Aged; M > F	Carbamazepine, phenytoin
Psychogenic			
Conversion	PG	None	Psychotherapy
Hypochondriachal	PG	None	Psychotherapy
Delusional	PG	None	Antipsychotics

OG, organogenic; PG, psychogenic; PS, psychosomatic.
*Includes hypertension due to pheochromacytoma, administration of pressor drugs, ingestion of tyramine in the diet, and essential hypertension.

ache in some cases is preceded by premonitory mood changes that may be pleasant or unpleasant. In classic migraine, the headache itself is usually on only one side of the head (from whence the name, migraine) and may vary in intensity from mild to severe. Nausea and vomiting may accompany the attack. The attacks often occur in flurries, alternating between the left and right hemispheres. The incidence of classic migraine headaches increases in women during pregnancy. In common migraine, headaches are often bilateral and dull, and nausea is less common and less severe. The attacks are periodic, not clustered. The frequency of common migraine headaches decreases during pregnancy but increases during periods of life transition. Common migraine is among the most prevalent forms of headache, while classic migraine is comparatively rare.

Cluster headaches are diagnostically distinct from migraine headaches, but are treated similarly. Cluster headaches are unilateral severe pains occurring in and around the eyes and are accompanied by tearing, a runny nose, and reddening of the eyes. Duodenal ulcers often accompany cluster headaches, supporting the theory that the condition is related to excess parasympathetic activity. Cluster headaches occur more often in males than in females.

Migraine occurs more frequently in females. It is rare before puberty, and when it occurs in young people it may disappear at puberty. It most often occurs in adolescence and in such cases is likely to persist for many years. Another modal age group for the appearance of migraine is during menopause, but in such cases it seldom lasts more than a few years.

Migraine tends to occur in persons having a personality profile marked by obsessive-compulsive tendencies and a great need for achievement. They may also exhibit a hypersensitivity to sensory stimuli and are more than normally likely to have allergies or epilepsy. They may be sexually maladjusted. Only a single rare subtype of migraine is genetically linked, but a familial history of migraine is often present.

There are three aspects to the treatment of migraine: symptomatic, prophylactic, and acute. Symptomatic treatment includes the inhalation of amyl nitrite or carbon dioxide for the relief of ocular and neurologic disturbances, and antiemetics or antispasmodics for the relief of GI problems.

Prophylactic treatment should center around an adjustment of life-style that reduces sources of stress and overwork. Anxiolytics may be prescribed as an aid in reducing the response to stressful conditions. Specific prophylactic chemotherapy for migraines entails the use of antiserotonergic substances. Of these, the best-known and most widely tested is methysergide (also spelled methysergid) (Sansert). Methysergide is the most efficacious treatment currently available but also has many side effects, including heartburn, diarrhea, nausea, vomiting, and GI cramps. Side effects in the CNS include light-headedness, nervousness, insomnia, euphoria, weakness, and loss of appetite. A rare but dangerous side effect is inflammatory fibrosis. A peculiar drug interaction involving methysergide is that it potentiates the effects of phenothiazines, necessitating a reduction in dosage of the latter. A drug employed widely in Europe and Australia, but not yet in the United States, is pizotyline (Pizotifen, Sandomigran). It is slightly less effective than methysergide, but is relatively devoid of side effects. Other antiserotonergic agents, including cyproheptadine (Periactin), methdilazine (Tacaryl), and methylergol carbamide maleate (Lysenyl), have been tested clinically for use in migraine. An antihypertensive drug, clonidine (Catapres), has been tested with some degree of success.

For acute treatment during migraine attacks, the drug of choice is ergotamine. Ergotamine is most effective if given early in an attack. The mechanism of ergotamine's action in migraine is not known with certainty, but current speculation is that it constricts dilated cranial vessels responsible for the headache. Methysergide given during an attack is not beneficial.

Biofeedback has proven effective in about 50 percent of patients with migraine. The technique employed involves detection of skin-surface temperature measured from a finger. The patient learns to warm skin temperature by assuming mental states that promote peripheral vasodilatation. This lowers blood pressure and relieves cerebrovascular distention. Later, when a vascular headache begins to develop, the patient resumes the mental posture learned during the training sessions.

The effectiveness of antiserotonin agents has led to development of two theories of migraine centering around levels of serotonin. The first of these stresses the role of plasma serotonin in controlling the tone of cerebral blood vessels. Serotonin is a potent constrictor of cerebral arteries. Just before migraine attacks, serotonin is released from blood platelets. This vasoconstrictor phase is associated with prodromata, including flash sensations, odd smells, and feelings of dread. This phase lasts about 10 minutes and gives way to a compensatory vasodilatation phase lasting a few hours, days, or even a week. This phase is associated with severe pain. Methysergide is believed to act as an antagonist at serotonin receptors in the blood vessels and thereby maintains tone in these vessels during precipitous changes in plasma serotonin concentrations.

The second theory focuses on serotonin's role in the CNS. The raphé system, which encompasses the bulk of the serotonin-containing pathways in the CNS, is known to be involved in habituation of sensations, including suppression of chronic pain sensations. According to this theory, temporary depressions of activity in this gating system result in migraine. Methysergide in this instance is viewed as a serotonin agonist, compensating for depressed serotonin levels.

Muscle Tension Headaches

Tension headaches are characterized by a dull, aching sensation, usually lasting 1 to 4 hours. These headaches are related to acute or chronic elevations in muscle tone, especially involving the muscles of the neck and cranium. Trigger factors are fatigue and emotional or physical stress. Tension headaches are best treated pharmacologically with centrally acting skeletal-muscle relaxants such as diazepam or meprobamate, often in combination with analgesics. Equagesic, for example, is a combination of meprobamate, ethoheptazine (a narcotic), and aspirin, marketed specifically for tension headaches. Another combination marketed for the same use is Fiorinal, which combines butalbital, a barbiturate, with aspirin, phenacetin, and caffeine. Nondrug approaches have also proved to be effective for treating tension headache. Relaxation therapy and biofeedback using myoelectric signals from the frontalis muscle of the forehead have been useful approaches.

Neuralgias

Neuralgias are paroxysmal discharges at the cranial nerves carrying somatic sensory sensations from the face and skull. The most common neuralgias involve the trigeminal and glossopharyngeal nerves. In trigeminal neuralgia, the second and third branches of the trigeminal (5th) cranial nerve are usually involved and occasionally all three. Neuralgias are characteristically recurrent episodes of sharp, agonizing pain that may last days, weeks, or months, separated by similarly variable periods of complete relief. A characteristic considered a critical diagnostic test for neuralgia is the presence of trigger zones on the surface of the face where light touch can elicit the sharp, shooting pains. The prognosis for neuralgias is poor. They tend to worsen with age and undermine psychological health and morale.

Trigeminal paroxysmal discharges usually arise from the descending nucleus of the nerve. This nucleus can be surgically destroyed, but this procedure may be curative or it may produce an untreatable chronic burning sensation. Normal analgesics are notably ineffective. Mephenesin carbamate has been employed with limited effectiveness. The best-known treatments are two antiepileptic agents, phenytoin (Dilantin) and carbamazepine (Tegretol). The former is tried first, since it is relatively free of serious side effects (Chap. 28) but is effective in less than 50 percent of patients. Carbamazepine is effective in 70 percent of cases and is almost considered a diagnostic test for true neuralgia. It has many adverse side effects, some of a quite serious nature. The worst of these are agranulocytosis, leukopenia, thrombocytopenia, and aplastic anemia. Frequent blood tests to monitor the development of side effects are an integral part of carbamazepine therapy. The CNS side effects may include extrapyramidal side effects, dizziness, fatigue, and insomnia. Carbamazepine may also be indicated in glossopharyngeal neuralgias refractory to phenytoin.

Implications for Psychotherapy
There are many varieties of headache and they serve many psychological and interpersonal functions. "Convenient" headaches, which terminate a party, help to avoid sexual encounter, or postpone work are commonplace. One can only marvel at the sensitive organismic mechanism that conveniently produces a pain response to such a variety of subtly toxic or unpleasant circumstances in life. Head pain is almost an archetypal example of the intersection of organic and nonorganic factors that underlie the thesis of this book. An illustration of the many possible theories follows:

A social scientist complained of recurrent headaches of incapacitating severity. (1) He had a long history of sinusitis (confirmed by x-ray on several occasions) that was exacerbated by weather changes. (2) He had a childhood head injury with extensive scar-tissue formation that had apparently left him especially sensitive to head pain and pressure. (3) At this particular time, he was engaged in some demanding research and writing to which he was committed but which he did not enjoy. (4) He was currently having headaches, during which, of course, it was impossible for him to work on the research. Here we see clearly the cooperation of organic and psychological forces.

The psychotherapist must not only be aware of the reality of the pain of which clients may complain, but also the organic bases. Since headaches may be an early symptom of the onset of various neuropathologic conditions, including malignant tumor, the psychotherapist should not hesitate to suggest a thorough medical investigation of the organic components.

In the event of a diagnosis of migraine, the cooperative involvement of medicine and counseling or psychotherapy is clearly indicated. Effecting the changes in life-style required to reduce stressors may necessitate family-unit or even network intervention. Should anxiolytics be employed, the discussion in Chapter 17 applies.

Neuralgia itself is refractory to psychotherapy, but the psychotherapist can serve supportively and aid in adjustment when the neuralgia remains refractory to drug treatment.

With clients already on drug treatment for migraine, cluster headache, or neuralgia, the psychotherapist must be alert to the possibility that drug side effects could be misinterpreted as psychogenic symptoms; psychiatric side effects have been reported with methysergide. Or side effects may substitute for the headache as a convenient justification for avoiding unwanted responsibilities. When "Not tonight, I have a headache," is replaced with "But I feel nauseated by my medicine," the significance of the pattern becomes undeniable even to the client, and a real therapeutic opportunity is created.

Drugs Used in the Treatment of Neuralgias and Certain Headaches

carbamazepine (Tegretol), a tricyclic antiepileptic: used in neuralgias (see text). Antiepileptic: 300 to 1,000 mg, 2,000 maximum. Neuralgia: typical: 600 mg.

cyproheptadine (Periactin), an antiserotonergic and antihistamine: prophylactic use in migraine. Typical: 16 to 20 mg. Extreme: 12 to 32 mg.

phenytoin (diphenylhydantoin, DPH) (Dilantin), a hydantoin antiepileptic, used in neuralgias. Typical: 300 to 500 mg. Extreme: 100 to 600 mg.

ergotamine (Ergomar, Gynergen), a vasoconstrictor: acute treatment of migraine. Typical: 1 to 2 mg per administration, no more than 6 mg per day, 12 mg per week.

methysergide (Sansert), an antiserotonergic: used prophylactically in migraine. Typical: 4 to 6 mg. Maximum: 8 mg.

Selected References and Further Readings

1. Elliott, F. A. *Clinical Neurology* (2nd ed.). Philadelphia: Saunders, 1971.
2. Gilman, A. G., Goodman, L. S., and Gilman, A. *The Pharmacological Basis of Therapeutics* (6th ed.). New York: Macmillan, 1980.
3. Raskin, H. Pharmacology of migraine. *Annu. Rev. Pharmacol. Toxicol.* 21:463–478, 1981.

Drugs and Consciousness VIII

℞

Thus far, we have discussed drugs that modify fundamental arousal state (Part Four), drugs that alter affect (Part Five), agents that alter extrapyramidal outputs (Part Six), and drugs used in the management of pain (Part Seven). We have seen in each of these cases examples of drugs that produce incidental effects on consciousness as well. Indeed, it would be difficult to cite an example of a drug that affects any of these aspects of brain function and is totally devoid of effects on consciousness, although the range of effects certainly varies from slight to profound. In this section, we will consider drugs that have little or no influence on affect or motor outputs and a variable effect on arousal state, but that are employed specifically for their ability to stabilize the electrical activity of the cortex, which is the underpinning of consciousness (Chap. 28). Once again, we will begin the section with a description of the neuroanatomic system involved, in this case the cortex, the seat of consciousness (Chap. 26), with special emphasis on the functional unit of the cerebrum: the cerebral cell column (Chap. 27).

Neuroanatomy of the Cerebral Cortex

26

In humans, the cerebral cortices constitute about 80 percent of the mass of the brain. Since the cortex is phylogenically the newest brain region, most behaviors and mental processes exclusive to, or most highly developed in, humans have been attributed to it. The surface area of the human cortex is about 200,000 square inches, and it varies in thickness from 1.5 cm in the visual area to about 4.5 cm in the motor area.

The cortex is primarily involved with the more complex and modifiable aspects of behavior. There is a firm correlation between the extent of cortical development of a species, its phylogenic position, and the degree of complexity and modifiability of its behavior.

Organization of the Cortex

The cerebral cortex is divided into two hemispheres that interconnect by a limited number of networks of crossing fibers called commissures. There are substantial differences between the two hemispheres with respect to their function (see p. 370).

Anatomists divide each hemisphere into lobes: the frontal, parietal, occipital, and temporal. The lines of demarcation between the lobes are in certain places quite distinct, following the bulges and fissures of the cortical tissue; at other points they are considerably less obvious. Each lobe is further divisible into gyri, which are the individual protrusions formed by the convolutions of the cortex.

The frontal lobe extends forward from the central sulcus and comprises the precentral gyrus and frontal regions. The parietal lobe lies directly behind the central sulcus and extends to the parieto-occipital fissure. The rearmost portion of the brain is the occipital lobe. The lateralmost portion of the cortex separated from the frontal lobe by the sylvian fissure is the temporal lobe. The cortical area is distributed approximately as follows: 41 percent, frontal; 21 percent, temporal; 17 percent, occipital; and 21 percent, parietal.

Brodmann has further distinguished various surface areas on the basis of cell types and characteristics. There areas are known by their Brodmann's numbers (Fig. 26-1, Table 26-1). The cortex is also organized vertically, consisting of differentiated layers of cells except in the frontal granular cortex and in certain portions of the temporal lobe. Other regions have been divided by various anatomists into six or seven layers. Both the vertical and surface mapping draw on a number of techniques and observations,

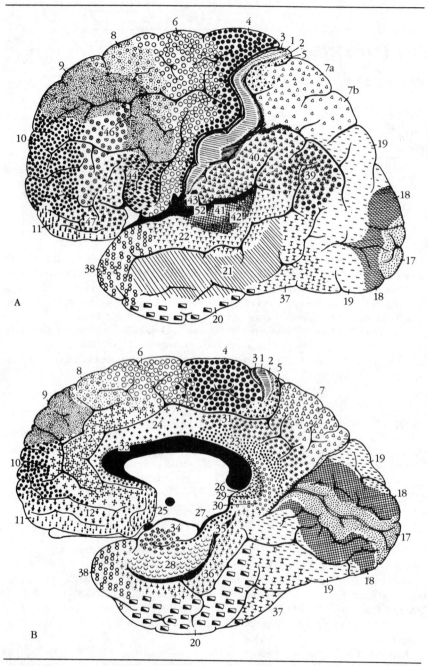

Fig. 26-1. Lateral (A) and medial (B) views showing cortical subdivisions, according to Brodmann. See Table 26-1 for key to areas. (From T. L. Peele. The Neuroanatomical Basis for Clinical Neurology (2nd ed.). © 1961 by McGraw-Hill Book Company, New York. Used with permission.)

Table 26-1. *Cortical areas*

Brodmann's area*	Name	Function
Frontal lobe		
4	Precentral gyrus	Primary motor cortex
6, 8, 9 (inferior portion)	Middle and superior frontal gyri	Premotor cortex: associative and supplementary motor cortex
44, 45	Prefrontal: inferior frontal gyrus, pars opercularis and pars triangularis	Motor speech (Brocas area)
46	Prefrontal: anterior part of middle frontal gyrus	Eye movements
47	Prefrontal: inferior frontal gyrus, pars orbitalis	Autonomic regulation
9 (anterior portion)	Prefrontal: anterior part of superior temporal gyrus	Volitional behavior, affective tone, conscious regulation of emotional behavior, delayed responding
10	Prefrontal: frontal pole	
11, 12 (anterior part)	Prefrontal: orbital gyri	
13	Prefrontal: gyrus rectus	
32	Superior frontal convolution	Possibly related to cingulate gyrus
Parietal lobe		
1, 2, 3	Postcentral gyrus	Primary somatosensory cortex
5, 7a, 7b	Superior parietal lobule	Sensory associative cortex
19 (anterior portion)	Preoccipital cortex	Optokinetic eye movements
43	Operculum	Gustatory sensibility
39	Angular gyrus	Verbal hemisphere: reading comprehension (39); language symbolism (40); logical, sequential thinking
40	Supramarginal gyrus	Nonverbal hemisphere: temporal and spacial ordering, body image; intuitive, holistic thinking
Occipital lobe		
17	Occipital pole	Primary visual cortex
18, 19 (occipital portion)	Lateral occipital gyri	Visual meaning, color vision, voluntary eye control
Temporal lobe		
41, 42, 52	Superior temporal gyrus	Primary auditory cortex
22		Speech comprehension (Wernicke's area), vestibular sensibility

Table 26-1 (continued)

Brodmann's area*	Name	Function
38	Temporal pole	Visceral control
21	Middle temporal gyrus	Formation of memories
20	Inferior temporal gyrus	Visual and auditory association
37	Fusiform gyrus	?
Limbic lobe		
	Amygdala	Defensive behaviors (aggression, avoidance), olfactory modulation of behavior, etc. (see Chap. 15)
	Hippocampus (Ammon's horn)	Short-term memory; selective response suppression (see Chap. 15)
	Dentate gyrus	Related to hippocampus
	Prepyriform cortex	Pyriform cortex: relay of olfactory signals to amygdala and hippocampus
28	Periamygdaloid cortex	
	Parahippocampal gyrus (entorhinal cortex)	
27	Presubiculum, subiculum, and prosubiculum	Related to hippocampus
34	Uncus	Olfactory sensibility
35	Perirhinal cortex	Transitional between entorhinal and neocortex
26, 29, 30	Isthmus	Connects cingulate gyrus and hippocampus
23, 24 (upper part), 31, 33	Cingulate gyrus	? (see Chap. 15)
32 and 24 (lower parts)	Subcallosal (paraterminal) gyrus	Septal region: consummatory reward, etc. (see Chap. 15)
25	Parolfactory region of Broca:	
	Posterior parolfactory gyrus	
	Anterior parolfactory gyrus	
12 (posterior portion)	Insula	Visceral sensibility
Central lobe		

*Numbers refer to areas illustrated in Figure 26-1.

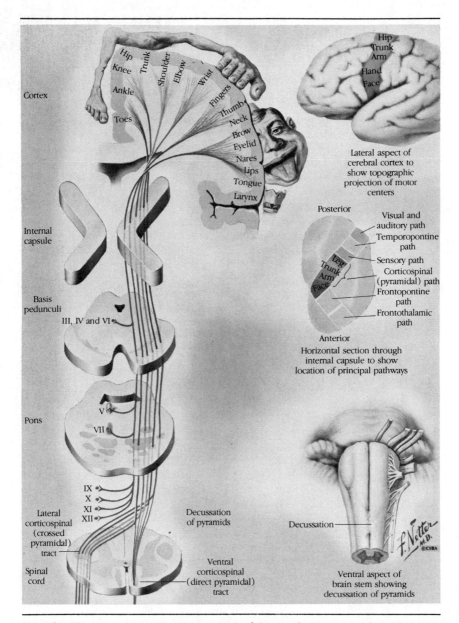

Fig. 26-2. *The pyramidal system at various levels of the CNS. (© Copyright 1965 CIBA Pharmaceutical Company, Division of CIBA-GEIGY Corporation. Reproduced, with permission, from the CIBA Collection of Medical Illustrations by Frank H. Netter, M.D. All rights reserved.)*

including appearance and distribution of cells, cell types, and results of myelin staining or metallic impregnation.

In addition, areas or layers may be mapped in terms of their projection pathways by observing the progression of nerve degeneration after lesions, a technique known as retrograde degeneration. This approach has led to the observation that there is an orderly arrangement of projection, or receptotopic organization, in each of the sensory modalities as well as the motor cortex. Figure 26-2 illustrates the motor homunculus, the orderly pattern of cortical regulation of the somatic musculature. The topology of the primary sensory cortex is the mirror image of the motor homunculus.

An additional, frequently useful distinction is made on the basis of functional differences between cortical areas. Areas that receive direct receptotopic projections in one or another sensory modality, or that project topographically to the somatic musculature, are known as the primary cortex. Other areas are designated the associative cortex.

The organization of the cortex was at one time considered to be primarily horizontal, in line with the view of the cortex as fundamental to all learning. Ironically, the subcortex was somewhat ignored until the 1950s, but it is now better understood than the cortex. The traditional concept of the Pavlovian school held that perceptual integration depended on transcortical irradiation of impulses from primary to associative areas. In general, however, vertical lesions (such as between primary visual and visual associative cortex) are less disruptive than horizontal lesions. Moreover, certain cells in the associative areas that respond to stimuli in more than one sensory modality do so with latencies so small that the sensory connections must arise directly from the subcortex. On the other hand, in recent years the pendulum has swung back somewhat, with physiologists once again elaborating the importance of transcortical connections, as emphasized by the so-called split-brain studies.

Sensory and Motor Functions of the Cortex

The gyrus lying immediately posterior to the central sulcus (areas 1, 2, and 3, Fig. 26-1), the postcentral gyrus, is the area of the cortex that serves as the terminus for sensory inputs to the somatosensory system. This system comprises two subsystems, the lemniscal system, which carries sensations of light touch, deep pressure, and joint movement, and the spinothalamic system, which delivers sensations of pain, cold, warmth, and diffuse touch. Cortical representation in the somatosensory system is mainly contralateral; that is, the left hemisphere receives information from the right side of the body and vice versa.

Much of the occipital lobe is connected with the visual system. The occipital pole (area 17, Fig. 26-1), or posteriormost region of the occipital lobe, constitutes the primary visual cortex. The cells of the retina are displayed receptotopically in the primary visual cortex. Destruction of a small region of this cortical area leads ultimately to degeneration in a similarly small area of the retina, even though a synapse is interposed between the two sites. The point-for-point representation can also be demonstrated by mapping evoked potentials generated in the visual cortex using a small-point light source aimed successively at various discrete points on the retina. Some cells of the visual cortex, however, respond only to stimulus complexes such as shadows, movement, and convexity. Some cells fire in correlation with psychophysical phenomena such as flicker fusion, afterimages, or binocular rivalry.

The auditory system has cortical representation in the temporal lobe, on the medial surface adjacent to the sylvian fissure (areas 41, 42, and 52, Fig. 26-1). Each frequency is spatially represented, and individual cells have a frequency to which they are most sensitive. The taste modality is represented in the somatosensory strip (postcentral gyrus) in the region corresponding to the tongue (area 43).

The primary motor cortex is located just anterior to the central sulcus in the precentral gyrus (area 4, Fig. 26-1). Actually, the distinction between the somatosensory and motor cortex is not absolute. Each has some of the other's function. The motor cortex is the origin and highest integrative level of the pyramidal motor system. Fibers arising from the precentral gyrus and other brain regions pass through the internal capsule at the level of the corpus striatum and form the pyramids, bulky structures that overlie the midbrain and hindbrain. The pyramids crisscross (decussate) at the level of the medulla, so that control of muscles on the right side of the body resides in the left hemisphere and vice versa, similar to the somatosensory system. Thence, the pyramidal fibers proceed (without synapsing) via the lateral and ventral corticospinal tracts of the cord and synapse at α-motor neurons at various levels. The pyramidal tracts represent a direct, rapidly conducting pathway for initiation of volitional movement. They are phylogenically recent, being found only in mammals.

The cerebral cortex also sends fibers to the corpus striatum. Through these connections, the cortex can modify extrapyramidal motor control, and the individual can volitionally modulate typically subconscious processes such as posture or gait.

Associative Cortex

The associative cortex consists of all portions of the cortex that are neither primary sensory nor primary motor cortex. Under pentobarbital anesthesia, these areas do not exhibit evoked responses to sensory stimulation, nor does electrical stimulation of the area produce a motor response. The associative regions are phylogenically late-occurring areas of neocortex and are also ontogenically late-maturing. Associative regions exhibit considerable plasticity of function and individual variation in localization of functions.

Frontal Associative Functions

The frontal associative regions consist of the premotor area, just anterior to the primary motor strip, and the prefrontal or granular cortex (areas 9–13 and 44–47, Fig. 26-1). The premotor area is closely associated with the motor cortex and controls coordinated patterns of muscular activity.

The prefrontal cortex is designated "granular" cortex because its vertical expanse is shallow and lacks differentiation. The prefrontal cortex is the neocortical area most closely associated with the limbic system. Efferents from the granular cortex travel to the hypothalamus, hippocampus, corpus striatum, and midbrain. It is probable that these connections provide for cortical suppression of limbic-regulated behaviors, for example, volitional suppression of a rage reaction. Lesions of the granular cortex produce a characteristic syndrome, called the frontal syndrome. Frontal animals are hyperreactive and demonstrate an inability to suppress ongoing behavior. The latter effect leads to deficits in behavioral tests requiring response suppression, such as alteration of noticing order, delayed responding, and delayed alternation. In frontally lobotomized or lobectimized human subjects, there is a lack of responsiveness to chronic pain, impairments in certain sensory motor functions such as visual searching, and a lack of volitional behavior.

An area of frontal cortex called Broca's area, adjacent to the temporal cortex, regulates motor aspects of speech (areas 44 and 45, Fig. 26-1). This area interconnects with an area of the temporal lobe proximal to the auditory associative cortex.

Parietal Associative Functions

Immediately posterior to the primary somatosensory cortex is the sensory association cortex (areas 5 and 7, Fig. 26-1). The posteriormost area is associated with the occipital lobe and control of eye movements such as following and fixation. Other parietal associative areas possess a particularly high degree of lateralization. In the dominant hemisphere (usually the left), much of the parietal associative cortex (areas 39 and 40) is involved with language—speech, reading comprehension, and writing skills. There is little, if any, verbal ability in the nondominant hemisphere, but the parietal lobe on this side is related to orientation in space and time. Lesions result in disorders of body image and inability to find one's way around, to count backward, or to order historical events.

Occipital Associative Functions

The associative areas of the occipital lobe (areas 18 and 19, Fig. 26-1) are related exclusively to visual associative processes, including color vision and opticokinetic responses. Lesions may produce, for example, visual agnosia, in which objects are seen but not named. Pathways from the frontal to the parietal lobes are involved with control of eye movements.

Temporal Associative Functions

The temporal lobe is closely related to the limbic system except for the insular and occipital regions, which are involved in coordination of hearing and language. The Klüver-Bucy syndrome, originally associated with temporal lobe lesions in general, but now related specifically to the amygdala, has been described in Chapter 15. Similarly, the hippocampus and associated cortex (areas 27, 28, 35, Fig. 26-1) are functional components of the limbic system and were treated in Chapter 15. Area 22 is often called Wernicke's area. Lesions in this region lead to an inability to comprehend spoken language. The remaining associative portions of the temporal lobe, the middle and inferior temporal gyri, are poorly understood as regards functional correlates.

Lateralization of the Cerebral Cortex

The two hemispheres of the human cortex have such limited interconnections that they may be properly considered two independent organs. A limited number of commissures, of which the corpus callosum is the most massive, interconnect and coordinate the activity of the two. The importance of the corpus callosum and the lateralization of the hemispheres can be demonstrated via the so-called split-brain technique discovered by Myers and Sperry in the early 1950s. They began their work with laboratory monkeys in which the corpus callosum had been surgically severed. Later, this procedure was adopted as a treatment for severe epilepsy in human patients, and these patients became subjects for experiments.

The first exciting discovery was that monkeys with split brains could learn discrimination tasks independently in the two hemispheres. Learning isolated in one hemisphere did not facilitate learning of the task in the other hemisphere. Furthermore, two different tasks could be learned simultaneously, one by the left and one by the right.

When human subjects with split brains were employed, the results were even more startling. Human subjects were unable to identify verbally pictures of objects or words flashed exclusively to the right hemisphere. On the other hand, the right hemisphere turned out to be superior in a spatial arrangement task requiring construction of a three-dimensional structure. In a simple comparative test, it was further discovered that the right hand of the split-brain subject retained full ability to copy words but could no longer draw a picture. With the left hand, the situation was the reverse—drawing ability was adequate, while ability to copy words was greatly impaired.

A more recent approach to the study of lateralization in normal human subjects is the observation of eye movement during various mental tasks. Bakan [2] discovered that subjects tended to gaze to the right while solving problems requiring verbal processes, while spatially related problems elicited a tendency to gaze to the left. Along the same line, Ornstein [4] studied EEG synchronization during verbal and spatial problem-solving and found increased synchronization (alpha activity) in the right hemisphere during verbal tasks and in the left during the spatial tasks. Since synchronization is indicative of decreased activity, these results parallel the split-brain data.

The earliest evidence concerning the specialization of function in the hemispheres actually predates split-brain work. It has long been a matter of record that in most patients surgical or accidental injury to the left hemisphere results in impairment or loss of verbal functions. On the other hand, right hemisphere damage seldom produces verbal deficits but leads to disturbances in spatial and temporal orientation, spatial manipulation, and body image. A patient with right parietal damage may be unable to find the way back to bed or to dress himself or herself.

Ornstein [4] believes that the left hemisphere is organized for linear thought processes and verbal logic, while the right hemisphere is oriented toward intuitive and aconceptual ideation. It appears from a study of war-injured veterans that the left hemisphere is more completely differentiated and specialized, whereas functions in the right hemisphere are more diffuse. This may provide an anatomic basis for the difference in functions.

Humans with split brains reportedly use significantly fewer qualifying phrases in their spontaneous speech. An interesting possibility, as yet untested, is that the cross-monitoring between the two hemispheres may play an instrumental role in self-consciousness in humans and thus the ability to make verbal adjustments in the course of conversation. Lateralization is far more pronounced in humans than in lower animals, both with respect to anatomic separation of the hemispheres and the degree of function specialization.

The relationship between handedness and cerebral dominance is consistent only in right-handed individuals, all of whom apparently have dominant left hemispheres. Left-handed individuals may possess verbal function in either or even in both hemispheres.

A determination of laterality is an integral part of an effective neuropsychodiagnosis. This begins with the diagnostic interview in which handedness as well as dominance of the eyes and legs is established by requesting the patient to perform simple tasks, such as writing, kicking, or looking through a microscope. Test of laterally specific brain functions can aid in localizing brain damage. A simple test developed by Heimburger and Reitan involves the testing of language and spatial manipulation tasks. For lateral motor evaluation, comparisons can be made between the left and right hands in grip strength or finger-tapping speed.

Deficits in right-left discrimination, dyslexia, and mixed dominance are frequently indicative of minimal brain dysfunction and are a diagnostic indication of this condition.

Selected References and Further Readings

1. Angevine, J. B., Jr., and Cotman, C. W. *Principles of Neuroanatomy.* New York: Oxford University Press, 1981.
2. Bakan, P. The eyes have it. *Psychol. Today* 4:64–67, 1971.
3. Carpenter, M. B. *Human Neuroanatomy* (7th ed.). Baltimore: Williams & Wilkins, 1976.
4. Ornstein, R. E. *The Psychology of Consciousness.* New York: Viking, 1972.

Toward a Neurophysiologic Basis of Mind

27

The problem of mind and its relationship to physical reality has enticed philosophers and scientists alike for several centuries. The issue might be put thus: Is the mind entirely a product of the workings of the brain? Or has it an independent existence, a life of its own? Descartes, the father of modern philosophy, chose the dualist point of view and thereby set off a dispute that has not abated in some 340 years. One can only smile at Descartes' compounding his error by maintaining that "although the soul is joined to the whole body, there is yet in that a certain part in which it exercises its functions more particularly than in all the others; . . . a certain very small gland [the pineal gland] which is situated in the middle . . . ." Spinoza, excommunicated from the synagogue in 1656 for his heretical views, saw mind and substance as two attributes of one substance. His contemporary, Leibniz, adopted a pluralist view, seeing mind and body as independent of each other, but equally dependent on one "master plan." In the eighteenth century, neither the empiricism of Hume nor the idealism of Kant puts the dispute to rest. Nineteenth century scientist-philosophers such as T. H. Huxley and G. H. Lewes began the process of applying the growing wealth of knowledge from biologic observation to the issue. Today, central-state identity theory, which postulates that mental states are identical to neurophysiologic events in the brain, is most widely accepted.

The adherent of the central-state identity theory might define *mind* or *minding* as the totality of all the neurophysiologic processes intrinsic to the brain by which we organize and find meaning in experience. Modestly satisfactory, if incomplete, explanations of many brain processes came out of the growing knowledge of the brain's functional neuroanatomy, neurochemistry, and neurophysiology. For example, the ability of the brain to function as a "reducing valve" for sensory experience is made comprehensible by our knowledge of brainstem gating mechanisms. And the modification of behavior as a result of positive and negative reinforcement is made comprehensible by the recognition of subcortically based reward and punishment systems.

On the other hand, at least one process has persistently evaded even modestly satisfactory explanation: awareness, or consciousness. This process is uniquely dear to the hearts of humankind because more than any other capability it seems to invest our lives with meaning. Consciousness—or at the very least, a qualitative enrichment of consciousness—is what sets humankind apart from the beasts. And consciousness lies at the root of sentience and self-identity. As long as this one, most special brain process lacks an adequate explanation in neurophysiologic terms, all pretensions to a successful reconciliation of the mind-body dilemma ring hollow. Now, recent developments in the study of the neurophysiology of the brain has set the stage for overcoming this last obstacle to solution of the mind-body problem.

The new development is a fundamental breakthrough in the understanding of the organization of the nervous system. Recent experimental observations have forced us to recognize that the nervous system is organized into functional modules that serve as information-processing systems. The design—and therefore the function—of modules differs from structure to structure and region to region within the brain. The simplest possible module is the single neuron, with its capacity to integrate, over time and space, inhibitory and excitatory influences exerted by the hundreds of nerve terminals converging on it. In the cerebral cortex, information-processing modules may comprise 50,000 or more individual neurons. Two functional capabilities are common to all modules: (1) the capacity to recognize one or more input combinations as sufficient to trigger its activity and (2) the ability to generate one or more output signals that influence other modules or effector cells. The module may perform simple or complex operations in generating its output pattern. The single-cell module is capable only of indicating the time period over which the sufficient combination of inputs is present. Complex modules of the cerebrum perform far more sophisticated forms of recognition, conduct elaborate operations utilizing the afferent complex, and generate complex output patterns for transmittal to widely divergent targets. The key to understanding a brain region lies in identification of the functional attributes and mechanisms characteristic of the modules of that region.

The region of the brain that appears to be fundamental to awareness is the cerebral cortex. We know this partly because of comparisons of the neuroanatomy of the brain across species. Such comparisons indicate that the cerebral cortex is the brain region that has undergone the greatest degree of change through the most recent stages of phylogenetic development. The trend has been toward expansion of the cerebral mass, especially associative regions, portions of the cortex not exclusively linked to a single sensory or motor system. It is natural to suspect that the most augmented region in the human brain relative to other species provides the anatomic substrate for many of the uniquely human behavioral and mental capabilities. Even more compelling is the evidence from clinical medicine that closely links disturbances of consciousness with anatomic and electrophysiologic disorders of the cerebrum.

A converging body of evidence from studies of the cerebral cortex [1, 2] indicates that much, or all, of the cerebral cortex is organized into functional units, or modules, that are vertically oriented columns of cells, transversing the six strata of the neocortex. Each column is about 250 μm in diameter and contains in the neighborhood of 10,000 cells. These columns are the fundamental processing units of the cerebrum. The beauty of this new bit of wisdom is that it renders feasible the task of developing a basic understanding of the functioning of the cortex. Where it once appeared that the task would require mapping in toto the interconnectivities of some 10 to 50 billion neurons, the task now seems to reduce into two manageable undertakings: the elucidation of the functional mechanisms of the cell column module and the illumination of supramodular control mechanisms. Although much further work will need to be done in the experimental arena, a preliminary model of cell-column function can be formulated by deduction of function from what is known of form. What we know of the form of these columns includes the characteristics of the lamina, the appearance, number, distribution, and intrinsic connectivity of the constituent cell types, and the kind and pattern of terminations of extrinsic fibers. A review of these matters of form is in order before turning to the model.

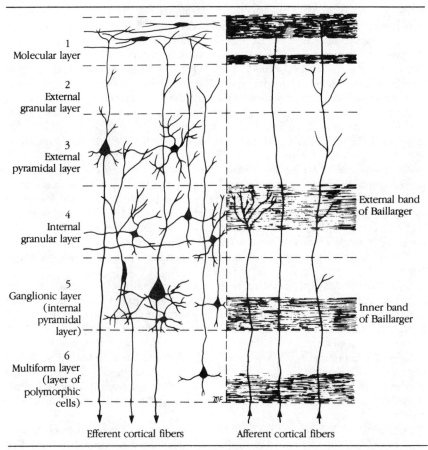

Fig. 27-1. *Laminar structure of the cerebral cortex and characteristic cell types. (From R. S. Snell. Clinical Neuroanatomy. Boston: Little, Brown, 1980.)*

Laminar Organization, Cell Types, and Extrinsic Connectivity

The cerebral cortex is generally organized into six layers (Fig. 27-1). In associative cortex, these layers are well articulated and distinctive. Layer I is called the *molecular,* or plexiform, layer. It contains few cell bodies, these few consisting of horizontal Cajal's cells and Golgi type II cells. The dendrites and axons of these two cell types form a dense mesh with tangentially oriented fibers from cells in lower layers. These fibers include the so-called apical dendrites of pyramidal cells and fusiform cells, and axons from Martinotti's cells, granule cells, thalamic association projections, and (rarely) transcortical projections. This layer is noteworthy for the extraordinary number of synapses.

Layer II is the *external granular* layer, which contains a large number of small pyramidal cells and a type of stellate cell called a small basket cell. The stellate cell processes are mainly arrayed within level II. The stellate cells form inhibitory axoaxonal synapses on descending axons of pyramidal cells. The pyramidal cell dendrites are of two types. Large, apical dendrites extend into the molecular layer, while shorter basal dendrites are arrayed at the same level as the cell body. Pyramidal cell axons descend through the six layers to serve as outputs, usually transcortical projections.

Layer III is the *external pyramidal* layer. It consists largely of pyramidal cells that increase in size toward the deeper aspect. The processes of these pyramidal cells exhibit the same pattern of projection as those of layer II pyramidal cells.

Layer IV is the *internal granular* layer. This layer features many closely packed stellate cells. Many of these have thick arrays of horizontally directed projections that compose the external Baillarger's band. Some of the stellate cells, called large basket cells, form tight inhibitory synapses on pyramidal cell bodies. This layer varies depending on the region of cortex. The density of stellate cells in this layer is greatest for primary sensory cortex (giving it a striate appearance), intermediate in associative cortex, and least dense in primary motor (hence agranular) cortex. A special type of stellate cell found in this layer is the spiny stellate (or granule) cell, which is excitatory and projects upward to contact upper-level stellate cells and pyramidal cell apical dendrites. Specific sensory afferents terminate in this layer principally on these spiny stellate cells. The majority of transcortical and transcallosal projections also terminate here.

Layer V is the *internal pyramidal* layer. Most prevalent here are medium-to-large pyramidal cells, whose apical dendrites project up to layer I. A dense array of basal dendrites extends laterally from the cell body, contributing to the interior Baillarger's band. The main axon trunk usually extends to the corresponding thalamic association nucleus. Collateral axons extend laterally and recurrently into higher layers.

Layer VI is called the *multiform* layer. In this layer are found additional pyramidal cells and fusiform cells. Large fusiform cells have been called modified pyramidal cells and have axonal and dendritic projection patterns similar to the pyramidal cells of layers V and VI. Also noteworthy in this layer are the Martinotti's cells that project upward to layer I.

To summarize: The *intrinsic* (or local-circuit) neurons are largely of the stellate type. Most, but not all, are inhibitory. The inhibitory stellate varieties include small and large basket cells and axoaxonal cells. These cells ramify in dense array, for the most part within the layer of the cell body. The granule cell is a distinctive stellate cell that is excitatory and projects upward. The Martinotti's cells are also intrinsic, lying in layer VI and projecting to layer I.

The *efferents* of the cortex are the main axon trunks of the pyramidal and fusiform cells. The upper level pyramidal cells (in layers II and III) contribute to transcortical connections by way of the white matter underlying layer VI. The lower level pyramidal and fusiform cells (in layers V and VI) project almost entirely to subcortical targets. Corticostriatal and corticorubral projections arise from the highest portion of layer V. Corticothalamic projections to the intralaminar nucleus originate in the middle of layer V. Corticofugal projections to the tectum, pons, and spinal cord derive from the lowest portion of layer V, while corticothalamic projections to the corresponding relay nucleus arise in layer VI.

Afferents to the cerebral cortex are of four types. Specific sensory afferents from thalamic relay nuclei and trancallosal afferents from contralateral cortex reach mainly level IV. Less abundant nonspecific (or associative) thalamocortical projections reach to level I. And regulatory afferent fiber systems reach the cortex from various subcortical nuclei. This last category includes norepinephrine-releasing fibers from the locus ceruleus that terminate diffusely in all layers; serotonergic fibers from the medial raphé terminating in all layers; dopamine-releasing fibers from mesencephalic nuclei to the · frontal cortex; cholinergic fibers from the substantia innominata, largely to layer VI; and histaminergic afferents of unknown distribution.

The neurotransmitters released by intrinsic neurons are more or less well established for some of the cell types. The inhibitory stellate cells probably release gamma-amino-butyric acid (GABA) in most cases; some may release taurine. The transmitters of the excitatory spiny stellate and Martinotti's cells are unknown. Pyramidal cell efferent fibers release glutamate (and possibly aspartate) in most or all cases. The transmitter released by thalamocortical projections is unknown.

An Organizational Hierarchy

The neurons of the cerebral cortex display a hierarchical organization into functional units. Vertically oriented groups of neurons, each group numbering in the order of 50,000 nerve cells, are organized around each afferent fiber that enters the cerebrum. These units are termed *minicolumns* and provide for initial processing and distribution of incoming signals. Minicolumns are organized in clusters of 100 to 500 into *columns* (also called macrocolumns or modules), which provide for recognition and representation of patterns of afferents and serve as output units. The column is the fundamental functional unit of the cerebral cortex. Columns are further organized into *matrices* or topographical arrays of two or more afferent projection fields. Several such matrices might constitute a cortical area, as specified by Brodmann (see Chap. 26).

A Model of the Cerebral Cell Column

The model proposed here draws heavily on descriptions of cerebral cell column design developed by Mountcastle [1] and on theoretical propositions articulated by Edelman [1]. The emphasis on representation as a second fundamental function of the columns in addition to recognition (proposed by Edelman) is developed for the first time here, though philosophical formulations invoking the concept of representation as fundamental to consciousness have been extant for at least 200 years, for example in Kant's transcendental idealism. The model proposed here adds a considerably more detailed, though still rudimentary, specification of the neural mechanism underlying each of the functions of columns.

Each column, or module, contains 100 to 500 minicolumns. Each minicolumn consists of an afferent fiber or a small group of afferents, together with a vertically oriented array of associated granule and pyramidal cells. In the model proposed here, the minicolumns serve as afferent distribution units, potential recognition units, and representational elements. Accordingly, minicolumns exhibit three distinct neuronal activity states. When impulse volleys reach a minicolumn along the transcortical or thalamo-cortical afferent projection fiber, the minicolumn enters into an *afferent-distribution* state. Spiny stellate cells distribute impulse activity to the apical dendrites of pyramidal cells to set the stage for representation. Spiny and aspiny stellate cells distribute impulse activity laterally to pyramidal cell bodies in minicolumns throughout the column. Activation of any one pyramidal cell within the column constitutes recognition, and the minicolumn to which the pyramidal cell in question belongs enters the *recognition* state. The set of minicolumns that were afferent-active at the point of recognition is stimulated by the recognition event to enter the *representation* state.

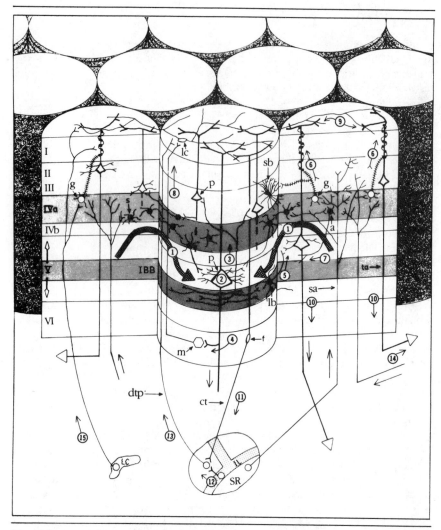

Fig. 27-2. *A semischematic depiction of several minicolumns belonging to the same column, a column lying in associative cortex, receiving transcortical and sensory afferents. The afferents received by a minicolumn vary from column to column based on brain region and zoning within regions, and they vary from minicolumn to minicolumn based on topographical representation. Open cell bodies indicate excitatory neurons; filled cell bodies indicate inhibitory neurons. AS, association nucleus of the thalamus; IBB, interior Baillarger's band; IL, intralaminar nucleus of the thalamus; LC, locus ceruleus; SR, sensory relay nucleus of the thalamus; a, axoaxonal cell; ct, corticothalamic tract; dtp, diffuse (nonspecific) thalamic projection; f, fusiform (modified pyramidal) cell; g, granule (spiny stellate) cell; gII, Golgi type II cell; lb, large basket cell; lc, longitudinal Cajal's cell; m, Martinotti's cell; p, pyramidal cell; s, stellate cell; sa, specific sensory afferent; sb, small basket cell; ta, transcortical association efferent.*

RECOGNITION-SELECTION: [1] An afferent complex is recognized if the sum of serial and parallel excitatory and inhibitory influences converging on any one pyramidal cell excites it. [2] Activation of one pyramidal cell within a minicolumn leads to activation of all pyramidal cells within the minicolumn by [3] impulses carried along recurrent axons. [4] Recognition also activates Martinotti's cells of layer VI. [5] Selection: The minicolumn stimulated first, or most vigorously, is selected from the repertoire of degenerate recognition units by a process of pericolumnar inhibition of neighboring minicolumns.

Afferent Distribution

Each column receives a convergence of many afferents consisting of sensory projections and association fibers from other cortical areas, both ipsilateral and contralateral. Thalamocortical afferents to a given module come from a cluster of thalamic cells (receiving a bundle of afferent fibers of a single modality and course) and release an unknown excitatory transmitter. Transcortical afferents release glutamate, an excitatory transmitter. In primary sensory cortex, afferents are largely sensory; in associative cortex, sensory afferents become increasingly sparse, while transcortical association fibers become increasingly dense, at each successive level in the cascade of distribution away from primary sensory areas.

The afferents terminate largely in layers III and IV, mainly on spiny stellate cells (Fig. 27-2). Some afferents also reach directly to pyramidal cell bodies and dendrites and to sparsely spiny, peptide-containing bipolar cells that appear to regulate cerebral blood flow in relation to module activity level. Associative areas may receive transcortical afferents from 10 to 30 different cortical areas.

The spiny stellate cells project mainly upward, distributing excitatory signals to stellate-type inhibitory cells, including chandelier and basket cells. Spiny stellate cells also terminate directly on the apical dendrites of pyramidal cells to subserve the representation function discussed later. Some spiny stellate cells, called double-bouquet cells, distribute afferent signals downward as well as upward.

Recognition

The inhibitory stellate cells, stimulated by minicolumn afferent activity, impinge directly or in series on dendrites and soma of pyramidal cells throughout the column. An afferent complex (reflected as a combination of afferent-active minicolumns) pro-

---

Fig. 27-2 (continued). REPRESENTATION: [6] A graded excitability state is generated by the action of a granule cell on apical dendrites of pyramidal cells within its receptive field (or minicolumn). This is the afferent-active state. [7] But extrinsic propagation of action potentials is prevented by inhibitory axoaxonal cells. [8] Representation is triggered by the recognition unit via the ascending axon of Martinotti's cell. [9] Representation: Activation of excitable dendrites of pyramidal cells (the subset of units belonging to minicolumns active at recognition) is brought about by the horizontal Cajal's cells. [10] Representation is signaled to other modules by layers II and III pyramidal cell axons to subserve successive abstraction. Representation is signaled by layer V pyramidal cells via corticifugal projections to subcortical centers. Axoaxonal inhibition is absent at this point.

REENTRANT SIGNALING: [11] Representation can be momentarily "fixed," past the period of recognition, by reentrant signaling. Propagation of a representation signal from the cell column to the thalamus momentarily increases excitability of the corresponding thalamic projection cell cluster. The period of increased excitability lasts about 200 msec. [12] Phasic pulses are received from the intralaminar nuclei. [13] A reentrant signal is projected to each cell column for which the corresponding thalamic cell cluster is in an excitable state. The pulse carried by the diffuse thalamic projection system activates the longitudinal Cajal's cell. [9] Representation is repeated—return to step 9. The cyclical loop (steps 9 through 13) may be disrupted in several ways: by occurrence of an afferent complex that inhibits the selected recognition cell; by transcolumnar inhibition by Golgi type II cells (distraction); or by an intrinsic adaptive mechanism.

ASSOCIATION AND COMMITMENT: [14] Transcortical signaling of representation provides for successive abstraction. Golgi type II cells in layer I may provide a means of controlling associations between columns within a given matrix. [15] Release of norepinephrine from axons originating in the locus ceruleus and terminating diffusely in all layers promotes adaptations favoring transmission at synapses active during behavioral patterns culminating in positive reinforcement.

duces "recognition" if the sum of serial and parallel excitatory and inhibitory influences converging on any one pyramidal cell within the column generates an action potential. All-or-nothing activation of one pyramidal cell activates the entire set of pyramidal cells within the same minicolumn by way of recurrent axon collaterals, as well as activating layer VI Martinotti's cells of that minicolumn. The recognition state persists as long as the requisite pattern of minicolumn afferent-active states continues.

Recognition capacity is degenerate, meaning that recognition can be achieved in more than one way. This is because any one minicolumn in the recognition state determines recognition. The minicolumn activated first, or most vigorously, is *selected* from the repertoire of possible recognition events by a process of pericolumnar inhibition (also called dynamic isolation). When a minicolumn has been activated to the recognition state, pericolumnar inhibition precludes recognition by other minicolumns. Pericolumnar inhibition is largely the work of large and small inhibitory basket cells and chandelier cells that arborize within a given layer, exerting an inhibitory effect on pyramidal cells of neighboring minicolumns. The minicolumn that is in the recognition state stimulates nearby basket and chandelier cells, and these in turn exert an inhibition on the basal dendrites of pyramidal cells in other minicolumns within the same module.

Recognition of patterns not previously, or infrequently, experienced occurs in "uncommitted" columns in the cortical region receiving the requisite set of sensory and transcortical afferents. Recognition by a given column generates transcolumnar inhibition of adjacent units, so that recognition of a given afferent stimulus complex becomes specific for one module within the matrix.

Recognition is signaled by Martinotti's cells in layer VI to initiate the representation process.

Representation

Concurrent with recognition-selection activity, minicolumns are engaged in preparing the column for representational activity. As a component of afferent distribution, spiny stellate cells relay impulse activity from matched sensory or transcortical afferents to apical dendrites of pyramidal cells. Spiny stellate axon projections wind around the apical dendrites of the pyramidal cells that lie within the minicolumn. The apical dendrites of these pyramidal cells extend to and bifurcate in layer I. Activity in the spiny stellate cells produces a long-lasting graded depolarization of the pyramidal cell apical dendrites, and this holds the pyramidal cells of the minicolumn in an especially excitable state. (These dendritic potentials, taken summatively for all pyramidal cells in the especially excitable state, constitute the major component contributing to recordings of cortical electrical activity that we call the electroencephalogram.) With a subset of the column's minicolumns in this especially excitable state, the column is primed for generation of a representation event.

Representation is triggered initially by the recognition process itself, subsequently by reentrant signaling from the thalamus. In the first instance, Martinotti's cells located in layers V and VI, activated by a minicolumn recognition event, project excitatory impulses to horizontal Cajal's cells in layer I. These horizontal cells project longitudinally in thick array to form dense plexuses with the dendrites of pyramidal cells. Impulse flow through the plexuses preferentially activates those pyramidal cell dendrites that are momentarily in the excitable state. Thus, pyramidal cells of minicolumns that are afferent-active at the instant that recognition occurs are a moment later excited into the representation activity state by plexal impulses. The firing of pyramidal cells of this subset of the column's total population of minicolumns is the mental representation of the afferent complex previously recognized by that module. The representation state for a minicolumn entails impulse traffic along pyramidal cell axons and continued pericolumnar inhibition of pyramidal cell basal dendrites. Following the momentary representation event, each minicolumn resumes an afferent-active or afferent-inactive state, depending on the status of afferent activity.

Phasic Reentrant Signaling

Representation of the afferent complex continues in the fashion described for as long as the afferent impulse complex is sustained in a condition that retriggers recognition or by a process of phasic reentrant signaling, which begins with activation of layer VI fusiform cells during representation. The fusiform cells are activated through their apical dendrites in layer I. The efferent signal of the fusiform cell, indicating representation, is conveyed to the corresponding relay nucleus of the thalamus. In response to this indication of representation, a reentrant pulse is returned to the module by way of the diffuse thalamocortical radiations. Phasic signals are pulsed out from the thalamus, along the diffuse projection system at a frequency determined by the thalamic pacemaker (intralaminar nuclei), to all columnar modules from which representation signals have been recently forthcoming. Diffuse thalamic-system pulses, generally about 10 per second in the waking state, project to layer I, to activate horizontal Cajal's cells (the same cells that were activated by Martinotti's cells during active recognition). Pyramidal cells that are still especially excitable from the preceding representation state are reactivated. This new representation event is again signaled to the thalamus by fusiform cells and results in generation of a new reentrant pulse. The cycle of representation → reentrant signaling → representation continues until interrupted. Cycle interruption may involve inflow of a stimulus complex that inhibits the selected minicolumn recognition unit (disrecognition); an intrinsic fade mechanism involving adaptations at a critical synapse; or inhibition by adjacent modules through Golgi type II cells in layer I (distraction). In this manner, the mental representation is "fixed" for a period of time until disrupted.

It can be postulated that phasic reentrant volleys are projected at each pulse point only to units from which a representation signal has reached the thalamus within an interval of about 200 msec or so. In such a case, reentrant signaling would be minimal and would be ineffective in fixing mental representations when the frequency of thalamic pulses fell below about 5 Hz, which occurs during slow-wave sleep or coma. But at pacemaker frequencies above about 5 Hz, selective reentrant signaling would produce a moment-to-moment "readout" of mental representations of each currently and recently recognized stimulus complex, as well as successive abstractions in associative regions. This phasic reentrant activation of mental representations would provide the continuity of mental state that is experienced as awareness.

Reentrant signaling is seen here as the *sine qua non* of consciousness, and it follows that consciousness is specifically associated with, and limited to, telencephalic regions subject to reentrant signaling. This would include much, but not all, of the neocortex, hippocampus, amygdala, and portions of the corpus striatum.

Successive Abstraction

Transcortical projections are organized to project, in a cascade or series of steps, away from primary sensory areas to associative areas of increasing distance from the primary sensory area. In primary sensory areas, afferent fibers entering a given column are nearly

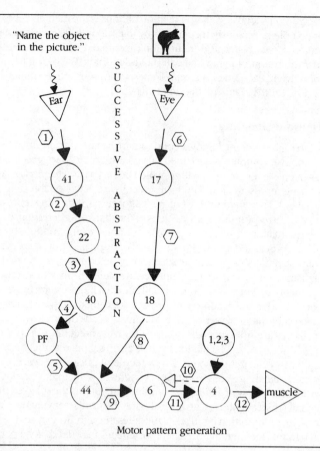

Fig. 27-3. Schematic representation of regional interactions of the cerebral cortex illustrating successive abstraction and response generation. The illustration depicts a hypothetical situation in which the subject is asked to name the object in a picture and then is shown the picture of a cow. This leads to the following sequence of brain activities: [1] Impulses from the auditory receptors, generated by the verbal instruction, project to primary auditory cortex, area 41, where the intensity of each frequency is represented. [2] Representation activity of various modules in area 41 is indicated as afferent activity to modules in area 22, associative auditory cortex. These area 22-modules recognize and represent sound qualities (patterns of rising or falling intensities or frequencies by time and binaural disparity). [3] An area-40 module recognizes the combination of sound qualities represented in area 22. Area 40 is involved in speech comprehension. The "meaning" of the sound quality pattern (i.e., words heard) is determined by associative connections with other modules in area 40. The multimodular representation of "meaning" is projected to the prefrontal cortex. [4] The instruction is evaluated in a series of prefrontal modular abstractions and is found consistent with the subject's internalized system of values and goals. [5] The output signal from the prefrontal lobe becomes part of a recognition complex for a module in the speech center and furnishes, in effect, a disposition or volition to fulfill the instruction. [6] Meanwhile, presentation of the picture triggers visual afferents to the visual cortex. Modules in primary visual cortex, area 17, recognize and represent, in topographical array, stimulus attributes, including movement and form. [7] A module in area 18, secondary visual cortex, recognizes the combination of attributes in the visual stimulus complex generated by the picture of the cow. [8] A speech-center module in a zone receiving prefrontal projections recognizes the combination of a visual representation afferent and a disposition to vocalize the

all sensory afferents, other afferent fibers being pyramidal cell axons from adjacent and nearby columns. Thus, the act of recognition by a module in primary sensory cortex is recognition of a sensory complex. Associative areas adjacent to primary cortex receive sensory afferents and rich complements of transcortical afferents from recognition units in primary cortex. Thus, the recognition function in modules of second-order regions is recognition of combinations of signals generated by first-order columns. Some columns may recognize a combination of sensory afferent and transcortical representations. Associative areas still further removed from primary sensory cortex receive predominantly transcortical afferents for evaluation and recognize representational patterns from second-order modules. Maps of cortical function and interconnectivity suggest at least four or five levels of abstraction and perhaps more (Fig. 27-3).

Columns are organized as matrices within a cortical region. A group of columns receives fiber bundles from two or more sources, projected topographically; the arrays are often oriented at right angles to each other to form a matrix. The third dimension, depth, is organized by output targets. A brain region (in the sense of a Brodmann's area) may contain many such matrices.

Outputs to the thalamus that provide for reentrant signaling arise from fusiform cells in layer VI. Transcortical outputs arise from upper-layer pyramidal cells. Corticifugal efferents to the brainstem and corpus striatum arise from layer V. The nature of output patterning remains to be determined. The module might, in some instances, transmit a single discharge, indicating that recognition or representation has occurred; in other instances, the represented pattern, in complete or abridged form, might be transmitted to efferent targets.

The activity of recognition units at second-order and higher levels of abstraction provides one basis for "learning" or recognizing associations that exist in nature as reflected in stimulus patterns. Abstraction requires only that the elements be repeatedly active as simultaneous mental representations, whether by status of active recognition or in the reentrant holding pattern.

There may be a second mechanism for linkage of modules within a matrix, at the same level of abstraction. The anatomic basis for this might be plexal connections, subject to regulation by Golgi type II cells. It was observed by Ramon y Cajal that the major difference in cell-type distribution patterns in human brains relative to other species is an increased abundance of these Golgi type II cells.

Column Commitment

Recognition-representation activity by a cell column gradually generates increasing commitment of a column to a specific afferent complex if recognition-representation of that complex recurs frequently. Heavily traveled synapses undergo adaptations that facilitate subsequent transmission. Adaptations promoting commitment are hastened,

---

Fig. 27-3 (continued). corresponding word. This leads to: [9] A signal to a module in premotor cortex, which activates the preestablished representation pattern of that column (for the production of muscle contractions and vocal-cord movement needed to vocalize "cow"). [10] The premotor module has been committed or preprogrammed as a result of experience and positive reinforcement to recognizing and representing the requisite pattern of motor-strip column activities. [11] The representation of this pattern is projected to modules of the precentral gyrus that recognize combinations of afferents from the premotor cortex and somatosensory cortex. Outputs from motor-strip modules activate effector cells.

moreover, when recognition-representation activity in a column shortly precedes articulation of a behavioral pattern that leads to positive reinforcement.

The locus ceruleus, the bed nucleus of the reward system, projects diffusely to all cortical regions. The influence of positive reinforcement is less potent in the case of the association process (successive abstraction) of the cortex (as evidenced by principles governing verbal learning) than in subcortical, especially limbic-system, regulation of behavior (operant conditioning). Nevertheless, some influence is observed. Positive reinforcement activates locus ceruleus projection fibers, causing release of norepinephrine and activation of adenyl cyclase in all cortical layers, but especially in layers II and III in the frontal cortex. Norepinephrine might then facilitate commitment of recently active recognition units by promoting morphologic changes in layer I neural plexuses favoring the discharge trail developed in the representational process.

Influences from Other Brain Regions

Cortical activity is subject to regulation by several extrinsic transmitter systems in addition to the norepinephrine inputs from the locus ceruleus. These include dopaminergic, cholinergic, serotonergic, and histaminergic networks. Dopaminergic inputs arise mainly from the midbrain dopamine nucleus, A_{10}, and project to the frontal lobe. The projection pattern is topographical and parallels the topographical projections to the frontal lobe from the mediodorsal nucleus of the thalamus. Most of the dopamine inputs terminate in layers V and VI.

Cholinergic inputs arise from a nucleus of the telencephalon called the substantia innominata, which lies just below the globus pallidus. This cholinergic pathway is considered to be the final link of the reticular activating system. The cholinergic fibers terminate in the lowest layers of the cortex, layers V and VI, especially to influence the fusiform cells of layer VI. These anatomic relationships suggest that this system is designed to interrupt ongoing reentrant signaling so as to clear modular activity for processing current-time sensory inputs, so that attention is shifted to external events.

Serotonergic inputs reach the cortex from the raphé nuclei. Their terminals reach all cortical layers and are largely inhibitory. These inputs presumably contribute to sleep generation.

Histamine has been found to stimulate receptors in the cortex. These receptors are principally of the H_2 variety. The histamine found in the cortex is largely associated with extrinsic histaminergic fibers.

In all probability, based on functional considerations, cell types and distribution, and patterns of interconnectivity, modules in some neocortical regions and in phylogenetically older cortical regions are organized quite differently than the module described here. Modules in granular frontal cortex and in the hippocampus and basal ganglia are presumably quite different from each other and from the model cell column postulated here and characteristic of associative cortex.

These atypical structures of the telencephalon (frontal lobe, hippocampus, basal ganglia) appear to influence the functioning of modules within associative cortex through transcortical and transthalamic mechanisms, and each of these structures is organized toward advancing a distinctive regulatory end. Influences related to intentional, mnemonic, and cognitive mechanisms originating in the prefrontal lobe, hippocampus, and corpus striatum respectively are superimposed on the current-time recognition-representation and phasic reentrant processes described in this chapter.

With these considerations in mind—and returning to the original challenge—a definition of consciousness, rooted in our understanding of neurophysiology, might be suggested: Consciousness is a phasic activation of a selected subset of the established repertoire of mental representations, each such representation being the acquired function of a particular cerebral cortical recognition-representation columnar module, with the subset activated by a given pulse being determined by a combination of current-time sensory stimulation, reentrant signaling, and intentional, mnemonic, and cognitive mechanisms.

This is a definition that a central-state identity theorist can live with for the time being.

Selected References and Further Readings

1. Edelman, G. M., and Mountcastle, V. B. *The Mindful Brain.* Cambridge: MIT Press, 1978.
2. Schmitt, F. O., Worden, F. G., Adelman, G., and Dennis, S. G. (Eds.). *The Organization of the Cerebral Cortex.* Cambridge: MIT Press, 1981.
3. Snell, R. S. *Clinical Neuroanatomy for Medical Students.* Boston: Little, Brown, 1980.

Epilepsy and Antiepileptic Drugs

28

Epilepsy is derived from a Greek word meaning "to seize." The term encompasses a group of related chronic disorders characterized by the occurrence of seizures. During the seizure, there is a loss or disturbance of consciousness, sometimes accompanied by convulsions. As many as 2 million Americans have epilepsy of sufficient severity to come to clinical attention. Some are gainfully employed; some require prolonged hospitalization. Epilepsy is a chronic disease that generally does not shorten life. Neurologic, psychiatric, or cognitive impairments are more or less likely to occur, depending on the type of epilepsy involved. Yet some of the greatest figures in history have been epileptics: Alexander the Great, Julius Caesar, Peter the Great, Mohammed, Byron, von Schiller, Mozart, Dostoevski, Balzac, and Handel. Epilepsy constitutes a grave health, social, and economic problem.

Physiologic Basis of Epilepsy

Epilepsy appears to be related, in most if not all cases, to the presence of a region of organic pathology. It has not been possible to demonstrate a pathologic focus in all cases, and clinicians have therefore categorized cases of indefinite cause as "idiopathic." It is probable, however, that in many or all such cases the focus is simply too deep in the brain interior to be observable on the EEG. The pathologic focus may originate from congenital defects, cerebral trauma, "ischemia" caused by lesions in cerebral blood vessels or insufficiency of blood supply, tumors, infections, childhood illnesses, or hypoxia at birth. If the damaged area is near the upper layer of the cortex, the EEG will show either an abnormal spike discharge, or abnormal slow-wave activity, or both.

Normally, the spread of electrical discharge from the focus is prevented by cerebral inhibitory mechanisms (Fig. 28-1). Physiologic changes may occur, however, that facilitate the spread of paroxysmal discharges and thus initiate a seizure. Among the changes known to induce seizures are fatigue, emotional stress, and changes in blood sugar levels, acidity, gas concentrations, or endocrine levels. In petit mal epilepsy, the seizure focus is located subcortically, typically in the thalamus or midbrain (Fig. 28-2). In positive-spike pattern, the focus is believed to be in the thalamus or hypothalamus.

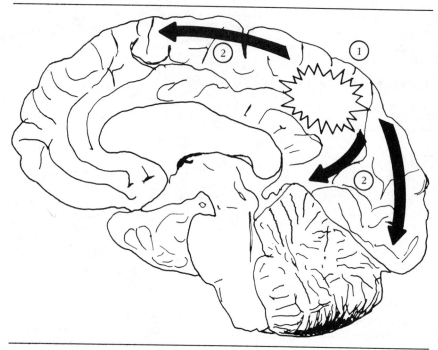

Fig. 28-1. *Pathogenesis of a grand mal seizure. A seizure focus [1] has developed as a result of localized brain damage due to organic causes such as hypoxia at birth or concussion. A reduction in cerebral inhibition permits the influence of the abnormal focal activity to spread [2] throughout the cortex.*

Types of Epilepsy

Grand Mal

Of the distinguishable forms of epilepsy, grand mal is the most common, occurring alone or in combination with other forms in 90 percent of all cases. A grand mal attack is sometimes preceded by an "aura," a vague premonitory symptom. Gastric and visual sensations, paresthesias, or vertigo are the most common types of aura. The aura is followed by the onset of convulsions during which the patient loses consciousness. Convulsions include a short-lasting tonic phase (about 3 to 15 seconds) and a longer-lasting clonic phase. In the tonic phase, muscles are strongly contracted. The legs extend, arms cross up over the chest, and the back arches. Respiration is impossible during this phase. In clonus, the limbs flail about vigorously, and the patient is at risk of concussion, injury to the limbs, or biting the tongue. Gradually, clonic bursts begin to subside, leaving the individual in a restful coma. Slowly, the patient regains consciousness and enters a period of postseizure depression. The interval between seizures may vary from more than a year to just a few minutes. When attacks come in continuous or rapid succession, the condition is called status epilepticus, which can be fatal if treatment is not quickly successful.

Grand mal epilepsy is more common in men than women (Table 28-1). Neurologic

③ EEG: ⋀⋀⋀⋀⋀⋀⋀

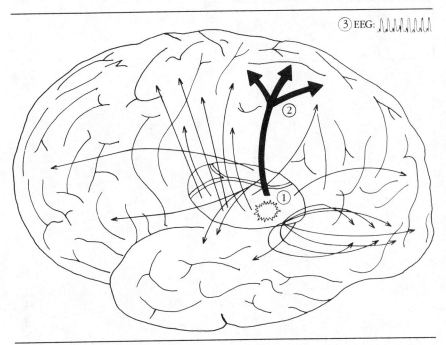

Fig. 28-2. *Pathogenesis of a petit mal seizure. In petit mal epilepsy, the seizure focus is subcortical [1]. Abnormal discharges from the focus cause the diffuse thalamic projection system to produce [2] a characteristic 3-Hz spike-and-dome pattern of electrical activity [3] in the cortex.*

concomitants, such as hemiplegia, hemiparesis, partial blindness, and speech impairments, occur in about 14 percent of patients. Psychiatric and cognitive concomitants barely exceed the frequency in the population as a whole (Table 28-1).

Several less common varieties of grand mal epilepsy can be distinguished on the basis of etiology even while presenting similar seizure manifestations (Table 28-1). The petit mal variant (not to be confused with petit mal epilepsy), also called Lennox-Gastaut syndrome, shows a diffuse EEG disturbance similar to petit mal in waveform, but slower. Neurologic, psychiatric, and cognitive correlates are frequent in this form of epilepsy. Infantile spasms and febrile convulsions are two varieties that occur only in infants. Infantile spasms is progressive, usually culminating in death within a few years. It is associated with bizarre, diffuse changes in the EEG and progressive mental deterioration.

In another variety of epilepsy called focal seizures, convulsive activity is limited to a particular part of the body or, at most, one side of the body. Typically, the attack arises from a focal discharge in the corresponding cortical area, but fails to spread throughout the cortex. If an aura is present, the nature of the aura is often a clue as to the location of the focus. If a seizure begins as a focal seizure, but then gradually expands into a full grand mal convulsion, the term *Jacksonian seizure* is applied. When the focus is located in the anterior part of the temporal lobe, the seizure pattern generally takes the form of the psychomotor type of epilepsy described subsequently.

Table 28-1. Forms of epilepsy

Type of seizure	Age and sex correlates, seizure characteristics, and EEG correlates	Aura	Incidence of mental concomitants		
			Neurologic	Psychiatric	Cognitive
Grand mal	Onset: modal age groups 0–2 and 12–18 yr; 59% males Major convulsions and postseizure depression Interval EEG may show spikes or may appear normal	+	+	0	0
Petit mal variant	Onset: 65% before age 5; 95% before 20; 58% males Seizures may be mild (loss of posture, myoclonic jerks) or severe (major convulsions); seizures are frequent Diffuse, spike and dome, < 3 Hz	0	+++	++	+++
Jacksonian and focal	Onset: 90% before age 10; 57% males Frequency and type of seizure dependent on site and focus; partial convulsion EEG shows localized abnormality	0 to +++	+++	+	+
Febrile convulsions	Onset: before age 5 Triggered by fever; significant hereditary factor; major convulsions	0	+	0	0
Infantile spasms	Onset: by age 4; 65% boys Major convulsions and progressive mental deterioration Hypsarrhythmia	0	++++	0	++
Petit mal (absences)	Onset: modal age is 5; 92% by age 15; 54% females Syncope, loss of muscle tone, muscle fasciculations 3-Hz spike and dome	0	0	+	0
Psychomotor (temporal lobe epilepsy)	Onset: usually 10–30 yr; 56% males Blackouts Anterior temporal lobe focus	+++	+	+++	+
Positive-spike pattern syndrome	Onset: modal age 12–18 yr; 55% males Major convulsions (55%); rage or tantrums (15%); syncope (30%); pain (20%) 6- and 8-Hz positive spikes at night	+++	++	+++	+
Myoclonus	Isolated muscle contractions, combined with grand mal in 63% of cases EEG often exhibits multiple spikes	0	+	0	+

0 < 8%; + 8–17%; ++ 18–30%; +++ 31–50%; ++++ > 50%

Petit Mal

Petit mal epilepsy differs considerably from grand mal. A current trend is to refer to petit mal as "absence seizures" or "absences," to strengthen the distinction from grand mal epilepsy and to reduce the stigma attached to the child from the use of the more emotionally laden term *epilepsy*. In petit mal, a characteristic pattern develops in the EEG, particularly in the posterior frontal region. The pattern, called the *spike and dome*, indicates the presence of an abnormal focus in the thalamus or midbrain, from whence the electrical disturbance spreads via the diffuse thalamic projections. Petit mal occurs mostly in children and more frequently in girls than boys (see Table 28-1). Attacks are typically of short duration, from 5 to 15 seconds, and consist of syncope, or temporary cloudings of consciousness. The patient may stare blankly or exhibit minor movements of the head or limbs. The patient is usually unaware of the attack and may become confused by the discontinuity of events. Psychiatric symptoms occur in 10 percent of petit mal patients, with an increased frequency in the category of behavioral problems, accounting for the difference in overall frequency of psychiatric symptoms relative to the overall population.

Psychomotor Epilepsy

Psychomotor, or temporal lobe, epilepsy is a form that is coming increasingly to the attention of psychotherapists because of the overlap between behaviors associated with it and so-called psychopathic behaviors. An examination of individuals convicted of motiveless crimes indicated that some 70 percent had abnormal EEGs. It is now known that the presence of an abnormal discharge focus in the anterior temporal lobe can elicit bizarre, antisocial conduct. Psychomotor seizures are characterized by complex but inappropriate activity about which the patient is usually amnesic. The acts may be innocuous, such as singing or undressing, or they may be violent and destructive. The patient may refuse help and not believe that episodes have indeed occurred. Psychiatric symptoms are three times more common in temporal lobe epilepsy than in grand mal.

Auras are common in temporal lobe epilepsy. Gastric auras are most likely (occurring in 11 percent of patients). Other forms of aura include déjà vu, visual, gustatory, auditory, or olfactory sensations, jamais vu, vertigo, nausea, paresthesias, dreamy states, or the lump-in-throat sensation. Motor manifestations common during psychomotor seizures include incoordination, aggression, staring, groping, lip-smacking, swallowing, chewing, crying, laughing, shouting, screaming, confused talking, and undressing. Psychiatric concomitants are varied: Personality or behavioral disturbances occur in about 20 percent of patients; excessive daytime sleepiness, depression, suicidal tendencies, anxiety, hallucinations, and paranoia each occur in about 2 to 3 percent of patients. In 70 percent of instances of psychomotor epilepsy, grand mal is also present.

A recent development in the understanding of epilepsy is the growing awareness that subictal (or subseizure) varieties of temporal lobe epilepsy frequently occur and are undiagnosed. Physical manifestations can include frequent muscle fibrillations, twitchings, or involuntary uncoordinated movements of the extremities. Behavioral and psychological manifestations may include depression, outbursts of temper, "hysterical" symptoms, hallucinations, obsessional thinking, or anxiety. Since EEG findings may well be negative, often only an inferential diagnosis based on responsiveness to antiepileptic medication can be made.

Positive-Spike Pattern

Electroencephalography may identify the existence of a condition characterized by the occurrence of 14- and 6-Hz positive spikes. This pattern is specific in its neurologic manifestations, but is variable in its behavioral concomitants. Psychiatric correlates occur in 38 percent of patients and neurologic correlates, in 21 percent (see Table 28-1). Outbursts of intense rage and hostile impulsiveness may be manifested; in other cases, affect may be severely blunted. There may be autonomic dysfunctions and feelings of bodily aches as well as behavioral disorders. It is easy for a psychotherapist to attribute such symptoms to psychogenic origins if the positive-spike pattern goes undetected.

Myoclonus

Myoclonus is another class of illnesses involving motor disturbances. Any discussion of myoclonus must necessarily begin with clarification of nomenclature, because *myoclonus* is a term of variable meaning to different clinical groups. The surest beginning is to define myoclonus phenomenologically as the occurrence of isolated, involuntary muscular jerks of a clonic type. The muscle activity may take the form of a twitch, a fasciculation, or an obvious contraction. The movements may occur singly or in brief showers lasting 3 to 6 seconds.

Myoclonias may be symptomatic, constituting but one manifestation of a multifaceted neurologic disorder, or they may be essential, being the predominant or only evidence of disorder. In the first category are myoclonias secondary to encephalitis (acute and slow viral infections), encephalopathies, intoxications (e.g., mercury, methyl bromide, penicillin, imipramine, tetanus toxin), degenerative dementias, lipidoses (such as Tay-Sachs disease), and seizure disorders. Both infantile spasms and petit mal variant are sometimes classified as myoclonic epilepsies. Myoclonus often occurs as a feature of grand mal or petit mal epilepsies.

Nearly 30 percent of cases are unrelated to epilepsy or other extrapyramidal syndromes. Among these essential forms of myoclonus is paramyoclonus multiplex, a hereditary and progressive degenerative disorder. In essential myoclonus isolated, clonic jerks are evoked by sensory stimuli, often with associated EEG spikes. The frequency of contractions increases in the morning, with fatigue and stress, and prior to the onset of menstruation. Because initiation of motor activity for the performance of delicate tasks also intensifies the myoclonic activity, these arrhythmic forms of myoclonus are often designated "action" or "intention" myoclonus.

The various forms of myoclonus may be limited or generalized in distribution, rhythmic or arrhythmic, symmetrical or asymmetrical, and may originate within the cortex, basal ganglia, brainstem, or spinal cord. Generally, the myoclonias of brainstem or spinal origin are rhythmic, while those originating in higher centers are arrhythmic.

Nocturnal myoclonus is a common phenomenon. Fasciculations and jerks of varying intensity occur in virtually all normal people during stage 1 of slow-wave sleep. If such myoclonic episodes are excessively intensive, the sleeper may be startled awake. Insomnia and excessive daytime sleepiness occur secondarily if such awakenings are frequent.

There is evidence that at least some forms of myoclonus are related to a deficiency of serotonin activity in the brain. A combination of the serotonin precursor, L-5-hydroxytryptophan, and carbidopa (a peripheral decarboxylase inhibitor) is often an effective treatment. Among the antiepileptics, only clonazepam and valproic acid are notably effective.

EEG Diagnosis of Epilepsy

A number of reflections of epilepsy may occur in the EEG. In some cases, it is possible to demonstrate the presence of an irritating focus either in the resting EEG, in a sleep

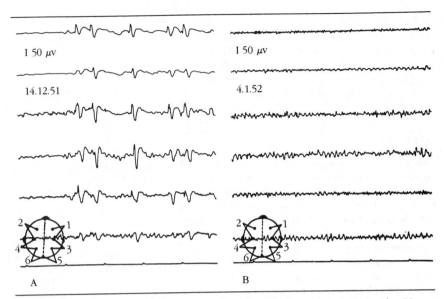

Fig. 28-3. *EEG tracing from six lead pairs showing focal discharges in a patient with a 32-year history of grand mal seizures. A. Before treatment. B. After treatment with phenytoin. (From R. R. Hughes.* An Introduction to Clinical Electro-Encephalography. *Bristol, Engl.: John Wright & Sons, Ltd., 1961.)*

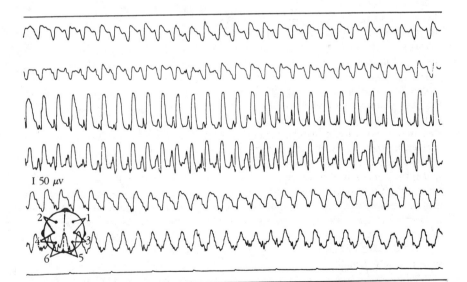

Fig. 28-4. *EEG tracing from six lead pairs showing typical petit mal spike-and-dome pattern. (From R. R. Hughes.* An Introduction to Clinical Electro-Encephalography. *Bristol, Engl.: John Wright & Sons, Ltd., 1961.)*

reading, or by "activation" of the EEG by metrazol, hyperventilation, photic stimulation, or a barbiturate. If an electrode is placed immediately above the focus, a sharp, biphasic spike is usually detected recurring at variable intervals (Fig. 28-3). An abnormal slow wave may be seen instead, but this usually indicates that the focus is slightly removed from the electrode placement, either laterally or at a depth.

Abnormal discharges may in some cases be observed at some distance from the focus because of transcortical interconnecting fibers. Sometimes, a "mirror" focus is found in the corresponding area of the opposite hemisphere. If the focus lies in the midbrain or upper hindbrain, it is impossible to localize it by means of the EEG, and this leads to a diagnosis of idiopathic or constitutional epilepsy, indicating an unknown cause. In such cases, there may be a diffuse distribution of abnormal slow spikes and waves because of projection from the subcortical focus via the diffuse thalamic projections.

The most dramatic and specific correlation between the EEG and a disease state is the occurrence of characteristic 3-Hz spike-and-dome discharges in petit mal. This complex consists of a sharp spike followed by a large-amplitude slow wave, which repeats with great regularity at a rate of 3 per second (Fig. 28-4). The pattern may occur diffusely and symmetrically throughout the cortex, but it is particularly prominent in the posterior portion of the frontal lobe. The bursts of spike-and-dome activity may vary in duration. When they exceed a few seconds in duration, they are accompanied by the lapses of consciousness characteristic of petit mal. The abnormal electrical activity in petit mal arises from disturbances in the thalamus.

The epileptic attack may itself be generative of subsequent abnormalities in the EEG in severe cases. During an attack, a mixture of sharp spikes and high-amplitude theta or beta activity can be observed. The period of postictal depression is accompanied by a markedly depressed EEG recording. Transient foci of irritation may arise as a result of brain damage occurring during the seizure, particularly in youthful epileptics. In cases of prolonged or frequent attacks, brain damage may result, with an accompanying generalized slow activity in the EEG.

Many cases of epilepsy are associated with organic brain damage related to any of a myriad of possible injuries or disease states, and EEG changes may accompany this brain damage independent of the associated epilepsy.

Excessive theta activity of a diffuse nature may occur in some cases of epilepsy, particularly, but not exclusively, in cases of temporal lobe epilepsy.

Antiepileptic Drug Therapy

Strictly speaking, the term *anticonvulsant* should be used to denote a drug (such as diazepam or certain barbiturates) that is effective in terminating the drug-induced or epileptiform seizure itself, while the term *antiepileptic* is used to denote an agent employed chronically to reduce the frequency of seizures in an epileptic. Commonly, however, the term *anticonvulsant* is employed for the latter as well as the former category of drugs.

Hydantoin Derivatives

Phenytoin (Dilantin) is the best-known and best-studied, most widely employed, and least toxic drug of the hydantoin group and will be discussed as its prototype. Another available hydantoin is mephenytoin (Mesantoin).

The development of phenytoin is one of the true success stories of the pharmaceutical industry. It resulted from a methodical, planned program of development and is close to being an ideal drug for grand mal epilepsy. Phenytoin exerts antiepileptic activity with little general sedation. The mechanism of action appears to be the stabilization of nerve cells by increasing the efflux of sodium ion from the cells. This increase in efflux is brought about by stimulation of the sodium pump (Fig. 28-5) and leads to hyperpolarization. The increased stability of cortical neurons reduces the spread of abnormal discharges from the seizure focus to surrounding cortical areas. Phenytoin is a primary drug choice in epilepsy other than petit mal, in which it is contraindicated (Table 28-2). Phenytoin is also employed for the treatment of positive-spike pattern and neuralgias.

The overall toxicity of the hydantoins is low in comparison with that of most other antiepileptics and with that of psychotropic drugs in general. In comparison with phenobarbital, phenytoin has the advantages of less sedation for a given level of efficacy and freedom from abuse potential. On the other hand, hypersensitivity reactions are somewhat more common with phenytoin. Phenytoin has a more narrow spectrum of effectiveness (being contraindicated in petit mal). Side effects, especially hyperplasia of the gums, are more frequent, though not notably severe, with phenytoin. Also, there is evidence of teratogenicity when phenytoin is used during pregnancy. In the case of antiepileptic drugs, the risk of teratogenicity must be weighed against the risk that seizures in the mother holds for the fetus.

Hyperplasia (softening and overgrowth of the gums) is the most common difficulty with phenytoin, occurring in about 20 percent of patients. It can be prevented or controlled in many cases by intensive oral hygiene, including increased brushing of the gums. Other, rarer symptoms include ataxia, sedation, hypocalcemia, and blurring of vision. Hydantoins may rarely produce blood dyscrasias. Hypersensitivity reactions are more frequent with mephenytoin than with phenytoin and take the form of skin rashes, granulocytopenia, and aplastic anemia.

Hydantoins are metabolized by the liver drug-metabolizing enzymes and also stimulate their activity. Consequently, phenytoin interacts with barbiturates and other drugs that are metabolized in the liver. This is the interaction that is often called *induction of liver enzymes* (see Chap. 7). A second type of drug interaction involving phenytoin is competition for plasma albumin protein-binding sites. A fraction (nearly 90 percent) of any dose of phenytoin is normally bound to inactive albumin-binding sites in the blood. Only the small, unbound fraction is free to exert pharmacologic actions on the brain. Other drugs, such as aspirin, that are likewise bound to these protein-binding sites increase the activity of phenytoin by competing for the limited number of inactive sites. When aspirin and phenytoin are used concurrently, each will increase the fraction of the other that is in the unbound and pharmacologically active state. Dosage adjustment must take into account interactions of this type, or toxicity will occur.

A third interaction of phenytoin with other drugs is additive CNS depression. Since phenytoin is essentially a depressant drug—albeit less sedating than many other antiepileptic drugs—it will produce additive CNS depression with any other CNS depressant used concurrently.

Barbiturates

Phenobarbital was the first effective antiepileptic having an acceptable level of toxicity. It is still widely prescribed and is the other primary drug of choice besides phenytoin for grand mal epilepsy. The overall incidence of side effects is a little less than with phenytoin, teratogenicity is less, and phenobarbital is not contraindicated in any form of epilepsy. On the other hand, the abuse liability and greater degree of sedation are limiting features of the barbiturates. The occurrence of tolerance creates a problem with

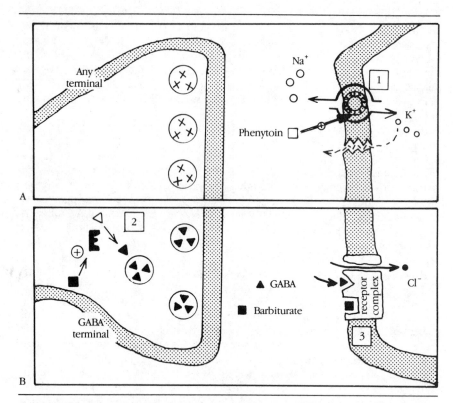

Fig. 28-5. *Neurochemical mechanisms of primary drug choices for grand mal epilepsy. GABA, gamma-aminobutyric acid. A. Phenytoin stimulates the Na^+-K^+ exchange pump to hyperpolarize nerve cells, increasing cortical inhibition. B. Barbiturates facilitate GABA synthesis and GABA binding, increasing inhibitory neurotransmission.*

respect to termination of drug treatment. Withdrawal of a patient from barbiturate medication must be accomplished slowly, since seizure liability increases during sedative-hypnotic abstinence.

Antiepileptic potency is usually evident at a dosage that produces an acceptable level of sedation. If higher dosages are required, phenobarbital can be given in combination with amphetamine, which has weak antiepileptic effects of its own, but—more important—counters the sedative effect of the barbiturate. The mechanism of the antiepileptic action of barbiturates is attributed to the actions of barbiturates on gamma-aminobutyric acid (GABA) transmission (Fig. 28-5).

Only the long-acting barbiturates are useful in epilepsy because of the chronic nature of the illness. In any case, phenobarbital and mephobarbital (Mebaral) seem to possess some special potency as antiepileptics because of the phenyl group that each contains. Another drug closely resembling phenobarbital but not, strictly speaking, a barbiturate is primidone (Mysoline). It has no special advantage over phenobarbital, but has proved to be effective in some cases of grand mal refractory to other treatments and is especially useful in psychomotor epilepsy (see Table 28-2). Side effects with phenobarbital are very rare. A rash develops in about 2 percent of patients. Primidone can

Table 28-2. Drug spectrum in the treatment of epilepsy

Type of drug	Type of seizure					
	Grand mal	Status epilepticus	Petit mal	Psychomotor	Myoclonus	Infantile spasms
Hydantoins	++++	0	–	+++	+	0
Barbiturates	+++	++	+	++	+	0
Primidone	+++	0	+	++++	+++	+
Oxazolidines	–	–	++++	0	0	0
Succinimides	0	0	+++	0	0	0
Diazepam	+	++++	+++	0	+++	+
Clonazepam	+	++++	++++	0	++++	++
Sodium valproate	+++	0	+++	+++	+++	+

+, efficacy in treatment; 0, no efficacy in treatment; –, contraindicated.

produce a number of side effects, including nausea, headache, rash, and sexual impotence. The barbiturates are employed primarily in grand mal and psychomotor epilepsy.

Barbiturates produce an additive CNS depression when given concurrently with any other CNS depressant, including alcohol, narcotics, and antihistamines. This can be of practical significance, since each of these is sometimes self-administered. Like phenytoin, barbiturates interact with drugs (such as anticoagulants) metabolized by liver drug-metabolizing enzymes, generally shortening the duration of their action.

Oxazolidones

The oxazolidones (or oxazolidinediones), as well as the succinimides, are used exclusively in petit mal epilepsy. The two currently employed oxazolidones are trimethadione (Tridione) and paramethadione (Paradione). Combination therapies involving amphetamine and oxazolidones are commonly employed to antagonize the sedation produced by the oxazolidones and because amphetamine has itself some effectiveness in petit mal. Side effects occur commonly and include nausea, vomiting, fatigue, light sensitivity, neutropenia, kidney damage, loss of hair, and, rarely, grand mal seizures.

Succinimides

Three succinimide derivatives—ethosuximide (Zarontin), methsuximide (Celontin), and phensuximide (Milontin)—have proved effective in petit mal. Ethosuximide has been employed successfully in positive-spike pattern. All produce drowsiness, but are slightly less toxic than the oxazolidones. Side effects that occur include rash, easy bruising, jaundice, swollen glands, persistent fever, and changes in urine output. There have been some reports of these drugs inducing dream-like states and psychotic episodes. Personality changes have been attributed to ethosuximide.

Benzodiazepines

The benzodiazepines were discussed in detail in Chapter 17. Among the benzodiazepines, diazepam (Valium) appears to have a special effectiveness in petit mal. Moreover, when given intravenously, it is considered the drug of choice in terminating seizures in status epilepticus.

A newer benzodiazepine, clonazepam (Clonopin), has been marketed expressly for use in epilepsy. It is both more effective and more toxic than diazepam. It is useful alone or in combinations for petit mal epilepsy and is the current drug of choice for myoclonus (see Table 28-2).

Valproic Acid

Valproic acid (dipropylacetate) (Depakene) is the newest entry in the antiepileptic market. It has a broad spectrum of usefulness (see Table 28-2), but is probably not the optimal choice for any one form of epilepsy. It elevates GABA levels, and this is the likely basis for its action. Early enthusiasm for the drug was based on the belief that valproic acid had relatively few adverse effects. The frequent incidence of hepatic toxicity (in about 15 to 30 percent of patients), occasionally leading to death, has proved to be a limiting feature. Other mild or infrequent side effects include gastrointestinal disturbances (anorexia, nausea, vomiting), alopecia, and an anticoagulant action. Teratogenicity has been reported.

Implications for Psychotherapy

A psychotherapist should know about epilepsy and antiepileptic drugs for a number of reasons: (1) Some forms of epilepsy may present themselves as psychological disturbances or learning disabilities. (2) Epilepsy may involve adjustment problems and a need for supportive therapy. (3) Antiepileptic medications may produce psychiatric side effects. (4) Some drugs used for psychiatric problems increase seizure liability. (5) The presence of temporal lobe epilepsy may predispose to an alcohol-induced or sedative-hypnotic–induced amnesic disorder. (6) Subictal epilepsy might predispose to abuse of depressants as a kind of self-medication. And (7) the presence of epilepsy may dictate limitations in the forms of nondrug therapy that can be employed.

The complications of drug dependency in the case of barbiturates were discussed in Chapter 11. Other antiepileptic agents are nonaddicting.

Complaints of apathy or lethargy may reflect the sedative action associated with all of these drugs. While sedation is rare with phenytoin, it may occur. Outright depression is seldom reported with the hydantoins, but may accompany treatment with other antiepileptic drugs. Impotence is a side effect of primidone and may have important psychological significance to the patient. The succinimides have been reported to cause anxiety, agitation, and hallucinations in some patients.

The need for awareness of the ways in which epilepsy may manifest itself, particularly manifestations that resemble psychopathologic symptoms, has been stressed throughout this chapter. The frequency with which subictal and temporal lobe varieties interpolate themselves into the domain of the psychotherapist is probably much greater than is commonly supposed. The therapist needs to be alert to signs of epileptiform activity and prepared to refer such patients to appropriate medical personnel.

If, on the other hand, inquiry reveals that antiepileptic medication has been prescribed for a client, consultation with the prescribing physician is requisite. The need for a cooperative effort betwen the psychotherapeutic and medical professions is nowhere more necessary than with epilepsy. Apart from the psychological complications directly attributable to epilepsy, personal adjustment difficulties are the rule rather than the exception, for the epileptic may suffer embarrassment, ridicule, fear of accidents, or confusion concerning time lapses. Drug therapy is the beginning of, rather than the conclusion to, successful treatment.

Drugs Useful in Epilepsy

clonazepam (Clonopin), a benzodiazepine: for petit mal, myoclonus, Lennox-Gastaut
    syndrome (petit mal variant). Starting dose: 1.5 mg daily. Maximum: 20 mg daily.
diazepam (Valium), a benzodiazepine: antianxiety, anticonvulsant, antiepileptic. Anti-
    epileptic: 4 to 40 mg. Status epilepticus: 5 to 10 mg per administration, IV or IM.
ethosuximide (Zarontin), a succinimide antiepileptic: for petit mal, positive-spike
    pattern syndrome. Typical: 500 to 1,000 mg. Maximum: 1,500 mg.
mephenytoin (Mesantoin), a hydantoin antiepileptic: for epilepsy, excluding petit mal.
    Typical: 200 to 600 mg. Extremes: 50 to 800 mg.
mephobarbital (Mebaral), a barbiturate antiepileptic: for grand mal and psychomotor
    epilepsy. Antiepileptic: 100 to 200 mg.

methsuximide (Celontin), a succinimide antiepileptic: mainly for petit mal. Typical: 300 to 900 mg. Maximum: 1,200 mg.

paramethadione (Paradione), an oxazolidine antiepileptic. Typical: 900 to 1,600 mg. Extremes: 250 to 2,100 mg.

phenobarbital (Luminal), a barbiturate antiepileptic: for grand mal, psychomotor, and other forms of epilepsy and status epilepticus. Typical antiepileptic: 100 to 300 mg. Status epilepticus: 200 to 320 mg per administration, IV or SQ.

phensuximide (Milontin), a succinimide antiepileptic: less potent than ethosuximide. Typical: 1,000 to 3,000 mg. Maximum: 4,000 mg.

phenytoin (diphenylhydantoin) (Dilantin), a hydantoin antiepileptic: for epilepsy (except petit mal), positive-spike pattern, neuralgias, cardiac arrhythmias. Typical: 300 to 500 mg. Extremes: 100 to 600 mg.

primidone (Mysoline), a barbiturate-like antiepileptic: particularly useful in psycho-motor epilepsy. Typical: 250 to 2,000 mg.

trimethadione (Tridione), an oxazolidine antiepileptic: useful principally in petit mal. Typical: 900 to 1,600 mg. Extremes: 250 to 2,100 mg.

valproic acid (Depakene), an antiepileptic: useful in grand mal and petit mal. Typical: 1,000 to 3,000 mg. Extremes: 1,000 to 5,000 mg.

Selected References and Further Readings

1. Calne, D. B. Treatment of epilepsy with valproate. *Clin. Neuropharmacol.* 4:31–38, 1979.
2. Gilman, A. G., Goodman, L. S., and Gilman, A. *The Pharmacological Basis of Therapeutics* (6th ed.). New York: Macmillan, 1980.
3. Hughes, R. R. *An Introduction to Clinical Electro-Encephalography.* Bristol, Engl.: Wright, 1961.
4. Jonas, A. D. *Ictal and Subictal Neurosis.* Springfield, Ill.: Thomas, 1965.
5. Small, L. *Neuropsychodiagnosis in Psychotherapy.* New York: Brunner/Mazel, 1973.
6. Van Woert, M. H., and Hwang, E. C. Biochemistry and pharmacology of myoclonus. *Clin. Neuropharmacol.* 3:167–184, 1978.

Appendixes

Psychotropic Drugs in Top 200 of All New and Refill Prescriptions in 1972 and 1981·

A

1981 Rank	Trade name (manufacturer)	Generic name(s)	Class(es)	1972 Rank
1	Valium (Roche)	Diazepam	Anxiolytic	1
4	Tylenol w/Codeine (McNeil)	Acetaminophen and codeine	Nonnarcotic and narcotic analgesic	142
12	Dalmane (Roche)	Flurazepam	Hypnotic	72
20	Darvocet-N 100 (Lilly)	Propoxyphene and acetaminophen	Narcotic and non-narcotic analgesic	—
29	Empirin w/Codeine (B-W)	Aspirin and codeine	Nonnarcotic and narcotic analgesic	—
34	Dilantin (Parke-Davis)	Phenytoin	Antiepileptic	43
36	Benadryl (Parke-Davis)	Diphenhydramine	Antihistamine, anti-parkinsonian	19
37	Tranxene (Abbott)	Clorazepate	Anxiolytic	—
39	(Generic)	Phenobarbital	Antiepileptic	15
42	Elavil (MSD)	Amitriptyline	Antidepressant	36
44	Librium (Roche)	Chlordiazepoxide	Anxiolytic	3
46	Fiorinol (Sandoz)	Butalbital and APC*	Sedative-hypnotic, two nonnarcotic analgesics and stimulant	29
48	Ativan (Wyeth)	Lorazepam	Anxiolytic	—
53	Mellaril (Sandoz)	Thioridazine	Antipsychotic	42
54	Zomax (McNeil)	Zomepirac	Nonnarcotic analgesic	—
66	Atarax (Roerig)	Hydroxyzine	Antihistamine sedative	165
73	Percodan (Endo)	Oxycodone and APC	Narcotic, two non-narcotic analgesics, and stimulant	60
74	Triavil (MSD)	Perphenazine and amitriptyline	Antipsychotic and antidepressant	52
79	Sinequan (Roerig)	Doxepin	Antidepressant	133

Appendix A (continued)

1981 Rank	Trade name (manufacturer)	Generic name(s)	Class(es)	1972 Rank
85	Darvon Compound-65 (Lilly)	Propoxyphene and APC	Narcotic, two non-narcotic analgesics, and stimulant	2
89	(Generic)	Meprobamate	Sedative-hypnotic	61
99	Haldol (McNeil)	Haloperidol	Antipsychotic	—
100	Serax (Wyeth)	Oxazepam	Anxiolytic	109
108	Thorazine (SKF)	Chlorpromazine	Antipsychotic	25
114	Talwin (Winthrop)	Pentazocine	Narcotic	55
115	Tenuate (Merrell-National)	Diethylpropion	Anorectic	70
125	Fiorinol w/Codeine (Sandoz)	Butalbital, codeine, APC	Sedative, narcotic, two nonnarcotics and stimulant	—
128	Compazine (SKF)	Prochlorperazine	Antipsychotic, antinausea	68
142	Equagesic (Wyeth)	Meprobamate, etho-heptazine, and aspirin	Sedative, narcotic, and nonnarcotic analgesic	—
146	Periactin (MSD)	Cyproheptidine	Antimigraine	111
147	Butisol Sodium (McNeil)	Butabarbital	Sedative-hypnotic	—
150	Tofranil (Geigy)	Imipramine	Antidepressant	82
151	Stelazine (SKF)	Trifluoperazine	Neuroleptic	71
157	Hydergine (Dorsey)	Dihydroergotoxine	Cerebral metabolism stimulant	—
160	Cogentin (MSD)	Benztropine	Antiparkinsonian	—
166	Vistaril (Pfizer)	Hydroxyzine	Antihistamine sedative	151
184	(Generic)	Amitriptyline	Antidepressant	—
194	Artane (Lederle)	Trihexyphenidyl	Antiparkinsonian	167

B-W, Burroughs-Welcome; MSD, Merck Sharp & Dome; SKF, Smith Kline & French; APC, aspirin, phenacetin, and caffeine.

*Excluding psychotropic drugs appearing in combinations for non-CNS purposes, such as cold and cough preparations, combinations for ulcers and asthma. Rankings taken from *Pharmacy Times.*

Some Adverse Reactions of Potential Psychotherapeutic Significance

B

The following adverse drug reactions, listed alphabetically, may be of significance to the psychotherapist. Included are emotional and behavioral symptoms that have been reported in reactions to psychotropic medication. The inclusion of a drug under an adverse reaction does not imply a causal connection, only that some investigators have reported such a reaction. The absence of a drug under any heading should not be taken to mean that the drug does not cause such a reaction. Nonpsychotropic drugs (peripherally active, exclusively or primarily) in common use are listed with asterisks under those adverse reactions that are often assumed by therapists to be essentially psychological in nature. The appearance of a class or chemical group name under an adverse reaction means that any member of that group may possibly be connected with that reaction.

This appendix is intended only as a general guide to possible drug involvement in psychiatric symptoms. Should the psychotherapist suspect an adverse drug reaction, medical consultation is, of course, in order.

aggression (anger, rage, etc.)
  amphetamines
  chlordiazepoxide
  diazepam
  levodopa
  meprobamate

agitation
  aminophylline
  amphetamines
  analeptics
  anticholinergics
  caffeine
  carbamazepine
  codeine
  dextromethorphan
  droperidol
  ketamine
  levodopa

  methylphenidate
  succinimides
  theobromine
  theophylline

akathisia (inability to sit still)
  butyrophenone neuroleptics
  phenothiazine neuroleptics

akinesia
  neuroleptics

amnesia
  anticholinergics
  diazepam
  MAO inhibitors
  methotrimeprazine

anger (see aggression)

anticholinergic syndrome
  atropine
  belladonna extract
  benztropine
  biperiden
  chlorpheniramine
  *cyclopentolate
  diphenhydramine
  ethopropazine
  marijuana
  *methantheline
  phenothiazines
  orphenadrine
  plants:
    bittersweet
    black henbane
    deadly nightshade
    jimson weed
    jerusalem cherry
    potato leaves, sprouts, tubers
  procyclidine
  promethazine
  *propantheline
  sleep aids
  tricyclic antidepressants
  trihexyphenidyl
  *tropicamide

anxiety
  caffeine
  cocaine
  droperidol
  *epinephrine
  flurazepam
  haloperidol
  *insulin
  *isoproterenol
  levodopa
  MAO inhibitors
  *quinine
  succinimides
  *sulfonylureas
  *tolazoline
  tricyclic antidepressants
  *vasopressors

ataxia
  amphetamines
  antihistamines
  anxiolytics
  barbiturates
  carbamazepine
  ethosuximide
  hydantoins
  levodopa

lithium
MAO inhibitors
methylphenidate
methsuximide
methysergide
primidone
tricyclic antidepressants

confusion
  analeptics
  anticholinergics
  *anticholinesterases
  *antidiuretics
  antihistamines
  aspirin
  carbamazepine
  clorazepate
  cocaine
  *digitalis
  ethopropazine
  flurazepam
  haloperidol
  indomethacin
  *insulin
  MAO inhibitors
  oxazepam
  phenmetrazine
  *sulfonylurea hypoglycemics
  tricyclic antidepressants
  tybamate
  *chloramphenicol

convulsion
  aminophylline
  analeptics
  antihistamines
  benzodiazepines
  chlorprothixene
  codeine
  levodopa
  lithium
  MAO inhibitors
  meperidine
  meprobamate
  neuroleptics
  propoxyphene
  tricyclic antidepressants

cough
  analeptics
  levodopa
  paraldehyde
  thiopental

delirium
  anesthetics

anticholinergics
antihistamines
barbiturates
benzodiazepines
*chloramphenicol
cocaine
levodopa
MAO inhibitors
meprobamate
*quinine
scopolamine
tricyclic antidepressants

depersonalization
indomethacin
methysergide
tybamate

depression
*amantadine
benzodiazepines
carbamazepine
*carbonic anhydrase inhibitors
*chloramphenicol
*corticosteroids
droperidol
*estrogens
haloperidol
indomethacin
isoniazide
levodopa
methadone
methsuximide
methysergide
*oral contraceptives
*propranolol
rauwolfia alkaloids
*sulfonamide antibacterials

dizziness
aminophylline
analgesics, strong
anticholinergics
antihistamines
anxiolytics
aspirin
carbamazepine
dextroamphetamine
dextromethorphan
diethylpropion
ethchlorvynol
ethosuximide
indomethacin
levodopa

lithium
MAO inhibitors
methsuximide
methylphenidate
methyprylon
methysergide
pentazocine
phenytoin
piperazines
tricyclic antidepressants

drowsiness
analgesics, strong
anticholinergics
anticonvulsants
antihistamines
anxiolytics
carbamazepine
levodopa
methysergide
neuroleptics
sedative-hypnotics
tricyclic antidepressants

dyskinesias
levodopa
methylphenidate
neuroleptics

dysphoria
narcotic analgesics

euphoria
amphetamines
analeptics
antihistamines
apomorphine
barbiturates
clorazepate
cocaine
*corticosteroids
diethylpropion
ethosuximide
flurazepam
haloperidol
ketamine
levodopa
MAO inhibitors
meprobamate
methylphenidate
methysergide
narcotic analgesics
scopolamine
tricyclic antidepressants
tybamate

excitement
  *acetazolamide
  amphetamines
  anesthetics
  antihistamines
  benzodiazepines
  chloral hydrate
  cocaine
  diethylpropion
  droperidol
  *ephedrine
  *epinephrine
  meperidine
  methylphenidate
  phenmetrazine
  *quinine
  scopolamine
  sedative-hypnotics
  tricyclic antidepressants

extrapyramidal reactions
  neuroleptics
  tricyclic antidepressants

fatigue (see lethargy)

fear (see anxiety)

hallucinations
  amphetamines
  analeptics
  anticholinergics
  chlordiazepoxide
  diazepam
  ketamine
  levodopa
  MAO inhibitors
  methylphenidate
  methysergide
  pentazocine
  *procainamide
  *propranolol
  *quinacrine
  succinimides
  tricyclic antidepressants

headache
  *allopurinol
  aminosalicyclic acid
  *antidiuretics
  antihistamines
  aspirin
  caffeine
  *carbachol
  carbamazepine

*carbonic anhydrase inhibitors
  *chloramphenicol
  *corticosteroids
  *epinephrine
  *hydralazine
  indomethacin
  *isoproterenol
  levodopa
  *mannitol
  *methoxamine
  *metronidazole
  *miotics
  *oral contraceptives
  perphenazine
  *probenecid
  *quinidine
  *streptomycin
  *sulfonamides
  *sulfonylureas
  theophylline
  tricyclic antidepressants

hyperactivity
  benzodiazepines
  *corticosteroids
  doxapram
  levodopa
  MAO inhibitors
  meprobamate
  phenobarbital

hypomanic reactions
  antidepressants
  levodopa

hysteria
  antihistamines

impotence
  alphamethyldopa
  amphetamines
  antihistamines
  antihypotensives
  *atropine
  carbamazepine
  chlordiazepoxide
  chlorprothixene
  cimetidine
  *guanethidine
  haloperidol
  MAO inhibitors
  *methantheline
  phenothiazine neuroleptics
  thiothixene
  tricyclic antidepressants

insomnia
  amphetamines
  anticholinergics
  antihistamines
  benzodiazepines
  caffeine
  chlorprothixene
  diethylpropion
  ephedrine
  levodopa
  MAO inhibitors
  meprobamate
  methylphenidate
  methysergide
  theophylline
  thiothixene
  tricyclic antidepressants
  tybamate

irritability
  *amantadine
  amphetamines
  antihistamines
  belladonna alkaloids
  benzodiazepines
  *corticosteroids
  droperidol
  *estrogens
  levodopa
  meprobamate
  *mithramycin
  *oral contraceptives
  theophylline

lethargy
  *acetazolamide
  *amantadine
  *antidiuretics
  *antihypertensives
  benzodiazepines
  carbamazepine
  chlordiazepoxide
  *cycloserine
  *digitalis glycosides
  *fluorouracil
  *insulin
  levodopa
  *lidocaine
  lithium
  *magnesium antacids
  MAO inhibitors
  *meclizine
  methysergide
  *mithramycin
  *mitotane

neuroleptics
  *phenindione
  phenytoin
  *propranolol
  *rifampin
  salicylates
  sedative-hypnotics
  *sulfonamides
  *sulfonylureas
  tricyclic antidepressants
  tybamate
  *vitamin A

libido changes
  *androgens
  antihistamines
  antihypertensives
  benzodiazepines
  cimetidine
  *corticosteroids
  levodopa
  *oral contraceptives
  tricyclic antidepressants

manic reactions
  analeptics
  *corticosteroids
  MAO inhibitors

muscle hypertension
  lithium
  promethazine
  trimeprazine

muscle spasm (and fasciculations)
  analeptics
  levodopa
  MAO inhibitors

muscle weakness (see akinesia)

narcosis (see stupor)

nervousness (see also anxiety)
  *amantadine
  amphetamines
  antihistamines
  *corticosteroids
  chlorprothixene
  *cyclopentamine
  diethylpropion
  ephedrine
  *flavoxate
  *lidocaine
  *methylhexaneamine

nervousness *(continued)*
  methylphenidate
  methysergide
  *nylidrin
  phenmetrazine
  *sulfonylureas
  tolazamide

ovulation, delayed
  neuroleptics

panic reaction (see agitation,
  anxiety, and confusion)

paranoid reaction
  amphetamines
  anticholinergics
  *corticosteroids
  levodopa
  methylphenidate

psychosis, acute intoxication
  *acetosulfone
  amphetamines
  analeptics
  anticholinergics
  bromides
  *corticosteroids
  droperidol
  isoniazid
  lithium
  methylphenidate
  *phenacemide
  *procainamide
  *quinacrine
  *sulfonamides
  *sulfoxone

rage (see aggression)

restlessness (see also akathisia)
  amphetamines
  anticholinergics
  apomorphine
  benzodiazepines
  cocaine
  *corticosteroids
  *epinephrine
  *isoproterenol
  levodopa
  MAO inhibitors

meprobamate
*nitroprussides
sedative-hypnotics
theophylline
tricyclic antidepressants
*vasopressors

ringing in ears (see tinnitus)

sedation (see drowsiness)

sexual behavior changes (see
  libido changes)

slurring, speech
  amphetamine
  diazepam
  flurazepam
  lithium
  methotrimeprazine
  oxazepam

stupor
  lithium
  narcotic analgesics

suicidal tendencies
  antidepressants
  *cycloserine
  levodopa

tics (see muscle spasm)

tinnitus
  indomethacin
  salicylates

tremor (see also muscle spasm)
  amphetamines
  antihistamines
  apomorphine
  belladonna alkaloids
  cocaine
  diazepam
  MAO inhibitors
  neuroleptics
  nicotine
  promethazine
  tricyclic antidepressants

vertigo (see dizziness)

Mr. G., a 55-year-old economist, was brought to the emergency room of South Hampton Hospital at noon by his 19-year-old son, in a state of agitation. His son indicated that the father has an alcohol problem, that he had been drunk the night before, and that he had begun acting "crazy" that morning.

Mr. G. is hostile to the staff, mutters to himself continuously, and appears confused and somewhat delirious. His blood pressure is below normal, and he experiences dizziness, nausea and anxiety.

The staff first obtains a drinking history. The son provides the following information: The drinking problem has existed for over 5 years. His father drinks whiskey every morning. The amount is unknown, since the father is very secretive about the drinking. The whiskey is kept hidden in the basement, and the father "takes the newspapers down to the basement" several times an evening. The son does not know if there have been any related medical problems, previous treatment, or history of delirium tremens. There is no other family source of information, since the mother is an institutionalized psychiatric patient.

A call to the family physician reveals that the drinking problem is of long standing. The patient has refused to undertake counseling, psychiatric treatment, or any other alcohol treatment program.

Mr. G.'s health has been good most of his life, but a physical examination a year ago revealed adult-onset diabetes mellitus. His medication now includes NPH insulin, 25 units every morning, and regular insulin according to a sliding scale based on the early evening urine test results.

Mr. G. has no history of seizures, associated with alcohol use or otherwise. He has no other drug prescriptions.

The staff orders a complete array of physical tests for evaluation of the patient's status. Urinalysis reveals the presence of acidosis and significant dehydration. Blood tests reveal conspicuously low blood sugar, reduced hematocrit, and prolonged prothrombin time. The ECG is normal. There is no evidence of significant infection. All other test values lie within the normal range.

1. What immediate treatment should be provided for Mr. G.? Be specific about any drug orders as to drug identity, dose, route, and frequency.
2. Should Mr. G. be admitted? Why?
3. What is the probable mechanism underlying each positive finding from the laboratory evaluation?
4. What are the factors contributing to the behavioral symptoms?
5. What interrelationships may exist between the alcohol use and the diabetes?
6. What are the symptoms of hypoglycemia, and how do they come about?
7. What steps would you recommend for achievement of a long-term resolution of Mr. G.'s problem?

Drug Report   D

You are dealing with a person in counseling and learn that he (she) is regularly using _____ . (Assume that if the drug is a prescription drug, the client has a prescription from a physician for the drug. If it is a social drug or drug of abuse, assume the client is self-administering it.) Being a conscientious therapist and well aware of the potential interactions of drugs with nondrug treatment programs, you refresh your knowledge of the drug by looking it up in such sources as the *Physicians' Desk Reference, AMA Drug Evaluations, Facts and Comparisons, Drugs and Therapy,* and *The Pharmacological Basis of Therapeutics.* Use the following spaces to indicate what you find out that is relevant to nondrug therapy.

1. What class does this drug belong to?

2. What, if anything, distinguishes this drug from other agents in the same category?

3. What are the clinical indications for this drug?

4. What are the psychiatric side effects (include behavioral, emotional, cognitive, and perceptual)? (*Note:* You lose points for including side effects that are completely unrelated to brain function.)

5. Does this drug interact in significant ways with any nonprescription drugs the client might be self-administering?

413

6. Does the client's use of this drug have any significant implications for you as counselor?

7. The dosage regimen for the drug in question in this client is _____. How does this compare with the normal and extreme ranges of total daily dosage for this drug?

8. Did you encounter any contradictory assertions among the drug information sources that you examined? If so, please quote the contradictory passages and give your opinion about why the discrepancy has occurred. Which viewpoint do you accept? Why?

Index

Index

Boldface page numbers indicate main entries.

Absence seizures. *See* Petit mal epilepsy
Abstinence syndrome. *See* Withdrawal
Abuse, drug, 6, 19, 131, 132, **145–157**, 307.
    See also Tolerance and dependence
    alcohol, 195–209
    anxiolytics, 273–274, 281
    education, 155–157
    narcotics, 341
    relationship to therapy, 8
    sedative-hypnotics, 187–188
Abuse liability, 147, 187, 191, 192, 211, 282,
    341, 342, 395, 399
Acetaldehyde, 199, 201
Acetaminophen, 120, 134, 151, 152, 207, 342,
    343, **351**, 352, 403
Acetophenazine, 265, 266, 297
Acetylcholine (ACh), **78–85**, 109
    in autonomic nervous system, 44, 49, 78
    in chronic organic brain syndrome, 21
    in corpus striatum, 82, 318
    and cyclic nucleotides, 108
    distribution, 55, 80–85, 164, 171, 248, 377,
        384
    and nicotine, 80, 81, 214, 215
    release, 75, 80, 100
    and response inhibition, 35, 85
    and scopolamine, 191
    and state-dependent learning, 38
Acetylcholinesterase (AChE), 44, 79, 80
Acetylsalicylic acid. *See* Aspirin
Action potential, 45, **65–66**, 71, 80, 86
Adaptations in neurotransmission, 76, 78, 81,
    88, 91, 92, 96, 98, 100, 259–261, 295–297,
    333, 340, 382
Addiction, **147–151**, 341, 345. *See also* Abuse,
    drug; Tolerance and dependence
Addison's disease, 19, 168
Additive drug effects, 119, 203, 204, 269, 339,
    350, 395, 398
Adenosine triphosphate (ATP), 70, 72, 106, 107

Adenyl cyclase, 31, 70, 72, 75, 77, 81, 87, 91, 94,
    96, 103, 106, 107, 108, 295, 384
Administrative routes, 116–118
Adrenocortical insufficiency. *See* Addison's
    disease
Adverse drug reactions. *See* Hypersensitivity
    reactions; Paradoxical reactions; Side
    effects; *and individual drugs*
Affect, 11, 237, 243, 285
Affective disorders, 127, 128, 130. *See also*
    Depression; Manic-depressive disorder
Affinity, 74–76, 77, 81, 88, 92, 96, 100, 103,
    113–115, 116, 340
Aggression, 57, 91, 93, 215, 232, 254, 276,
    324, 405
Agonists, 74–76, 81, 88, 92, 96, 100, 104, 113,
    114, 116, 119, 340, 343, 358
Akathisias, 149, 178, 263, 269, 325–327, **329**, 405
Akinesias, 321, 323, 325–327, 405
Akineton. *See* Biperiden
Alcohol, 120, **195–209**
    abuse, 1, 4, 8, 145, 148, 150–154, 156, 177,
        187, 188, 193, 273, 274, 277, 287, 301, 329,
        341, 356, 399
    dehydrogenase, 94, 199, 201
    excitation with, 196, 197, 198, 202
    and the liver, 134
    mechanism of action, 184, 196, 198
    as primary reinforcer, 39
    psychosis, 20, 168, 270
    and sleep, 185
    and state-dependent learning, 38
    and therapy, 6, 411
Alcoholism, 155, 201–202, 208
    and benzodiazepines, 277, 283
    and hypoglycemia, 19
    and lithium, 307
    and LSD, 230
    in therapy, 4, 9
    and tremor, 326

Alcohols, 183, 190
Aldehyde dehydrogenase, 94, 201, 206
Allergies, 355, 356, 357
  drug. *See* Hypersensitivity reactions
Alpha blocking, 167, 169, 215
Alpha motor neurons. *See* Motor neurons, alpha
Alpha (α) waves, 165, 167–173, 295, 371
Alprazolam, 281, 283
Alzheimer's disease, 18, 20, 21, 287
Amarita muscaria, 231
p-Aminophenol, 351, 352
Amitriptyline, 5, 95, 120, 126, 140, 268,
  297–299, 403, 404
Amnesia, 85, 202, 203, 405
Amobarbital, 38, 120, **189**, 193
Amotivational syndrome, 232, 235
Amoxapine, 298, 300, 301, 302
Amphetamine(s), 120, **213–216**, 224
  abuse, 146, 148, 150–153, 156, 211
  and antiepileptics, 396, 398
  and desynchronized (D) sleep, 177
  and hyperkinesis, 23, 218
  and neurotransmitters, 75, 86, 89, 90, 91
  psychosis, 223, 265
  and state dependency, 38
Amygdala, 59, 91, 92, 97, 239–241, **247**, 248,
  250, 277, 315, 370, 381
  basolateral, 33, 247
  corticomedial, 33, 247
Amytal. *See* Amobarbital
Analeptics, 100, 186, 196, 211, 221–223, 340
Analgesics, 119, 188, 356. *See also* Narcotic
  analgesics; Nonnarcotic analgesics; *and
  individual drugs*
Anesthetics, 5, 38, 153, 189, 343
Anorexia, 5, 211, 213, 219, 341
Anorexia nervosa, 131
Antabuse. *See* Disulfiram
Antagonism, drug, 74, 75, 81, 86, 88, 92, 96, 100,
  104, 113, 114, 116, 119, 358
Antiandrogens, 127, 131
Antianginal drugs, 149
Antianxiety drugs. *See* Anxiolytics
Anticholinergic
  drugs, 85, 156, 191, 203, 228, 231, 248, 262,
    264, 287, 321, 323, 328–330, 406
  effects, 38, 234, 263, 266, 294, 295, 300, 301,
    322, 406
Anticonvulsants, 5, 280, 393, 399. *See also*
  Antiepileptics
Antidepressants, 5, 12, 126, 127, 130, 132, 133,
  151, 152, 177, 203, 211, 259, 289, **293–302**
  atypical, 300–301
Antiepileptics, 5, 391, 392, **393–400**
  barbiturates as, 189
  benzodiazepines as, 281
  case example, 23
  depression caused by, 287
  drug interactions of, 119, 395, 398
  in hypertonias, 325
  overdoses, 152

screening with pentylentetrazol (PTZ), 221
  withdrawal, 149
Antihistamines, 5
  for allergies and colds, 342, 355, 356
  as anxiolytics, 276, 282
  depression caused by, 287
  drug interactions of, 119, 188, 196, 203, 398
  overdoses, 152
  in parkinsonism, 322, 323
  as sleep aids, 191, 194
  tricyclics as, 295, 301
Antihypertensive drugs, 149, 265, 287, 299, 356,
  357
Antiinflammatory drugs, 119, 188, 347, **348–354**
Antimanic drugs, 5, **305–311**
Antiparkinsonian agents, 133, **321–324**, 328
Antipsychotics. *See* Neuroleptics
Antipyretics, 347, **348**, 349, 351, 352, 353
Anxiety, 17, 19, 127–131, 133, 148, 168, 178,
  180, 181, 222, 230, 231, 261, 269, **273–276**,
  285, 300, 323, 329, 335, 341, 391, 399,
  406
Anxiolytics, 5, **276–284**
  abuse, 1
  and cyclic AMP, 107, 108
  and depression, 287
  and disinhibition, 41
  extent of use, 6, 130, 131, 193, 274, 289
  interactions of, 119, 133, 203, 297
  and neuroleptics, 41, 261, 269
  in organic brain syndrome, 21
  and therapy, 8, 12, 135, 275, 359
Apathy, 17, 19, 288, 323, 399
APC. *See* Aspirin; Phenacetin; Caffeine
Apneas, sleep, 178, 179, 180
Apomorphine, 90, 91, 92
Arcuate nucleus, 93, 163
l-Aromatic amino acid decardoxylase, 85, 94,
  323, 392
Arousal, 93, 159, 161–164, 169–172, 345, 361
Arousal response. *See* Alpha blocking
Artane. *See* Trihexyphenidyl
Arteriosclerosis, 18, 20, 199, 200, 261, 321
Ascendin. *See* Amoxapine
Aspartate, **101–104**, 109, 318, 377
Aspirin, 44, 119, 120, 151, 152, 207, 342, 343,
  347–352, 358, 395, 403, 404
Aspirin-like drugs, 347–353
Associative cortex, **369–370**, 374–385
Atarax. *See* Hydroxyzine
Ataxia, 196, 232, 280, 281, 283, 310, 324–327,
  406
Athemol. *See* Theobromine
Ativan. *See* Lorazepam
Atropine, 38, 85, 322
Attention deficit disorder. *See* Hyperkinesis
Auditory system, 56, 60, 367, 382
Aura, 388, 390, 391
Autism, 131, 171, 265
Autoimmune hypothesis, 257
Automatism, drug, 186

Autonomic nervous system, 47, **48-49**, 153, 221, 231, 262, 265, 273, 274, 349
Autoreceptors, 72, 76, 77, 94, 174, 297
Aventil. *See* Nortriptyline
Avoidant disorder, 131, 275, 276
Axon, 62, 65

Baclofen, 326, 330
Barbiturates, 183, 184, 185, 189
  abuse, 132, 148, 150-153, 154, 187, 188, 192
  compared with anxiolytics, 1, 41, 98, 277
  compared with neuroleptics, 257
  and epilepsy, 393, **395-398**, 399, 400
  interactions of, 119, 192, 203, 215, 230, 231, 300
  in liver disease, 134
  receptor, 100
  and sleep, 177, 192
  for tension headache, 342, 358
  and therapy, 8, 130, 275
Basal ganglia, 59, 165, 315, 384
Behavior therapy, 11
Belladonna alkaloids, 322
Bemagride, 38
Benadryl. *See* Diphenhydramine
Benzamides, 267
Benzedrine, 213. *See also* Amphetamine(s)
Benzodiazepines, 190-191, 276, **277-284**
  abuse liability, 132, 148, 150, 151, 152
  and akathisias, 325, 329
  clearance by liver, 133
  and desynchronized (D) sleep, 185
  and disinhibition, 41
  neurochemical mechanism, 75, 98, 100, 107, 184
Benzphetamine, 213
Benztropine, 91, 262, 322, 328, 330, 404
Beta (β) waves, 165, 167-171, 173, 215, 229, 295, 393
Biofeedback, 171-172, 356, 358
Biperiden, 322, 330
Bipolar II. *See* Manic-depressive disorder, atypical
Bipolar disorders. *See* Manic-depressive disorder
Birth
  defects, 395, 399
  injuries, 16
Blood-brain barrier, 73, 117, 118, 323
"Blue heaven," 189
Bouton, 66, 67
Bradykinin, 347, 348, 349
Brain waves. *See specific wave frequencies* (*e.g.,* Alpha (α) waves)
Brodmann areas, 363-366, 382
Bromides, 183, 188
Bruxism, 178, 180
Bubartal. *See* Butabarbital
Buffered aspirin, 350
Bufotenin, 227, 231
Butabarbital, 404

Butalbital, 341, 358, 403, 404
Butazolidin. *See* Phenylbutazone
Butisol. *See* Butabarbital
Butyrophenones, 92, 134, 259, 267, **268**, 270

Cafergot, 212
Caffeine, 5, 120, **211-212**, 224
  abuse, 150, 151, 156, 223, 356
  in APC combinations, 343, 351
  and headache, 356, 358
  in hyperkinesis, 218
  as phosphodiesterase inhibitor, 107
  as primary reinforcer, 39
  in respiratory depression, 196
  and therapy, 6, 8
Calcium, 31, 45, 67, 70, 71, 73-75, 80, 86, 94, 104, 184, 185
Calmodulin, 92
Cannabis, 5, 6, 117, 228, **231-235**
  abuse, 132, 146, 150-154, 156, 230
  and state-dependent learning, 38
Carbamazepine, 120, 356, 359, 360
Carbidopa, 134, 323, 330, 392
Cardiazol. *See* Pentylenetetrazol
Caroxazone, 301
Catapres. *See* Clonidine
Catecholamines, 44, 74, 78, 265, 301. *See also* Dopamine; Epinephrine; Norepinephrine
Catechol-O-methyl transferase (COMT), 86, 90
Caudate, 33, 59, 81, 83, 315
Celontin. *See* Methsuximide
Central nervous system, 50-60
Central-state identity theory, 373, 385
Central tegmental tract, 55, 87
Cerebellar peduncles, 54, 55, 56, 318
Cerebellum, 53, 55, 56, 81-83, 87, 88, 99, 100, 315, 317, **318**, 321, 325
Cerebral cortex, 59-60, **363-372**, **374-385**
  cell columns, 371, 374, **377-385**
  and degeneration, 18
  and desynchronized (D) sleep, 175
  and EEG, 162, 163
  and epilepsy, 387, 388
  layers, 363, 367, 374, **375-377**, 378-381
  and neurohormones, 81, 83, 87, 88, 97, 99, 100, 101, 103, 376-377, 384
  and other brain regions, 57-60, 239, 247, 250, 317, 318, 319, 325
  and plasticity, 35-37
  and sedative-hypnotics, 183, 196
  and self-stimulation, 33
  trauma, 16, 18, 168
Cerebral spinal fluid, 118, 291, 298
Cerebral-vascular insufficiency, 18, 168, 287, 321, 387
Cerebrum. *See* Cerebral cortex
Chemoreceptor trigger zone, 56, 340
Children and drugs, 131-132, 223, 263, 275, 276, 391. *See also* Autism; Hyperkinesis
Chloral hydrate, 38, 120, 159, 185, 188, 189, 193

Chlordiazepoxide, 5, 44, 148, 277, 281, 283, 403
  and arousal systems, 169
  and cyclic AMP, 108
  in delirium tremens, 148, 208, 209
  with MAO inhibitors, 300
  pharmocokinetics, 120, 134
  as primary reinforcer, 39
  and state dependency, 38
p-Chlorophenylalanine, 44, 94, 95, 97, 121
Chlorpheniramine, 191
Chlorphenoxamine, 322, 330
Chlorpromazine, 5, 20, 44, 91, 120, 131, 137,
  257, 258, 264, 265, 268, 306, 404
Chlorprothixene, 268, 271
Chocolate, 212
Choline, 21
Choline salicylate, 350, 353
Choreas, 324, 325, 326, 327
Cigarettes. *See* Tobacco
Cingulate gyrus, 59, 81, 84, 97, 163, 239, 240,
  250
Cirrhosis. *See* Liver cirrhosis
Clinical evaluation of drugs, 141–142
Clinoril. *See* Sulindac
Clonazepam, 120, 281, 325, 326, 392, 397–399
Clonidine, 76, 88, 148, 357
Clonopin. *See* Clonazepam
Clorazepate, 277, 281, 283, 403
Clozapine, 267, 268
Cluster headaches, 5, 356, **357**, 359
CNS, 50–60
Coca, 218
Cocaine, 5, 39, 44, 86, 117, 119, 132,
  150–152, 156, 211, 214–216, **218–221**,
  230, 300
Codeine, 39, 120, 340, **341–343**, 345, 347, 403,
  404
Coffee, 145, 212, 218, 223
Cogentin. *See* Benztropine
Cognitive functioning, 21, 170, 288, 323, 339,
  384, 385, 389, 390
Cola, 212
Colliculi, 55, 57, 87, 162
Colonil. *See* Diphenoxylate
Compazine. *See* Prochlorperazine
Compensatory mechanisms in neurotrans-
  mission, **76–78**, 91, 259–261, 295–297
Compliance, 135–136
Conditional behavior, 241, 242–244
Conditional stimuli, drugs as, 37–39
Conditioned avoidance response, 40, 41, 242
Conditioned emotional response, 41
Conditioning, 15, 30
Conduct disorder, 131, 261
Conduction, 64–66
Consciousness, 59, 361, **373–385**, 387, 388, 391
Convulsants. *See* Analeptics
Convulsions, 406. *See also* Electroconvulsive
  therapy; Epilepsy
Corpus callosum, 370
Corpus striatum, **315–317**
  and neurotransmitters, 82, 87, 88, 91–93, 96,
  97, 99–101

and other brain regions, 53, 58, 59, 170, 250,
  268, 318, 319, 321, 322, 324, 325, 369, 381,
  382, 384
Cortical evoked response, 166, 167, 230, 367
Corticosteroids, 20, 86, 149, 188, 356
Cough suppressants, 340, 342
Counterconditioning, 30, 275, 276
Coupling proteins, 70, 75, 76, 77, 81, 88, 92,
  96, 98, 100, 115, 340
CPZ. *See* Chlorpromazine
Cranial nerves, 48, 51, 52, 56, 57, 89
Creutzfeldt's disease, 18, 327
Cross-tolerance, 187, 203, 228
Cuneiform nucleus, 54, 55, 57, 82, 84, 318
Cushing's syndrome, 19, 168
Cyclic AMP, 70, **106–108**, 109, 198, 213–215,
  278, 280, 295
Cyclic GMP, 104, 108
Cyclothymic disorders, 128, 130, 305
Cycrimine, 322, 330
Cyproheptidine, 131, 357, 360, 404
Cytology of neurons, 61–63

Dale hypothesis, 66–67
Dalmane. *See* Flurazepam
Dantrium. *See* Dantrolene
Dantrolene, 326, 330
Darvocet. *See* Propoxyphene; Acetaminophen
Darvon. *See* Propoxyphene
Darvon compound. *See* Propoxyphene; Aspirin;
  Phenacetin; Caffeine
Daxolin. *See* Loxapine
Degradation, transmitter, 70, 73, 74, 75, 77, 78
Déjà vu, 10
Delirium tremens, 152, 187, 202, 203, 265, 327,
  328, 411
Delta (Δ) waves, 165, 168, 171–173, 175, 387
Demerol. *See* Meperidine
Dendrites, 62, 65
Dependence. *See also* Tolerance and de-
  pendence
  physiologic, 147, 150, 151, 187, 192, 220,
  222, 229, 234, 277, 341, 345
  psychological, 76, 147, 150, 151, 187, 192,
  216, 220, 222, 229, 234, 277, 341, 345
Depersonalization, 17, 228, 230, 407
Depletion, 74, 75
Depressants, 18. *See also specific drug classes*
Depression, 17, 20, 254, **285–293**
  agitated, 285, 291
  atypical, 285, 286, 288, 291
  drug-induced, 148, 149, 191–193, 220, 223,
  276, 287, 301, 323, 391, 393, 398, 407
  drug treatment of, 126, 133, 211, 293–302, 307
  endogenous, 127, 128, 168, **289–290**
  major, 130, 268, 286, **287–289**
  with melancholia, 285, 286, 290, 300
  norepinephrine and, 89, 286, **291–292**, 293
  and pain, 335
  postictal, 388, 393
  reactive, 127, 128, 285, 286, **289–290**
  residual, 189, 191
  respiratory. *See* Respiratory depression

retarded, 285, 291
secondary, **285-287**, 307
and serotonin, 286, **292-293**
and sleep, 180-181
Depressive neurosis. *See* Dysthymic disorder
Desipramine. *See* Desmethylimipramine
Desmethyldiazepam, 120
Desmethylimipramine, 134, 302
Desoxyn. *See* Methamphetamine
Desynchronized (D) sleep, 45, 56, 170-180, 184, 185. *See also* REM
Desyrel. *See* Trazodone
Dexedrine. *See* Dextroamphetamine
Dextroamphetamine, 39, 213, 224
Dextromethorphan, 340, 342
Diabetes mellitus, 18, 411
Diacetylmorphine. *See* Heroin
Diagnosis, 16-20, 24, 126-129, 274-276
Diazepam, 5, 9, 108, 120, 134, 140, 179, 216, 277, 281, 283, 297, 326, 358, 403
as anticonvulsant, 207, 209, 393, 398, 399
Dibenzodiazepines, 267, 268
Dibenzoxazepines, 267
Didrex. *See* Benzphetamine
Diencephalon, 32, 34
Diet
    deficiencies in, 18, 75, 199, 200
    essential constituents of, 71, 94
Diethylpropion, 213, 224, 404
Dietrol. *See* Phendimetrazine
Diffuse thalamic system (DTS), 84, 153, **161-165**, 171, 172, 174, 180, 221, 277
    and epilepsy, 389, 391, 393
    and hyperkinesis, 216, 223
    and other brain regions, 36, 166, 169, 170, 247, 251, 378-381, 384-385
Diflunisal, 350, 353
Dihydroergotoxine, 21, 404
Dihydromorphinone, 342, 343, 345
Dihydroxyphenylalanine. *See* L-Dopa
Dilantin. *See* Phenytoin
Dilaudid. *See* Dihydromorphinone
2,5 Dimethyl-4-ethylamphetamine (DOM, STP), 227
Dimethyltryptamine (DMT), 227, 231
Diphenhydramine, 126, 191, 322, 330, 403
Diphenoxylate, 342
Diphenylbutylamines, 259, 267
Disipal. *See* Orphenadrine
Disorientation, 17, 19, 85
Dissociation, learning. *See* State-dependent learning
Disulfiram, 12, 86, 204, **205-206**, 208, 209
Ditran, 38, 228, 231
Dolobid. *See* Diflunisal
Dolophine. *See* Methadone
DOM. *See* 2,5 Dimethyl-4-ethylamphetamine
L-Dopa, 21, 44, 73, 85, 86, 120, 134, 211, **322-324**, 325, 328, 330
Dopamine, **89-93**, 109
    and benzodiazepines, 278, 280
    and cerebral cortex, 165, 377, 384
    and corpus striatum, 319, 322, 323, 324, 328

hypothesis, 256
levels, 73
and narcotics, 76, 341
and neuroleptics, 258, 259, 261, 263, 264, 268, 278
and other neurotransmitters, 75, 85-87, 94, 100, 107, 108
nuclei, 55, 57, 93
and nucleus accumbens, 250
receptors, 72, 76, 92
and stimulants, 214, 215
Dopar. *See* L-Dopa
Dopram. *See* Doxapram
Doriden. *See* Glutethimide
Dorsal longitudinal fasciculus, 34, 250
Dorsal thalamus. *See* Thalamus
Dose-response relationship, 44, 115-116
Down-regulation of receptors, 78, 292, 295, 340
Down's syndrome, 19
Doxapram, 221, 340
Doxepin, 126, 298, 299, 302, 403
Doxylamine, 191
Dreaming, 173, 174-180
Droperidol, 343
Drug-induced psychopathology, 7, 19, 130, 203
"Drug of choice," 153-154
DTS. *See* Diffuse thalamic system
Dual arousal model, 161, **169-172**, 218
Dual memory theory, **30-31**
Dual process theory, 169, 313, **319**
Dyskinesias, 407
    tardive, 91, 263, 270, 323, 325-327, **328-329**
    withdrawal, 149, **328-329**
Dyslexia, 17
Dystonias, 325, 326, 327

ECT. *See* Electroconvulsant therapy
EEG. *See* Electroencephalograph
EEG activation. *See* Alpha blocking
Effector proteins, 71, 73, 75, 81, 88, 92, 96, 98, 100, 104, 106, 114, 115, 340
Efficacy, 113-115, 116
Elavil. *See* Amitriptyline
Electroconvulsant therapy, 30, 293, 297, 308
Electroencephalograph, 44, 165-168, 170, 171, 380
    clinical applications, 167-168, 172
    drug effects on, 191, 196, 211, 215, 229, 265, 277, 295, 300, 307, 322, 340
    and epilepsy, 4, 18, 221, 387, 389-391, **392-393**, 394
    and hyperkinesis, 216
    and neurotransmitters, 84, 85, 97
    and sleep, 172-174, 176
    synchronization, 371
    thalamic control of, 161, 162
Emphysema, 222
Encephalitis, 19, 326, 392
Endocrine system, 307, 309
    and CNS, 59, 91, 287
    and EEG, 168

Endoplasmic reticulum, 61, 105, 106
Endorphin(s), 105, 340
Enkephalins, 105, 334, 335, 340
Enuresis, 127, 132, 180, 299
Ephedrine, 224
Epicritic system, 51, 333
Epilepsy, 17, 18–19, 134, **387–400**
    and amphetamines, 211, 215
    and benzodiazepines, 277
    and biofeedback, 172
    and chronic medication, 6
    and EEG, 168, 172, 179, 221, **392–393**
    and migraine, 357
    and phenothiazines, 265, 270
    and psychotherapy, 3, 4
Epinephrine, 38, 44, 57, 85, 93, 106, 109
Epithalamus, 58
Equagesic, 358
Equanil. *See* Meprobamate
Equifinality, 15
Erections, penile and dreaming, 174, 180
Ergotamine, 356, 357, 360
Ergotropic process, 45, 319
Eskalith. *See* Lithium
Ethchlorvynol, 120, 184, 190, 192, 193
Ethoheptazine, 342, 345, 358, 404
Ethopropazine, 322, 330
Ethosuximide, 120, 398, 399
Ethyl alcohol. *See* Alcohol
Etiology of psychopathology, **14–25**
Etrafon, 268, 271. *See also* Amitriptyline;
    Perphenazine
Extrapyramidal system, 52–53, 54, 56–59, 313,
    315–319, 369
    disorders, 18, 313, **321–330**, 392
    drug effects on, 5, 138, 262–266, 270, 273,
        277, **326–329**, 408
    and transmitters, 82, 83, 91, 106

Family therapy, 3, 9, 22, 24, 208
Febrile convulsions, 389, 390
Fenamates, 351, 352
Fenoprofen, 351, 352, 353
Fentanyl, 343
Fetal alcohol syndrome, 201
Fiorinol, 342, 358. *See also* Butalbital; Aspirin;
    Phenacetin; Caffeine
Firing rate, neuronal, 74, 76
Flashback, 229
Fluid mosaic, **63–64**, 69, 70
Fluphenazine, 265, 266, 270, 271
Flurazepam, 120, **190–191**, 194, 403
Focal seizures, 389, 390
Fornix, 33, 36, 84, 240, 241, 247, 249
Freud, Sigmund, 22, 44
Frontal lobe, 59–60, 91, 92, 239, 241, 363, 365,
    369–370, 377, 384, 393
Functional disorders, 128, 313, 321, 329,
    334–335

GABA, 44, 72, 75, **98–101**, 109, 184, 185, 214,
    215, 221, 261, 278–280, 324, 377, 396, 398

GABA-modulin, 98, 100, 105, 278, 279
Gamma-aminobutyric acid. *See* GABA
Gangliosides, 71
Gating, 57, 58, 105, 230, 334, 335, 358, 373
Generalization, 37–39. *See also* State-
    dependent learning
General paresis. *See* Syphilis
Genetic factors, 15–16, 18–19, 324, 357, 392
Geniculate bodies
    lateral, 55, 81, 162, 163, 174, 175
    medial, 55, 162, 163
Gilles de la Tourette's syndrome, 127, 132,
    261, 268, 329
Globus pallidus, 33, 59, 82, 83, 101, 163, 244,
    250, 315, 317, 318, 384
Glucocorticoids. *See* Corticosteroids
Glutamate, **101–104**, 109, 377, 378
Glutethimide, 44, 120, 188, 190, 194
Glycine, 101, 102, 109, 214, 215, 278
Gold compounds, 349
Golgi bodies, 61, 105, 106
Grand mal epilepsy, 19, **388–389**, 390–400
"Grass." *See* Cannabis
Grave's disease. *See* Hyperthyroidism
Growth hormone, 244, 247, 263, 267
Guanethidine, 86, 87, 90

Habenulae, 58, 84, 99, 106, 239, 240
Habituation, 242, 334, 358
Halazepam, 281, 283
Half-life, 119, 120–121, 343
Hallucinogens. *See* Psychedelics
Haloperidol, 38, 91, 120, 259, 261, 263, 264,
    267, 268, 306, 308, 324, 325, 329, 404
Hangover, 202, 356
Harmine, 231
Headache, 132, 148, 149, 206, 222, 274, 277,
    310, 322, 331, 335, 351, **355–360**, 398, 408
    drugs used in, 5, 342, 347, **351–360**
Hemp, 233. *See also* Cannabis
Heroin, 39, 120, 132, 146, 154, 216, 342, 343,
    345
Hexamethonium, 81
Hippocampus, **247–248**
    and ACh, 81–84, 165
    and benzodiazepines, 277
    and conditioning, 32, 33
    and memory, 35, 36, 234
    and nicotine, 221
    and other brain regions, 59, 239, 240–244,
        249, 366, 369, 370, 381, 384
    and transmitters, 97, 99, 101, 103
Histamine, **103–105**, 107–109, 348, 356, 377,
    384
Homeostatic processes, 58, 244
Homicides, drug, 153, 195
Huntington's chorea, 18, 324, 327, 328
Hydantoins, **393–395**, 399, 400
Hydergine. *See* Dihydroergotoxine
Hydrocodone, 345
Hydromorphone. *See* Dihydromorphinone

5-Hydroxyindoleacetic acid (5-HIAA), 94, 95, 286, 293, 298
5-Hydroxytryptamine (5-HT). *See* Serotonin
5-Hydroxytryptophan (5-HTP), 21, 94, 95, 97, 307, 392
Hydroxyzine, 191, 276, 282, 283, 403, 404
L-Hyoscine. *See* Scopolamine
Hyperactivity, 17, 23, 408. *See also* Hyperkinesis
Hyperkinesias, 325, 326, 327
Hyperkinesis, 127, 131, 171, 172, **216–218**, 307
  and minimal brain dysfunction (MBD), 17
  and therapy, 9, 223, 224
  use of stimulants in, 12, 211, 215, 218
Hypersensitivity reactions, 262–263, 294, 310, 395
Hypersomnias, 178, 180, 288, 300, 306
Hyperthyroidism, 19, 168, 180, 325, 326
Hypnotics. *See* Sedative-hypnotics
Hypochondriasis, 17, 335, 356
Hypoglycemia, 18, 19, 168, 204, 208, 287, 326, 356, 412
Hypomanic episodes, 301, 305, 306, 311, 408
Hypopituitarism, 168
Hypotension, orthostatic (postural), 262, 263, 266, 294, 295, 323, 340, 345
Hypothalamus, 52, 58–59, **244–247**, 336, 337, 348
  and neurohormones, 81–84, 87, 88, 91–93, 97, 103
  and neuroleptics, 262–264, 266
  and other brain regions, 36, 163, 165, 239, 241, 248–250, 317, 335, 369
  and positive-spike pattern syndrome, 387
  and self-stimulation, 33, 34, 35
Hypothyroidism, 19, 168
Hypoxic drive, 186
Hystadyl. *See* Methapyrilene

Ibuprofen, 120, 134, 351–353
Identified patient, 3, 22
Idiosyncratic reactions, 185, 202
Imbalance hypotheses, 171
Imipramine, 5, 38, 75, 95, 120, 179, 275, 297, **298–299**, 404
Imodium. *See* Loperamide
Indocin. *See* Indomethacin
Indole alkylamines, 227, 231
Indolics, 267, 271
Indomethacin, 351, 352, 353
Infantile spasms, 389, 390, 392, 397
Insight, 11, 12
Insomnia, 12, 172, 173, 178, 180, 181, 270, 281, 286, 288, 306, 341, 357, 392, 409
Insulin, 19, 288, 289
Interactions
  alcohol, 203–207
  barbiturates, 188, 398
  drug-drug, 119–121, 141, 268–269, 347, 350, 395
  drug-therapy, 6–9
Interpersonal flexibility, 13

Interpersonal systemic process, 1, 15, **22–23**, 334–335
Intoxication, acute drug, 19, 20, 187, 190, 192, 193, 195, 196, 202, 204, 205, 234, 306, 341, 352, 392
Intralaminal nuclei, of thalamus, 33, 162, 163, 317, 379, 381
Ionamin. *See* Phentermine
Isocarboxazid, 86, 95, 137, 300, 302
Isomers, 213
Isoniazid, 134
Isonicotinylhydrazide (INH), 215

Jacksonian seizures, 389, 390
"Jag," salicylate, 350
Jet lag, 180

Kidneys and drugs, 119, 120–121, 307, 309, 398
Klüver-Bucy syndrome, 241, 247
Korsakoff's syndrome, 36, 152, 200, 201
Krebs' cycle, 98

Language, 17, 60, 370, 371, 383, 384
Larodopa. *See* L-Dopa
Lateralization, 17, **370–371**
Learning, **27–42**
  in cerebral cortex, 37, 381–384. *See also* Memory
  and dreams, 180
  and drugs, 8
  prepared, 243–244
  styles, 27–28
Levodopa. *See* L-Dopa
Levorphanol, 345
Libido, 198, 281, 294, 324, 409
Librax. *See* Chlordiazepoxide (with Clidinium)
Libritabs. *See* Chlordiazepoxide
Librium. *See* Chlordiazepoxide
Lidocaine, 218
Lidone. *See* Molidone
Limbic system, 32, 37, 59, **239–251**
  and ACh, 45, 82, 83, 84
  and drugs, 221
  and other brain regions, 60, 163, 170, 315, 319, 339, 366, 369, 370, 384
  and transmitters, 87, 106
Lioresal. *See* Baclofen
Lipid solubility, 117–118
Lithane. *See* Lithium
Lithium, 5, 12, 44, 107, 108, 120, 130, 133, 140, 203, **305–311**, 326
Lithonate. *See* Lithium
Liver
  cirrhosis, 134, 153, 195, 199, 200
  and drug metabolism, 119, 120–121, 134, 188, 192, 202, 203, 205, 307, 351, 395, 398
  toxicity, 134, 199–201, 351, 398
Locus ceruleus, 54, 57, 83, 87, 89, 107, 174, 175, 249, 376, 379, 384
Lomotil. *See* Diphenoxylate
Long-acting barbiturates, 189, 395–398

Loperamide, 243
Lorazepam, 120, 277, 281, 284, 403
Loxapine, 267, 271
Loxitane. *See* Loxapine
LSD. *See* Lysergic acid diethylamide
Ludiomil. *See* Maprotiline
Luminal. *See* Phenobarbital
Lysenyl. *See* Methylergol carbamide maleate
Lysergic acid diethylamide, 5, 12, 44, 120, 173,
    215, 227, **228–230**, 231
    abuse, 146, 150–152, 156
    and neurotransmitters, 94, 95, 96
    psychosis, 228–229, 235, 265

Maintenance, drug, 140, 254, 270, 298, 310,
    343–345
Major tranquilizers. *See* Neuroleptics
Mamillary bodies, 34, 36, 163, 239, 240, 241,
    246, 247
Mania, 180, 254, 268, 301, **305–306**, 307, 311
Manic-depressive disorder, 5, 261, 285, 286,
    305–306, 307, 310
    atypical (bipolar II), 305, 307
    diagnosis of, 126, 130
    lithium in, **305–311**
    and sleep, 180, 181
MAO, 44, 75, 85, 86, 90, 94, 95, 258
MAO inhibitors, 5, 44, 86, 119, 134, 140, 177,
    291, 292, **299–300**, 301
Maprotiline, 298, 302
Marijuana. *See also* Cannabis
    Tax Act, 44
Marplan. *See* Isocarboxazid
MDA. *See* Methoxyamphetamine
Meberal. *See* Mephobarbital
Meclofenamate, 351, 352, 353
Meclomen. *See* Meclofenamate
Medial forebrain bundle, 33–35, 82, 83, 178,
    241, 319
Medulla oblongata, 51, 53–57
    and motor systems, 315, 318, 369
    and narcotics, 340
    and neurotransmitters, 82, 89, 93, 97
    and periventricular system, 34
Mefenamic acid, 351, 352, 353
Melancholia. *See* Depression, with
    melancholia
Mellaril. *See* Thioridazine
Membranes, cell, 63–64
Memory. *See also* Learning
    long-term, 30, 31, 244, 248
    short-term, 30–31, 244, 248
Meningitis, 19, 355, 356
Mental health, 12–13
Mental retardation, 17, 19, 20, 131, 287
Meperidine, 119, 120, 134, 300, 342, 343, 345
Mephenesin, 223, 359
Mephenytoin, 393, 399
Mephobarbital, 189, 194, 396, 399
Meprobamate, 5, 44, 120, 134, **277**, 282, 284,
    404
    abuse liability, 132

and disinhibition, 41
and headache, 358
interactions with other drugs, 188, 205
as sedative-hypnotic, 190, 194
and state dependency, 38, 41
variability of absorption, 140
Meretran. *See* Pipradrol
Mesantoin. *See* Mephenytoin
Mescaline, 38, 227, 231, 235, 265
Mesencephalon. *See* Midbrain
Mesoridazine, 265, 266, 271
Metabolism
    cerebral, stimulators of, 21, 130
    disturbances of, 7, 18, 208, 287, 326
    drug, **118–119**, 188, 192, 202, 203, 205
Metalanguage, 28–29
Methadone, 12, 39, 120, 131, 132, 148, 342,
    343–345, 346
Methadrine. *See* Methamphetamine
Methamphetamine, 39, 120, 211, 224
Methapyrilene, 191
Methaqualone, 120, 132, 190, 192, 199
Methdilazine, 357
Methedrine. *See* Methamphetamine
Methohexital, 275
Methoxyamphetamine (MDA), 227
3-Methoxy-4-hydroxyphenylglycoaldehyde
    (MHPG), 291, 298
Methsuximide, 398, 400
Methylergol, 357
Methyl-para-tyrosine, 44, 85, 86, 177, 325
Methylphenidate, 120, 213, 215
    in chronic organic brain syndrome, 21
    in hyperkinesis, 9, 215, 218, 224
    as primary reinforcer, 39
    state dependency with, 38
Methyprylon, 190
Methysergide, 96, 149, 356–358, 360
Metrazol. *See* Pentylenetetrazol
Mianserin, 300, 301
Midbrain, 32–35, 51, 55, 57–59, 87, 95, 170,
    315, 369, 384, 387, 391, 393
Migraine, 6, 127, 133, 335, **355–358**, 359, 360
Milontin. *See* Phensuximide
Miltown. *See* Meprobamate
Mind-body problem, 373–374
Minicolumns, 377
Minimal brain dysfunction, 15, 17, 19, 20, 131
Minor tranquilizers. *See* Anxiolytics
Mitochondria, 61, 85
Moban. *See* Molidone
Modeled behavior, 27
Modulatory proteins, 70, 75, 76, 77, 88, 92,
    96, 98, 100, 115, 184, 185, 278, 279
Modules, 374. *See also* Cerebral cortex, cell
    columns
Molidone, 267, 271, 308
Monoamine oxidase. *See* MAO
Mood, 242, 243
Morning glory seeds, 231
Morphine, 38, 39, 93, 120, 132, 134, 339,
    340–346

Motor neurons
  alpha, 47, 369
  gamma, 47, 53, 318
Motrin. *See* Ibuprofen
Multa loca tenens principle, 121
Multiple sclerosis, 20, 287, 325, 327
Muscle relaxants, 191, 277, 280, 356, 358
Myelination, 62–63, 333, 367
Myoclonus, 178, 325–327, 390, **392**, 397–399
Myopathies, 199, 200, 208
Mysoline. *See* Primidone
Myxedema. *See* Hypothyroidism

Nalfon. *See* Fenoprofen
Naloxone, 120, 340, 343, 346
Narcan. *See* Naloxone
Narcolepsy, 178, 180, 211
Narcotic analgesics, 5, 331, 334, **339–346**
  abuse of, 146, 148, 150–152, 156
  compared with sedative-hypnotics, 183
  depression caused by, 287
  as discriminative stimuli, 38
  and disinhibition, 41
  and dopamine, 76, 91
  and extrapyramidal disorders, 326
  in headache, 355, 358
  interactions, 196, 203, 347, 350, 398
  and the liver, 134
  mechanisms, 78
  and medulla, 56
Narcotic antagonists, 340, 343, 346
Naproxen, 351, 352, 353
Naproxyn. *See* Naproxen
Nardil. *See* Phenelzine
Navane. *See* Thiothixene
NE. *See* Norepinephrine
Nembutal. *See* Pentobarbital
Neocortex. *See* Cerebral cortex
Nerve cell, **61–67**
Neuralgia, 5, 98, 356, **358–359**
Neuroanatomy, 43, 45, **46–60**, 373
Neurochemistry, 43, 44, **69–111**, 373
Neuroglia, 62, 63, 99, 101, 103
Neuroleptics, 5, **257–272**
  clinical indications, 126, 130, 259–262, 263,
    276, 287, 289, 343, 356
  contrasted with anxiolytics, 41, 276
  and dopamine, 75, 91, 92
  dosage, 140
  and extrapyramidal disorders, 324–329
  impotence, 137
  interactions, 203, 297, 309
  and learning effects, 40, 41
  mechanisms, 12, 76, 108, 257–259
  in organic brain syndrome, 21
  and polypharmacy, 133
  and self-administration, 39
  withdrawal, 149
Neuron, 61–67
Neuropathology, 8, 388, 390
Neuropharmacology, **43–45**
Neurophysiology, 45, **61–67**, 373

Neuropsychodiagnosis, **16–20**, 24, 128, 371
Neuroregulators, 61, 67, 105
Neurosis, 127, 130–132, 265
Neurotransmission, 66–67, **69–111**
Neurotransmitters, 61, 65, 66–67, **69–111**
Nicotine, 6, 214, 215, **221–222**
  abuse, 147, 148, 150, 151, 156, 223, 274
  as primary reinforcer, 39
  and state dependency, 38
  and therapy, 8
Nightmares, 179, 180
Night terrors, 179, 180, 277
Nigrostriatal pathway, 91, 93, 259, 324
Nisoxetine, 300
Nitoman. *See* Tetrabenazine
Noludar. *See* Methyprylon
Nomifensine, 300
Nonbarbiturate hypnotics, 151, 152, **190–191**
Nonnarcotic analgesics, 5, 132, 339, **347–353**,
    355
Norepinephrine, **85–89**, 109
  and cerebral cortex, 376, 379, 384
  and drugs, 198, 214, 215, 258, 259, 295–299,
    300, 307
  and extrapyramidal system, 318, 319
  and hyperkinesis, 218
  hypothesis, 291–292
  and learning, 31, 38
  nuclei, 55, 57
  and pain gating, 334
  receptors, 72, 76, 87, 88
  and reward, 35
  and septal region, 249
  and sleep, 174, 177, 180
  and sympathetic nervous system, 49
  and other transmitters, 75, 100, 107, 108,
    171, 337
Norpramin. *See* Desmethylimipramine
Nortriptyline, 120, 134, 298, 299, 302
Nucleus
  accumbens, 83, 91, 92, 249, 250, 268
  linearis, 57, 93
  reticularis pontis caudalis, 55, 56, 174, 175
  reticularis pontis oralis, 55, 164
  ventralis, posterolateralis, 162, 163
Numorphan. *See* Oxymorphone
Nutrition. *See* Diet
Nystagmus, 156, 230, 231
Nytol. *See* Pyrilamine

OBS. *See* Organic brain syndrome
Obsessive-compulsive disorder, 130, 275, 276,
    287, 357
Occipital lobe, 60, 363, 365, 370
Ocular effects of drugs, 156, 340, 341
Occulomotor nucleus, 57, 175
Olfactory sense, 52, 59, **239–240**, 243, 247, 248
Olivary complex, 54, 55, 56, 318
Opiates, 72. *See also* Endorphin(s); Narcotic
    analgesics
Opium, 183, 339, 341, 346
Optimil. *See* Methaqualone

Organic brain syndrome, 127, 129, 138, 168, 253–255, 287, 306
  acute, 18, 128, 130
  chronic, 17, 18, 20–21, 128, 130, 261, 270
Organic process, 1, **15–21**, 22, 23, 289, 313, 321–327, 334, 359
Orphenadrine, 322, 330
Ouabain, 86
Overdose, drug, 150, 151, **152–153**, 341, 350, 351
Oxazepam, 120, 134, 277, 281, 283, 284, 404
Oxazolidones, 134, 215, 397, **398**, 400
Oxycodone, 343, 346, 403
Oxymorphone, 346
Oxyphenbutazone, 351, 352, 353

Pacemaker, thalamic, 163, 170, 175, 184, 248, 278, 280
Pagitane. *See* Cycrimine
Pain, 333–335
Panic attacks, episodal, 130, **274–275**, 287, 299
Papaverine, 21
Parachlorophenylalanine, 44, 94, 95, 97, 121
Paradione. *See* Paramethadione
Paradoxical reactions, 21, 138, 281, 282
Paradoxical sleep. *See* Desynchronized (D) sleep
Paramethadione, 398, 400
Paramethoxy-amphetamine (PMA), 227
Paranoia, 128, 130, 138, 168, 230, 253–255, 288, 306, 324, 391, 410
Parasomnias, 178, 179, 277
Parasympathetic nervous system, 19, 50, 357
  and ACh, 78, 322
  and nicotine, 221
Parenteral drug administration, 116, 117
Paresis. *See* Syphilis
Parest. *See* Methaqualone
Parietal lobe, 60, 363, 365, 370
Parkinsonism, 287, **321–324**
  drug-induced, 262–264, 294, 295, **327–328**
  drug treatment of, 6, 211, 321–324, 328
Parnate. *See* Tranylcypromine
Parsidol. *See* Ethopropazine
Patient variables, 137–138, 282
Paxipam. *See* Halazepam
PCP. *See* Phencyclidine
PCPA. *See* p-Chlorophenylalanine
Peganone. *See* Ethotoin
Pemoline, 21, 39
Pentazocine, 120, 134, 342, **343**, 346, 347, 404
Pentobarbital, 38, 120, **189**, 194, 204
Pentothal. *See* Thiopental
Pentylenetetrazol, 21, 38, 211, 216, **221**, 224
Peptides, 67, **105–106**, 109, 334
Percodan. *See* Oxycodone; Aspirin; Phenacetin; Caffeine
Periactin. *See* Cyproheptidine
Peripheral nervous system, 47–49, 221
Periventricular
  gray, 33, 54, 56–58, 87, 91
  system, 34, 35, 184, 246, 278, 280
Permissive theory of depression, 292–293, 307

Permitil. *See* Fluphenazine
Perphenazine, 264–266, 268, 271, 272, 403
Personality disorders, 127, 128, 131, 180, 307
Pethidine. *See* Meperidine
Petit mal epilepsy, 19, 387, 389, 390, **391**, 392–395, 397–400
Petit mal variant, 389, 390, 392
Pertofran. *See* Desmethylimipramine
Peyote, 231
Phenacetin, 342, 343, 351, 353, 358
Phenaphen, 342
Phencyclidine (PCP), 132, 150–152, 156, 228, **230–231**
Phencyclohexyl derivatives, 228, 230
Phendimetrazine, 213
Phenelzine, 300, 302
Phenergan, 342
Phenindamine, 191
Phenmetrazine, 213
Phenobarbital, 20, 38, 120, 189, 194, 215, 395, 396, 400, 403
Phenothiazines, 5, 92, 131, **265**, 266–268, 270, 271–272
  amino-alkyl, 265, 266
  and liver function, 134
  and mania, 305
  and methysergide, 357
  piperadine, 265, 266, 267
  piperazine, 259, 265, 266, 270
  and psychedelics, 229, 230
  and state-dependent learning, 38
  and tricyclic antidepressants, 293
Phenoxene. *See* Chlorphenoxamine
Phensuximide, 398, 400
Phentermine, 213
Phenyl alkylamines, 227, 231
Phenylbutazone, 351, 352, 353
Phenylephrine, 87, 88, 213
Phenylpropanolamine, 213
Phenytoin, 3, 5, 44, 134, 152, 188, 325, 356, 359, 360, **393–397**, 398–400, 403
Phobias, 37, 130, 172, **274–276**
Phosphodiesterase, 70, 72, 75, 107, 108, 213–215, 278, 280
Phospholipids, 63, 117
Physiochemical inputs, 52
Pick's disease, 18
Pimozide, 267
Pineal gland, 58, 373
Pipanol. *See* Trihexyphenidyl
Piperacetazine, 265, 266, 271
Piperidinediones, 183, 184, 190, 192
Pipradrol, 39
Pituitary gland, 244, 246, 263, 273
Pizotifen. *See* Pizotyline
Pizotyline, 357
Placebos, 129, 135, 142
Placidyl. *See* Ethchlorvynol
Plasma
  levels of drugs in, 140, **141**, 299, 308, 310, 344
  protein binding, 119, **120–121**, 350, 395
Pleasure center. *See* Septal region

Plegine. *See* Phendimetrazine
PMA. *See* Paramethoxy-amphetamine
Polypharmacy, 133-134
Pons, 34, 35, 51, 55, **56-57**, 58, 82, 87, 89, 95, 99, 315
Ponstel. *See* Mefanamic acid
Positive spike pattern syndrome, 17, 19, 168, 265, 387, 390, **391-392**
Postictal depression, 388, 393
Postictal headaches, 356
Postsynaptic potentials, 65, 66, 70-72, 80, 81, 88, 96, 100, 103, 104, 165, 184, 185
Posttraumatic stress disorder, 130, 276
"Pot." *See* Cannabis
Prazepam, 277, 281, 284
Precursors, transmitter, 21, 73, 74, 78
Prefrontal cortex, 84, 365, 369, 383, 384
Preludin. *See* Phenmetrazine
Prepared learning, 243-244
Presamine. *See* Imipramine
Presenile dementia, 17, 18
Primary reinforcers, drugs as, 39, 147, 283, 301, 345
Primidone, 3, 121, 396, 397, 399, 400
Probenecid, 94, 95
Prochlorperazine, 261, 264-266, 271, 404
Procyclidine, 322, 330
Prodromal symptoms
  of migraine, 355
  of schizophrenia, 255
Prolactin, 92, 263, 264
Prolixin. *See* Fluphenazine
Propagation, of action potential, 65-66
Propanediols. *See* Meprobamate
Propoxyphene, 121, 132, 134, **342-343**, 346, 347, 403, 404
Propranolol, 309, 310, 325
Proprionic acid derivatives, 351, 352, 353
Prostaglandin E, 72, 107, 108, 333, 340, 347-349, 351
Protein kinase, 70, 108
Protein synthesis, 78
  inhibitors of, 31, 40
Protopathic system, 51, 333
Protriptyline, 121, 298, 299, 302
Pseudocholinesterase, 78
Psilocin, 227, 231
Psilocybin, 5, 227, 231
Psychedelics, 5, 150, **227-237**
Psychoanalysis, 11
Psychogenesis. *See* Psychological process
Psychological health, nature of, 12-13
Psychological process, 1, 15, 21-22, 23, 289, 359. *See also* Functional disorders
Psychomotor epilepsy. *See* Temporal lobe, epilepsy of
Psychopathology, 11, **13-25**, 126
Psychopharmacology, 43, 44, **125-143**
Psychosis, 127-130, 132, 253, 287, 288
  brief reactive, 132, 255
  toxic, 19, 130, 150, 151, 193, 215, 220, 221, 223, 228, 235, 253, 265, 270, 410
Psychosomatic disorders, 128, 131, 132

Psychotomimetics. *See* Psychedelics
Psychotropic drugs, 5-6
Ptosis, 156, 232
PTZ. *See* Pentylenetetrazol
Punishment mechanisms, 32-35, 45, 57, 87, 247, 250, 277-278, 373
Putamen, 59, 250, 315, 317
Pyramidal cells, 375-376, 377-382
Pyramidal system, 55, 56, 60, 101, 315, 368, 369
Pyridoxine (vitamin B_6), 324, 325
Pyrilamine, 191, 194

Quaalude. *See* Methaqualone
Quide. *See* Piperacetazine

Raphé nuclei
  function, 58, 251, 317-319, 334, 358, 377, 384
  location, 54, 57
  and psychedelics, 229
  and serotonin, 93, 95-98
  and slow-wave sleep, 173, 174, 175
Rapid eye movement. *See* REM
RAS. *See* Reticular activating system
Rauwolfia alkaloids, 265
Rauzide. *See* Reserpine
Receptors, 44, 63, 71-73, 105, **113-115**
  acetylcholine, 45, 71, 79-81
  alpha-noradrenergic, 44, 75, 76, 85, 87, 88
  benzodiazepine, 184
  beta-noradrenergic, 44, 76, 85, 87, 88, 107, 108
  dopamine, 72, 76, 90-91, 259, 324, 328, 341
  excitatory amino acid, 104
  GABA, 72, 98-99, 100
  histamine, 103, 384
  muscarinic, 80, 81, 322
  nicotinic, 80, 81, 115
  noradrenergic, 72, 76, 259, 295-297
  opiate, **340**, 341
  pain, **333**, 334, 335, 339, 347, 348, 349
  presynaptic, 70, 72, 74-76, 77, 87, 88, 91, 259, 261, 295, 297, 300
  serotonin, 72, 94-96, 358
Recognition by cell columns, 374, 377, **378-380**, 381, 382, 384, 385
Recognition proteins. *See* Receptors
"Red devils," 189
Red nucleus, 53, 55, 57, 58
Reentrant signaling of cell columns, 379, **381**, 382, 384
Release, transmitter, 66-67, 70, **71**, 74, 75, 79, 80, 86-87, 90, 94, 95
REM
  changes with age, 176
  density, 175, 177, 218, 286
  deprivation, 175, 177
  elevation, 148, 185, 186
  latency, 175, 286
  rebound, 177, 181, 185
  sleep. *See* Desynchronized (D) sleep
  suppression, 184-186, 188, 191-193, 215, 281, 283, 323, 345

Representation by cell columns, 377, 378, **380-381**, 382, 384, 385
Reserpine, 44, 265, 271
 and desynchronized (D) sleep, 177
 and disinhibition, 41
 and extrapyramidal disorders, 324, 325, 330
 and manic-depressive disorder, 306
 and neurotransmitters, 74, 86, 87, 90, 94, 95
Respiratory center, 56, 82, 186, 212
Respiratory depression
 and alcohol, 196
 and barbiturates, 186
 and narcotics, 340, 341
 stimulants in, 211, 221
Resting potential, 45, 64, 73
Restoril. *See* Temazepam
Reticular activating system, 81, 82, 163, **164-165**, 318, 319
 and alpha blocking, 169
 descending, 53, 318, 319
 and diffuse thalamic system (DTS), 170, 171, 172
 and drugs, 191, 215, 216, 223, 258, 280
 and other brain regions, 57, 251
Reticular formation, 32, 35, 55-59, 164-165, 170, 174, 175, 244, 248, 318, 319, 321
 and drugs, 184, 196
 and transmitters, 82, 83, 89
Reuptake of neurotransmitters, 67, 73-75, 86, 87, 90, 91, 95, 214, 295, 297, 298
Reward mechanisms, **32-35**, 45, 89, 147, 247, 373, 374
 consummatory, 34, 248, 249
 preconsummatory, 34
Rhinencephalon, 32, 35, 239
Ribonucleic acid, 40, 70
Ribosomes, 61
Rigidity, 321, 323, 325, 326, 327
Ritalin. *See* Methylphenidate
RNA. *See* Ribonucleic acid
Routes of administration, 116-118
"Rush," 216, 343, 345

Salicylamide, 350, 353
Salicylates, 134, 349-350, 352-353
Salsalate, 350
Sandomigran. *See* Pizotyline
Sandoptal. *See* Butalbital
Sansert. *See* Methysergide
Sauce-béarnaise effect, 243
Schizoaffective disorder, 132, 255, 268, 307
Schizophrenia, **253-257**
 and amphetamine toxic psychosis, 223
 chronic medication of, 133
 and differential diagnosis, 17, 20, 128-130, 287, 288, 306, 324
 and dopamine, 57, 93, 256
 and EEG, 168, 172
 and neuroleptics, 5, 12, 126, 137, 261, 265, 269, 328, 329
 organic factors in, 15-16, 17, 25, 250, 256-257

 and pain, 335
 and polypharmacy, 134
 and sleep, 180-181
 triggered by antidepressants, 127
Schizophreniform disorder, 132, 255, 306
Scopolamine, 38, 191, 194
Secobarbital, 38, 121
Seconal. *See* Secobarbital
Secondary amines, 298
Secondary reinforcement, 40
Sedative-hypnotics, 5, 140, 183-194
 abuse, 133, 146, 148, 150-152, 274, 287, 301
 anxiolytics as, 190, 276, 277, 278
 cannabis as, 231
 and conditioned avoidance response, 40
 and desynchronized (D) sleep, 177, 179
 and extrapyramidal symptoms, 326, 328
 and organic brain syndrome, 21
 and other depressants, 119, 203
 and reticular activating system (RAS), 319
 as reinforcers, 39
 and respiratory depression, 56
 and therapy, 6, 137
 withdrawal compared with narcotics, 341
Seizures. *See* Epilepsy
Self administration, 39, 151
Self-change processes, 30
Self-regard, 12, 13, 17
Self-stimulation, 32-33, 45
Senility, 18, 20, 261, 325
Sensory systems, 50-52
Separation anxiety, 131, **274-275**, 299
Septal region, **248-250**
 and benzodiazepines, 277
 and neurohormones, 82-84, 91, 97, 101, 103
 and nicotine, 147
 and other brain regions, 59, 163, 165, 239, 241, 242, 246, 335
 and self-stimulation, 33, 34
Sequential design, 141
Serax. *See* Oxazepam
Serentil. *See* Mesoridazine
Serotonin, 44, **93-98**, 109, 121
 and blood vessels, 348
 and corpus striatum, 318, 319
 and depression, 292-293, 295, 297-301
 and evoked response, 166
 and headaches, 357-358
 levels, 73, 78
 and LSD, 229-230
 and other neurohormones, 87, 107, 108, 337
 and pain gating, 334
 pathways, 251, 377, 384
 receptors, 72, 94-96, 358
 and reserpine, 265
 and slow-wave sleep, 171, 173-175
Serpasil. *See* Reserpine
Set-point, 337, 349
Sexual function, 17, 41, 131, 244, 246, 265, 267, 270, 287, 301, 357, 398, 399, 408
Shock treatments. *See* Analeptics; Electro-convulsant therapy

Short-term memory. *See* Memory, short-term
Side-effects, 1, 7–8, 133, 139. *See also specific drugs*
Sinemet, 323, 330
Sinequan. *See* Doxepin
Sinus headaches, 355, 356, 359
Skinnerian conditioning. *See* Conditioning, operant
Sleep, 99, **172–181, 184–186**, 213. *See also* Desynchronized (D) sleep; Slow-wave sleep
  deprivation, 175, 177, 286
  disturbances, 17, 127, **178–181**, 286, 288, 306
  induction, 189, 192
  spindles, 172, 173
  sustaining, 189, 192
  walking, 179, 180, 277
Sleep-Eze. *See* Pyrilamine
Sleepiness. *See* Somnolence, excessive
Sleep-wake cycle, **172–175**
Slow waves. *See* Delta (Δ) waves
Slow-wave sleep, 97, 172–177, 184, 381
Smoking
  cocaine, 219–220
  marijuana, 232, 234
  tobacco, 30, 145, 146, 204, 206, 222
Social variables in drug response, 136–137
Sodium-potassium exchange pump, 45, 65, 69, 70, 72, 198, 307, 308, 395, 396
Sodium salicylate, 350, 353
Sodium thiosalicylate, 350, 353
Solacen. *See* Tybamate
Somatic nervous system, 47–48, 318
Somatosensory system, 47–48, **333–334**, 365, 367, 383
Sominex, 191
Somnafac. *See* Methaqualone
Somnifacients. *See* Sedative-hypnotics
Somnolence, excessive, 178, 180, 295, 301, 391, 392
Sopor. *See* Methaqualone
Soporifics. *See* Sedative-hypnotics
"Speed," 213
Spike-and-dome discharges, 390, 391, 394
Spinothalamic, 333, 339
Split-brain, 370, 371. *See also* Lateralization
State-dependent learning, **37–39**
  and antidepressants, 301
  and anxiolytics, 41, 275–276
  and narcotics, 345
  and psychedelics, 236
  and sedative-hypnotics, 193
  and stimulants, 223
Status epilepticus, 149, 388, 397, 398
Steady potential, 36, 166, 167
Stelazine. *See* Trifluoperazine
Stereotypy, 93
Stimulants, 5, **211–225**, 366. *See also* Analeptics
  abuse, 148, 150–152, 341
  as antidepressants, 301

in chronic organic brain syndrome (OBS), 21
and hyperkinesis, 131, 218
and sleep, 178, 179
STP. *See* 2,5 Dimethyl-4-ethylamphetamine (DOM, STP)
Strategy, drug administration, 140–141, 282, 298–299, 307–310
Strychnine, 44, 101, 215, **223–224**
Substance P, 106, 334
Substantia gelatinosa, 334, 335, 339
Substantia innominata, 82, 83, 101, 249, 250, 377, 384
Substantia nigra, 33, 53–55, 57, 58, 91, 93, 317, 322, 324
Subthalamic nucleus, 53, 58, 59, 82, 83, 317, 325
Subthalamus, 58, 59, 165, 244, 315
Successive abstraction, 379, 381–383, 384
Succinimides, 134, 215, 397, **398**, 399, 400
Sudden infant death, 180
Suicide, 152, 153, 188, 192, 195, 270, 277, 288, 289, 301, 350, 391, 410
Sulfonamides, 20
Sulindac, 351, 352, 353
Sulpiride, 267, 268
Supersensitivity, 328
Surmontil. *See* Trimipramine
SW sleep. *See* Slow-wave sleep
Sympathetic nervous system, **48–49**, 50
  and drugs, 213, 221, 326
  and neurotransmitters, 44, 78, 85, 88, 92
Synapse, 45, 61, 69
Syndrox. *See* Methamphetamine
Synergic autonomy, 13
Synergistic drug interaction, 119
Synthesis, neurotransmitter, 69–71, 73–79
Syphilis, 19, 321, 324, 326, 355

Tacaryl. *See* Methdilazine
Tachyphylaxis, 76, 115, 146
Talwin. *See* Pentazocine
Tandearil. *See* Oxyphenbutazone
Taractan. *See* Chlorprothixene
Taste, 52, 56, 243–244
Tea, 145, 212, 218, 223
Tectum, 34, 57
Tegmentum, 35, 91, 164, 317
  dorsal, 55
  lateral, 55, 93
  ventral, 33, 55, 57, 82, 83
Tegretol. *See* Carbamazepine
Telencephalon, 59
Temazepam, 190, 194
Temperature, body, **336–337**, 348
Temporal lobe, 19, 60, 363, 365–366, 367, 370
  epilepsy of, 203, 389, 390, **391**, 393, 396–400
Tenuate. *See* Diethylpropion
Tepanil. *See* Diethylpropion
Teratogenicity. *See* Birth defects
Tertiary amines, 298, 299
Tetrabenazine, 95, 324, 325, 330

Tetrahydrocannabinol, 5, 121, 146, 228, 231, 232
Thalamocortical projections, 375–378, 381, 382. *See also* Diffuse thalamic system
Thalamus, 58
  anterior, 33
  and epilepsy, 387, 391, 393
  motivational centers, 33, 34, 35
  and neurotransmitters, 81, 83, 84, 87, 96, 97
  and other brain regions, 51, 161–165, 239, 240, 244, 248, 317–319, 334, 378–382, 384–385
THC. *See* Tetrahydrocannabinol
Theobromine, 211, 212
Theophylline, 107, 211, 212, 224
Therapist effectiveness, 28–29, 138–139, 282
Theta (θ) waves, 165–168, 171, 173, 248, 249, 393
Thiamine, 148, 207, 209
Thiopental, 189, 194
Thioridazine, 21, 131, 207, 263–265, 270, 297, 324, 328, 403
Thiothixene, 264, 267, 268, 270, 272, 297
Thioxanthines, 268, **269**, 270, 271–272
Thorazine. *See* Chlorpromazine
Tics, 277, 324–329, 410
Tindal. *See* Acetophenazine
Titration of drug dose, 140
Tobacco, 117, 145, 146, 156, **221–222**
Tofranil. *See* Imipramine
Tolectin. *See* Tolmetin
Tolerance, 146, 150, 185, 202, 211, 215, 216, 219, 222, 229, 294. *See also* Tolerance and dependence
  acute, 188, 220
  cross-tolerance, 187, 203, 228
  drug disposition, 146, 188, 202, 341
  negative, 146, 234
  pharmacodynamic, 76, 91, 146, 188, 202, 341
Tolerance and dependence, **145–146**, 180. *See also* Tolerance
  with alcohol, 201–202
  with amphetamines, 215–216
  with anxiolytics, 281
  with barbiturates, 187–188, 395
  with cannabis, 234
  with cocaine, 220
  with LSD, 229
  with narcotics, 91
  with neuroleptics, 262
  with nicotine, 222
Tolmetin, 351, 352, 353
Tourette's syndrome, 127, 132, 261, 268, 329
Toxicity, psychological, 135
Tranquilizers, 196, 319
  major. *See* Neuroleptics
  minor. *See* Anxiolytics
Transcendental meditation, 171
Transcortical projections, 103, 375–382, 384, 393

Transfer of learning. *See* State-dependent learning
Transmethylation hypothesis, 256–257
Tranxene. *See* Clorazepate
Tranylcypromine, 5, 39, 86, 95, 300, 302
Trazodone, 300, 301, 302
Tremin. *See* Trihexyphenidyl
Tremor, 202, 206, 213, 273, 274, 309, 310, 313, 321, 323, 324, 329, 410
Triavil, 268, 271. *See also* Amitiptyline; Perphenazine
Tricyclic antidepressants, 5, 44, **293–299**
  and adaptive mechanisms, 76
  administrative strategy, 133, 134, 140
  extrapyramidal effects of, 326, 327
  and norepinephrine, 78, 86, 291
  in organic brain syndrome, 21
  and other drugs, 300, 309
  responsiveness to, 290, 298
  and serotonin, 95, 298–299
  withdrawal, 148
Tridione. *See* Trimethadione
Trifluperazine, 265, 266, 272, 404
Triflupromazine, 264, 272
Trihexyphenidyl, 322, 330, 404
Trimethadione, 216, 398, 400
Trophotropic process, 45, 319
Tryptophan, 73, 94, 95, 97
Tuinal, 193. *See also* Amobarbital; Secobarbital
Tumor, 14, 287, 321, 326, 355, 356, 387
Two-disease theory of depression, 292, 293
Tybamate, 284
Tybatran. *See* Tybamate
Tylenol. *See* Acetaminophen
Tyramine, 86, 300, 356
Tyrosine hydroxylase, 85

Unconditional stimuli, drugs as, 40
Unisom. *See* Doxylamine

Vagusstoff, 78
Valium. *See* Diazepam
Valproic acid, 121, 134, 392, 397, 398
Vasodilators, cerebral, 21
Vasomotor center, 56
Verbal ability, 36
Vesicles, synaptic, 45, 69–71, 79, 85, 90, 106
Vesprin. *See* Triflupromazine
Vestibular system, 52, 53, 56
Vestran. *See* Prazepam
Viloxazine, 300
Vistaril. *See* Hydroxyzine
Visual system, 51–52, 60, 363, 367, 370, 383
Vital centers, 54, 56, 58
Vitamin(s)
  B_1 (thiamine), 148, 207, 209
  B_6 (pyridoxine), 324, 325
  B_{12} (cyanocobalamin), 20
  C (ascorbic acid), 207, 209
  in chronic organic brain syndrome (OBS), 21

K, 350
nicotinic acid, 201
Vivactil. *See* Protriptyline

Wernicke's area, 370
Wernicke's encephalopathy, 200, 201
Wilpo. *See* Phenteramine
Wilson's disease, 18, 325, 327, 330
Withdrawal, 19, 145, **146-149**. *See also*
    Tolerance and dependence
  alcohol, 148, 202, **207-208**, 281
  anxiolytics, 1, 148, 277, 281, 283
  barbiturates, 148
  cannabis, 234
  and desynchronized (D) sleep, 177
  narcotics, 148, 340, **341**, 343, 344
  nicotine, 148

sedative-hypnotics, 148, 185, 187, 328
stimulants, 148, 215, 216

Xanax. *See* Alprazolam
Xanthines, 107, 108, 152, **211-213**, 214, 215,
    218

"Yellow-jackets," 189
Yin-yang hypothesis, 108
Yohimbine, 75, 88

Zactane. *See* Ethoheptazine
Zarontin. *See* Ethosuximide
Zomax. *See* Zomepirac
Zomepirac, 351, 352, 353, 403
Zona incerta, 53, 91, 317